THE
PERRIN
TECHNIQUE

SECOND EDITION

Dedication

This second edition of my book is dedicated to:

All the severe ME/CFS and fibromyalgia patients around the world who are suffering from these cruel conditions, unable to read this book, listen to any music, enjoy the company of friends, eat normal food, watch a film on TV, have a decent night's sleep, and who are, or have been, stuck in bed often in a darkened, silent room existing day after day, month after month and year after year in pain and with dozens of severe physical and cognitive symptoms…

Linda, Jacques, Bliss, Elizabeth, Dave, Beverley, Tatiana, Freya, Joanna, Jean and her three brave sons Felix, Francis and Fabian, and all the 25% group plus the #MillionsMissing worldwide network

… this is for you!

THE PERRIN TECHNIQUE

SECOND EDITION

How to diagnose and treat chronic
fatigue syndrome/ME and fibromyalgia
via the lymphatic drainage of the brain

DR RAYMOND PERRIN

DO, PhD

Osteopath and Neuroscientist

Foreword by Dr Adrian Heald

BOOKS

Hammersmith Health Books
London, UK

First published in 2021 by Hammersmith Health Books
– an imprint of Hammersmith Books Limited
4/4A Bloomsbury Square, London WC1A 2RP, UK
www.hammersmithbooks.co.uk

The information contained in this book is for educational purposes only. It is the result of
the study and the experience of the author. Whilst the information and advice offered are
believed to be true and accurate at the time of going to press, neither the author nor the
publisher can accept any legal responsibility or liability for any errors or omissions that
may have been made or for any adverse effects which may occur as a result of following
the recommendations given herein. Always consult a qualified medical practitioner if
you have any concerns regarding your health.

British Library Cataloguing in Publication Data: A CIP record of this book is available
from the British Library.

Print ISBN 978-1-78161-149-4
Ebook ISBN 978-1-78161-150-0

Commissioning editor: Georgina Bentliff
Designed and typeset by: Julie Bennett, Bespoke Publishing Ltd
Cover design by: Madeline Meckiffe
Index: Dr Laurence Errington
Production: Helen Whitehorn, Path Projects Ltd
Printed and bound by: TJ Books, Cornwall, UK

Contents

List of Illustrations

Chapter 11

Acknowledgements

Gratitude is not only the greatest of virtues, but the parent of all others.
Marcus Tullius Cicero (106 BC – 43 BC)

Throughout the last three decades there have been many people to whom I owe an enormous debt of gratitude; first in enabling me to finish my thesis in July 2005, and subsequently the first edition of *The Perrin Technique* in 2007, and now this second edition 14 years later.

I would like to pay tribute to the benefactors, scientists, colleagues, patients, family members, staff and friends who have all played a pivotal role in my years involved with ME/CFS and fibromyalgia research.

Firstly, I would like to express my heartfelt thanks to The David and Frederick Barclay Foundation (now The Barclay Foundation) for providing the funds for my earlier research. Since the establishment of the Fund for Osteopathic Research into ME (FORME) in February 1995 there have been some exceptional members of the public who have served as trustees of FORME. I thank them all, especially co-founders Riaz Bowmer and Ruth Behrend, as well as past chairpersons Darren Mercer, Chris March, Kelvin Heywood, Steve Briggs, Ian Trotter and Tina Rushton. My special thanks go to the present chair Bev McDonald and her daughter Liv and the rest of the committee, Peter Gittings, Barry Geden, Laurent Heib and Nigel Brockwell, plus the continued support from Gill and Andrew Finch and all the Hodgkinson family.

Let me extend my thanks, too, to my first ME/CFS success, Pete, who in 1989 insisted that I begin this long road of research, and to my many patients who, over the past 30 years have contributed advice, encouragement and research funds. I remember the late Dr C Royde, a Manchester general practitioner, who, in the early days of my research, gave me encouragement and advice from an orthodox medical perspective and checked my earliest work. Thanks also to Dr Anne Macintyre and to Dr Andrew Wright for their invaluable information and inspiration in my earlier work.

Many thanks to Professor Jack Edwards, who initially took me under his wing in my early years at Salford University's Department of Orthopaedic Mechanics, for his patience, guidance and for his meticulous checking of my thesis. Thanks, too, to health psychologist Dr Pat Hartley, joint supervisor with Professor Edwards, for her guidance.

My main supervisor during the doctoral research, neurotoxicologist Dr Vic Pentreath, was a source of immense support and, without his cajoling, positive advice and cheerful disposition, I may never have persevered.

Let me thank Professors Alan Jackson and Jim Richards, who have both imparted a mere fraction of their practical skills and immense knowledge in neuroradiology and biomechanics respectively, which are incalculably useful. Merci beaucoup to my friend and colleague across 'the Pond', osteopathic physician Dr Bruno Chikly, for his incredible insight and knowledge of the lymphatic system.

Thanks to my fellow research collaborators who, together with Professor Richards, helped with the diagnostic study; namely Lucy Hives, Alice Bradley, Dr Bhaskar Basu, Dr Annice Mukherjee and Dr Tarek Gaber, Dr Chris Sutton, Professor James Selfe, Kerry Maguire and Gail Sumner, and my new research team led by Dr Adrian Heald of Salford Royal Hospital and The University of Manchester's Dr Lisa Riste. Thanks also to Adrian for his kind words in the forward and to Lisa for the beautiful poem which appears in the front of this book.

Thanks to all the contributing patients who have shared their stories and all the Perrin Technique practitioners' worldwide who have faithfully plied their trade and directed their patients to the right path in their journey of recovery. Thanks also to patient advocates and campaigners, Cathy Vandome, Emma Franklin, and Faye Chown for their social network campaigns around the UK and across the world.

I am also very grateful to the following:

My colleagues Sophie, Ian, Gail, Elisa, Collette, Sylveen, Rakhee, Mark, Lucy and Antionette at my London and Manchester clinics for helping with all my patients over the years.

Dr Margareta Griesz-Brisson, the most amazing neurologist whom I have had the honour to work with in Harley Street, London, for her encouragement and insight.

My practice manager Elaine Coleman, for her superb clerical and organisational skills plus the wonderful pastoral care she excels in when dealing with all the patients that contact and visit my clinic.

Melissa, for modelling her healthy spine and my patients-turned-models for the photographs in this book.

My father, Bernard Perrin, and my father-in-law, Colin Fretwell, for their proofreading skills. My nephew, Simon Klein, for his computer skills in my initial work.

Thanks go to my publisher Georgina Bentliff whose continued encouragement and patience over the past few years have helped me complete this edition. Also to my editor, Carolyn White, plus the editor of the first edition, Anne Charlish, and all the staff at Hammersmith Health Books for helping to bring my work to a much wider audience.

My sons Jonny, Max and Josh all deserve a mention as they still have to manage with a dad who is often too engrossed in his work to be of much use. Last, but never least, I must pay tribute to my wife Julie who is a true jewel. Through her own long battle with ME/CFS, Julie has empathised with my patients and patiently supported my work week by week, year by year and continues to do so as I spend much of my time in clinic or at research meetings spreading the word across the medical and scientific world.

About the author

Raymond N Perrin DO PhD is a Registered Osteopath and Neuroscientist specialising in Myalgic Encephalomyelitis/Chronic Fatigue Syndrome. His present academic posts include Honorary Clinical Research Fellow at the School of Health Sciences in the Faculty of Biology, Medicine and Health at the University of Manchester, Manchester, UK and Honorary Senior Lecturer in the Allied Health Professions Research Unit, University of Central Lancashire, Preston, UK. He is also Research Director of the FORME Trust and Founder and Clinical Director of the Perrin Clinic™ Treating a patient for back pain in 1989 led him to the concept that there was a structural basis to ME/CFS. He has spent over 30 years conducting clinical trials, researching the medical facts and sifting the scientific evidence while successfully treating an increasing number of ME/CFS and fibromyalgia sufferers and teaching fellow osteopaths, chiropractors and physiotherapists the fundamentals of the Perrin Technique.

For his service to osteopathy, Dr Perrin was appointed a vice-patron of the University College of Osteopathy (formerly the BSO) and was the winner of the inaugural Research and Practice Award from the Institute of Osteopathy in 2015.

Invisible symptoms

By Dr Lisa Riste

My chronic fatigue syndrome
Is sometimes called ME
The thing that's most frustrating
Is that others cannot see

They can't imagine the fatigue
That seeps deep into my core
Leaves me without energy
Flat-lining on the floor

When I walk around a bit
It's like I'm wading through mud
But I try to keep on moving
I just really wish my body would

My muscles ache from activity
Doesn't matter what I try
I try to avoid 'boom and bust'
'Cos tomorrow I'll know why

Although I spend hours sleeping
I always wake up feeling tired
It's like I'm battling nightly
Holding back the Sandman's tide

And when I do eventually
Escape off into my dreams
It's into a world of nightmares
With scenes that are surreal

And though I've been labelled
'Depression' was their name
But with these invisible symptoms
You'd feel pretty much the same

So whilst my body's switched off
Wish I could read or watch TV
But brain fog forces me to pause
Then replay the story of my ME

Dr Lisa Riste is a research fellow at the University of Manchester. Her poem is based on the combined symptoms of the hundreds of patients spoken to over the years in two major NHS trials in the North West of the UK.

Foreword

In this Second Edition of his comprehensive review of the treatments available for ME/chronic fatigue syndrome (ME/CFS), Dr Perrin has given the reader fresh insights into the ways that this complex condition can be managed, based on more than 30 years of clinical work and research in this area.

Dr Perrin has described all of the theories relating to the underlying mechanisms so far implicated in the development of ME/CFS, while also looking in an evidence-based way at the treatments available across the world. It is particularly helpful to have case histories built into the narrative, which bring a revealing and moving human perspective to the work.

In the time of Coronavirus-19, when a significant number of people are experiencing long-term fatigue-related symptoms following a Coronavirus infection, and in some cases developing post-Coronavirus-19 ME/CFS, this work is particularly pertinent.

There is a clear exposition of the differential diagnoses to be considered. The role of nutrition and lifestyle in addition to formal therapeutic strategies is clearly explained. The 'question and answer' and 'A to Z of symptoms' sections towards the end of the book are both very helpful for clinicians and patients alike. Above all, Dr Perrin's book provides a torch to light the path towards more effective treatments for this condition, including the adoption in due cause of the Perrin Technique by the National Health Service in the UK and by other publicly-funded health services/ insurance-funded health programmes across the world.

For anyone who is involved in the diagnosis and management of ME/CFS, this is an essential read and a seminal reference text.

Dr Adrian Heald
Consultant Physician
Salford Royal Hospital, UK

Dr Adrian Heald is currently lead physician of the Chronic Fatigue Service at Salford Royal NHS Foundation Trust where he is a Consultant Physician in Diabetes and Endocrinology. He is also an Honorary Research Fellow at the University of

Manchester and Visiting Tutor at St Peter's College, Oxford. He obtained his medical degree from St Peter's College, Oxford and trained at the John Radcliffe Hospital, Oxford. He then moved to Manchester, where he qualified in psychiatry before broadening his field of expertise to cover endocrinology. He is a member of the Royal College of Psychiatrists and the Royal College of Physicians, and was awarded a DM Thesis by Oxford University in 2005.

Dear Reader,

If you are a patient reading this book and wish to start the Perrin Technique, please try to find a practitioner near to you who is a trained and licensed Perrin Technique practitioner if possible. If there are none in your neighbourhood, seek out a practitioner trained and experienced in both cranial techniques and manual therapy but preferably an osteopath, physiotherapist/physical therapist or chiropractor. They should be able to follow the instructions in this book and help. It is better not to rely just on the self-massage and exercises. Although they may help, it is always best to do the whole treatment programme under the direction of a qualified practitioner to improve your outlook and to confirm the diagnosis.

I wish you every success with your treatment and progress to better health.

Raymond Perrin

Introduction

Thou shalt make me hear of joy and gladness; that the
bones which thou hast broken may rejoice.

The Bible, Psalm 51:8

Case: Jen's story

Dr Perrin's treatment was a ray (no pun intended) of light in the darkness of my world.

I became ill when I was 12 and was forced to drop out of school. By 15, I had spent four months in hospital, and when I was released, it was because the doctors could do nothing else for me. I was unable to eat, speak, or move. I was completely bedbound, tube-fed, isolated, and in constant pain. My paediatrician had very little hope that I would ever recover and said that I was the sickest patient on his caseload. My future looked bleak.

My best friend, who also had ME, recommended Dr Perrin's treatment after she had recovered under his care. I was almost 18 at the time and had spent three years in bed, so we were desperate for any kind of treatment. Prior to Dr Perrin's treatment, I had been recovering, but progress was glacially slow. I was able to speak, eat and drink when I met him, but I was still bedbound, unable to turn myself over in bed, and taking a cocktail of medication, some of which were to counter the side effects of other medications to deal with pain and nausea.

Everything that he explained when he came made sense. I fitted all of the risk factors of people likely to get ME and all of the physical indicators. He was able to explain my symptoms before I told him them: right down to why I had stretch marks on my legs (which he hadn't seen). It was refreshing to listen to someone who understood my illness, believed in it, and knew how to treat it.

The treatment itself started off as somewhat scary. After my first treatment, my brother came to see me and said that I looked spaced. I was. All of a sudden, brain fog was worse than ever all over again, and I was slipping back to where I had been when I was at my worst. If my friend hadn't done the same treatment and come out of the other side, I would never have continued with it. I had muscle spasms, experienced every illness I'd ever had in reverse order, and I was back to not being able to speak. It was awful to lose what I had so painstakingly gained little by little over several years.

But then, after about a month, I started getting better. Not at the previous glacial pace, but quickly. On my 18th birthday, just nine months after starting the treatment, and after over three years of being bedbound, I took my first steps. I was no longer taking medication for pain, and I was going from strength to strength.

I've never looked back since starting the treatment. My improvement was constant and now, although I might have to be careful not to overdo it, nobody would ever guess I had been so ill. I would recommend this treatment to anyone with ME.

Jen Turner
Lancaster, Lancashire, UK

The second edition of my book continues to describe a journey of discovery that started as a consequence of an event in 1989, which some would say was fate, others luck. A simple appointment for back pain led to a former cyclist changing my life forever and helping to improve the lives of countless people around the world. This book has been written as an informative guide for people who suffer from myalgic encephalomyelitis (ME) also known as chronic fatigue syndrome (in this book

ME/CFS), and in this edition I also welcome readers with fibromyalgia syndrome (FMS), to understand how it is very much a disorder on the same spectrum as ME/CFS, with some differences. I also reveal the trials and tribulations of the innovative research into the disease that led to the formation of the Perrin Technique and how research around the world over the last decade has validated everything I wrote in the first edition.

Many ideas have been put forward to explain the cause of chronic fatigue syndrome (ME/CFS) but, as yet, nobody has offered a universally accepted theory that has led to a successful treatment programme. As an osteopath, trained in the manual diagnosis and treatment of the body, I have discovered a probable physical cause of the disease. The details of my theory are contained within this book, interspersed with the background story of the research itself.

There was little known evidence in 1989 for the concept of ME/CFS having physical causes, and thus I have spent over 30 years researching the medical facts, conducting three clinical trials and discovering plenty of scientific evidence linking ME/CFS with emerging scientific studies to support my hypothesis. The results of this continuing research will help you to understand the underlying cause of the disorder and, more importantly, how to help beat the condition.

The first edition of The Perrin Technique, published in 2007, has been read by thousands of patients whose main comment was that 'It makes sense'. However, this means very little in the scientific world. Many theories have been eventually shown to be wrong however real they might have seemed at the time. An example of this is the static or stationary universe theory, which was a model proposed by Albert Einstein in 1917. It was later disproved by Edwin Hubble who showed that the universe is constantly expanding, demonstrating that even scientists as great as Einstein can sometimes be wrong.

What is needed is evidence that stands up to scientific scrutiny and debate as well as the rigour of well-conducted controlled clinical trials. This second edition provides much new evidence to support the theories hypothesised in the first edition. This latest evidence will hopefully satisfy even the most sceptical reader that my theories are not just some 'wacky' ideas of an alternative quack but based on sound research and backed by the current medical understanding of how the body actually works.

I'm no Einstein and I haven't all the answers for everybody and, most importantly, I am not offering a cure. ME/CFS and fibromyalgia syndrome are chronic illnesses and chronic in medical terms means lifelong. What I can say is that this approach helps most sufferers of ME/CFS and fibromyalgia improve their quality of life. Some improve a little and some become symptom free. Some have had no symptoms for over 25 years since receiving their treatment; however, the process that led to the disease can reoccur so the patient, once better, needs to follow the guidelines included in this book to hopefully prevent any relapse from happening.

In this new edition every section and chapter of the book begins with stories written by patients in their own words who have been helped by the Perrin Technique. With their permission their real names and their hometowns have been included to add veritas to their testimony.

I have also included a much more comprehensive guide to the manual treatment of ME/CFS and fibromyalgia that should prove helpful to both practitioner and patient. This approach to fighting the disease has already helped thousands around the world and will, I hope, improve the health of millions of sufferers in the future. I have also written an explanatory guide to other approaches in the diagnosis and treatment of these complex disorders.

For those readers who are not familiar with all of the medical and scientific terms in the book, there is an updated glossary at the end. This should enable the patient, as well as the practitioner, to fully understand my approach and to benefit from treatment for the debilitating conditions of ME/CFS and FMS.

In this new edition there is also an FAQ (frequently asked questions) section in Chapter 11 and an appendix entitled 'The ABC of symptoms' (page 367), which is a comprehensive list of all the possible symptoms that can present in patients with ME/CFS and FMS. I am constantly asked by patients: 'I have a symptom that my doctor can't explain… could it be due to my illness or is it due to something completely different?'. Together with a short explanation for each symptom when viewing these conditions as neurolymphatic disorders, I hope the 'ABC of symptoms' will be an invaluable quick reference guide to clinicians and patients alike.

Raymond Perrin
Manchester, UK, July 2020

Chapter 1

The basics: How the Perrin Technique works

Success is neither magical nor mysterious. Success is the natural consequence of consistently applying the basic fundamentals.
Jim Ron (1930–2009) American entrepreneur and author

Case: Olivia's story

When I think back to early 2004, I was a healthy 12-year-old girl with a passion for life. I took part in many extra-curricular activities and was thoroughly enjoying my first year at secondary school. I loved being outdoors and was naturally very energetic. I was in the school netball team, often played in football matches, went swimming, attended weekly dance lessons and regularly went quad-biking on the weekends – I felt like I had unlimited energy.

It was during the summer holidays that year that I became rundown with a virus; it cleared up after a week or so. Not long after that I had a quad-bike accident, I was thrown off the vehicle at speed. The new school term started a couple of days later. By the second day, I felt too fatigued to play in the school football team and I noticed I didn't have the strength to walk to school assembly. Simple things suddenly became a real struggle. The following morning, I was unable to get out of bed. The return to the school routine seemed to be the straw that broke the camel's back. I was overcome with exhaustion and my body ached all over. This was September 2004 and I wouldn't return to school again until September 2006.

My mother took me to see my GP, as well as a private consultant. After numerous and extensive blood tests all came back clear, both came to the conclusion that I was suffering from post-viral fatigue and expected me to be back at school soon. Many months later, and continuing to deteriorate, my GP diagnosed me with ME/CFS. I was told there was no cure and sent on my way feeling helpless and in absolute despair. The realisation that this was how my life was going to be was unimaginable.

Given the severity of the symptoms, I was confined to my bed. Most days I didn't have the ability to speak, my mind felt numb and unable to form thoughts. I couldn't lift my own spoon for breakfast. A slice of apple was too heavy for me to pick up to eat. Visual stimulation was now extremely difficult. I was no longer able to watch TV, listen to music or engage in any conversation. Listening to noise was impossible, it was a sensory overload. I was also overly sensitive to smells. There was such unrelenting pain and I had insomnia. Thinking back, I didn't clean my own teeth for about 12 months; how could I grip the brush or raise my arm? Bathing also took a back seat; I didn't shower for many months as the task was just too much.

In the summer of 2005, with no improvement in my symptoms whatsoever, a friend of a friend recommended the Perrin Technique to my mother as it was helping someone they knew. We booked a visit to The Perrin Clinic and despite how unbearable the trip would be for me, my mother and I knew it was essential to try and find help. At my first appointment, Dr Perrin confirmed the diagnosis of ME. In addition, he had a wealth of knowledge about the condition and was able to explain the science behind all of the complicated symptoms I was experiencing. More than that, he had answers and a treatment programme to alleviate the symptoms. There was finally hope that one day my life would return to normal; it was a huge relief to finally meet someone who fully understood the condition.

Treatment at The Perrin Clinic started off at once a week. My sister printed a daily checklist to ensure I adhered to the many elements of the treatment protocol (self-massage, rotation exercises, supplements, contrast bathing).

Slowly my symptoms started to improve, and a milestone change was going from not having enough energy to even speak, to being able to engage in conversation with my family. I could feel my personality gradually returning. My sleep began to return to normal. My cognitive function was improving: I noticed I became bored with resting.

Pacing is a crucial aspect of the Perrin Technique and even though I felt I was now able to do more, I had to be extremely careful to keep activity to an absolute minimum so as not to affect my recovery. The most important thing I learnt from Dr Perrin was the 50% rule – to do only half of what I was capable of, and that if doing something twice over will exacerbate symptoms, then doing it once is too much (this wasn't easy to stick to, but effective!).

It was Spring 2006 and with invaluable advice from Dr Perrin, a plan was put in place for my return to education. I initially began with a visit from a home tutor, once a week, which allowed flexibility in case I became fatigued. After this went well, I was finally well enough to begin thinking about returning to school. My visits to the clinic gradually reduced as I improved, and I maintained the daily home treatment routine. In September the same year I started at school with a one-hour lesson a week, ensuring that lesson was held on the ground floor. I very gradually built this up, an hour at a time each week, and didn't take part in any physical activity such as PE. By the New Year I was in school full-time, albeit on a reduced timetable as I took a couple less GCSEs than I had originally planned to prioritise my health.

However, it wasn't all plain sailing, balancing school and pacing. With me now attending lessons it was important to be careful about other strains, so I asked for help carrying my bag and books between lessons. It was also arranged with the school that I was exempt from homework assignments; then I could rest after school. I restricted my social life; I wouldn't often go out but when I did, I used a wheelchair. All of this was to ensure I kept within the 'doing half' rule, to avoid bringing on an onset of symptoms and undoing the progress I was making with the treatment – every little truly did help.

It was a great feeling to be back in school full-time. I was slowly able to have an increase in social activity and live life like a normal teenager. It was great to be able to spend time with my friends, building relationships that I had not been well enough to keep up with for a long time. I enjoyed simple things such as being able to chat on the phone; previously mental activity such as this would have drained me.

By July 2008, I was thrilled to have successfully sat my GCSEs and was back to quad-biking again on weekends. I still received treatment but only visited the clinic once every couple of months. It was at this time I felt confident enough in my abilities to take part in a school trip to Kenya – a four-week expedition that would include building schools, camping, climbing Mount Kenya and extensive travelling around the country. In particular, summiting Mount Kenya gave me a huge sense of relief and achievement. Afterwards I didn't feel any ME symptoms; I was just like everyone else. I remained vigilant, however, to lessen the strain wherever possible (not carrying my own luggage, sitting out of strenuous labour, having a rest day on the mountain).

Although I had made so much progress, I did have a relapse later that same year. There was the emotional toll of my parents' divorce combined with the stress of A levels which triggered symptoms again. I was disappointed but had improved before, using solely the Perrin Technique, so had faith that it would definitely be possible again. I decided to put my studying on hold indefinitely until I was discharged from The Perrin Clinic. It was a very difficult decision to prioritise my health rather than trying to keep up with my peers, but it was worth the sacrifice to one day be free of ME. Within six months I had recovered from the relapse and ever since then I have been symptom free.

It has been seven years since my last appointment at The Perrin Clinic, which was a huge milestone in my life. After being discharged I finally felt free to push my body to its limits without the return of any symptoms. I was so excited to be able to work full-time. I have held positions that involve long commutes, stressful environments and, at times, 24-hour shifts, all without needing any treatment whatsoever. I have been able to take holidays and do lots of travelling, finally able to live life to the full. It is the best feeling in the world. I enjoy every moment, knowing how different my life is because I found the Perrin Technique.

I am so grateful for the work of Dr Perrin; with the Perrin Technique you can live in hope. I have seen first-hand how, for those who are aware of the Perrin Technique, ME is no longer seen as a prison-sentence – the despair is replaced with hope and there is a life out there ready to be taken back.

Olivia McDonald, Lancashire, UK

If you don't enjoy reading or, because of ME/CFS or fibromyalgia you are unable to concentrate on long texts, this one chapter is for you. It sums up my theory of diagnosis and treatment of these complex diseases. After this chapter, I advise those needing to keep their reading to a minimum to skip to Chapters 10 and 11, which include the Perrin Technique treatment plan (Chapter 10). This will hopefully guide you, the patient, along your own individual road to recovery.

If, after reading this and the final chapter, you wish to fully understand the complexities of diagnosis, pathophysiology and treatment of ME/CFS and fibromyalgia, the rest of the book is waiting to be read. I endeavour to keep the explanations as simple as possible in this first chapter.

Case: Mr E

My theory for the diagnosis and treatment of ME/CFS started with one patient: this case was the first and perhaps the most dramatic of all the ME/CFS patients I have treated. In 1989 an executive, who shall be referred to as Mr E, walked into my city-centre practice, in Manchester, where I ran a clinic specialising in treating sports injuries. He had been a top cyclist, racing for one of the premier teams in the north west of England.

He had suffered from a recurring, low back pain, which, after examination, I had diagnosed to be a strain of the pelvic joints. While treating his pelvis, I noted that his dorsal spine was particularly restricted. I enquired whether or not he had any problems in his upper back, and he acknowledged that for years, during his cycling, he had experienced a dull ache across his shoulders and at the top of his back. This in itself was nothing significant, as it was very common to find cyclists with pelvic problems and a stiff and disturbed curvature in the thoracic spine (the upper part of the backbone between the waist and the neck). What was interesting was the fact that, for the past seven years, Mr E had been diagnosed with ME/CFS.

Mr E complained of tingling in both hands and a 'muzzy' feeling in his head. He suffered general fatigue and an ache in his knees, as well as the pain in his back and shoulders. He had been forced to stop racing since the onset of the disorder.

This patient was one of many who came to me after being diagnosed by their doctor, or specialist, as suffering from ME/CFS. As I have said, he originally attended for treatment to his lower back. At that time, although I had helped other patients with ME/CFS, I had done no research into the disease, and I had no specific treatment programme for the disorder.

With only five treatments, Mr E's back was better, but, most incredibly, the signs and symptoms of ME/CFS had drastically improved. He was symptom-free after a mere two months from the start of treatment. After many years he continued to remain healthy and the last news I heard of him was that he had moved to Holland, cycling with the same power and zeal that he used to enjoy prior to his illness.

It was after helping this patient that I realised that there must be a correlation between the mechanical strain on the thoracic spine and ME/CFS. Although I had not set out to help the fatigue signs and symptoms in this patient, I had done exactly that by improving the posture and increasing movement in the spine. My thoughts turned to the other ME/CFS patients that I had treated for back pain and biomechanical strain. The restriction of the dorsal spine was a common factor that could not be ignored.

Since 1989, thousands of patients with signs and symptoms of ME/CFS have visited my clinic and also practices all over the world run by practitioners trained in the Perrin Technique. None of them has presented with exactly the same symptoms but all have shared common structural and physical signs. This cannot be dismissed purely as coincidence. So, what is really going on?

The Perrin Technique: the facts

Fact 1: Fluid flow

A fluid flows around the brain and continues up and down the spinal cord: this is the cerebrospinal fluid (see Figure 1). This fluid has many functions – for example, as a protective buffer to the central nervous system and for supplying nutrients to the brain. However, one function has been discussed in osteopathic medicine since the 1860s[1] but has received significant scientific attention only in recent years[2, 4, 5, 6, 7, 8, 9, 10, 11, 12, 13, 14, 15], and that is the role it plays in the drainage of large molecules, including many poisons (toxins), out of the central nervous system into the lymphatic system.

The lymphatic drainage of the central nervous system was actually postulated as early as 1816 when the Italian anatomist Paolo Mascagni speculated that there were lymphatic vessels at the surface of the human brain[16].

This system, which I have referred to since 1989 as 'neuro-lymphatic drainage', has now been proven to exist by a brilliant group of scientists in the USA and Europe who have termed this drainage 'the glymphatic system', as it has been shown to drain toxins from cells known as the 'glia' of the brain to the lymphatics[17, 18, 19, 20].

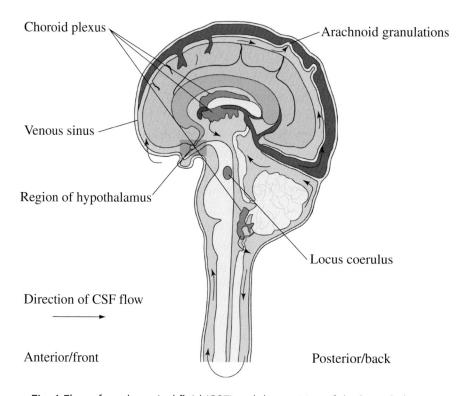

Fig. 1 Flow of cerebrospinal fluid (CSF) and the position of the hypothalamus. CSF diffuses superiorly around the brain and inferiorly around the spinal cord, flowing down the subarachnoid space (SAS) to a cistern at the base of the cord and then most travels back to the brain. However not all of the CSF in the lumbar cistern returns to the cranium; some is absorbed into lymphatics along the perivascular spaces in the spinal nerve roots.

In fact, not only is there visual evidence of the drainage system detailed in the first edition of this book, but actual lymphatic vessels have been discovered in the membranes of the brain in both animal and human studies, which can now be visualised by MRI scanning – see Figure 17 (page 233)[21].

Fact 2: Getting the toxins out

The lymphatic system is an organisation of tubes around the body that provides a drainage system secondary to the blood flow. Why does the body need a secondary system to cope with poisons or foreign bodies in the tissues? Are the veins not good enough? The answer in one important word is 'size'. The blood does process poisons and particles which enter the blood circulatory system via the walls of the microscopic blood vessels known as the capillaries. Their walls resemble a fine mesh which acts as a filter, thus allowing only small molecules to enter the bloodstream itself. When the blood reaches the liver, detoxification takes place, cleansing the blood of its impurities.

Larger molecules of toxins often need breaking down before entering the blood circulation, and they begin this process of detoxification in the lymph nodes on the way to drainage points just below the collar bone into two large veins (the subclavian veins), with most of the body's lymph draining into the left subclavian vein (see Figure 2).

The capillary beds of lymphatic vessels, known as terminal or initial lymphatics, take in any size of molecule via a wall that resembles the gill of a fish, opening as wide as is necessary to engulf the foreign body. The lymphatics also help to dispose of some toxins and impurities through the skin (via perspiration), urine, bowel movements and our breath. Once toxins have drained into the subclavian veins, they eventually find their way into the liver and, as is the case with normal circulatory toxins, are broken down by the liver[22].

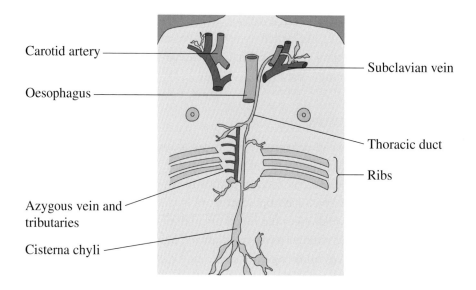

Carotid artery

Oesophagus

Subclavian vein

Thoracic duct

Ribs

Azygous vein and tributaries

Cisterna chyli

Fig. 2 The thoracic duct (the central lymphatic drainage system into the blood).

Fact 3: The pumping mechanism

Since 1622, when Italian physician and anatomist Gasparo (Gaspere) Aselli (1581–1626) discovered the lymphatic system, it was thought not to have a pump of its own. Its flow was believed to depend on the massaging effect of the surrounding muscles and the blood vessels lying next to the lymphatics, akin to squeezing toothpaste up the tube. However, now we know that the collecting vessels and ducts of the lymphatic system have smooth muscle walls[23] and Professor John Kinmonth, a London chest surgeon, discovered in the 1960s that the main drainage of the lymphatics, the thoracic duct, has a major pumping mechanism in its walls[24, 25, 26] and that this is controlled by the sympathetic nervous system[27]. If there is a disturbance of the sympathetic nervous system, the thoracic duct pumping mechanism may push the lymph fluid in the wrong direction and lead to a further build-up of toxins in the body.

Fact 4: The sympathetic nervous system

The sympathetic nervous system is part of the autonomic nervous system, which deals with all the automatic functions of the body. Although it is known for being the system which helps us in times of danger and stress, often referred to as the 'fight or flight' system, the sympathetic nervous system is also important in controlling blood flow and the normal functioning of all the organs of the body, such as the heart, the kidneys and the bowel. We know it is vital for healthy lymphatic drainage. In ME/CFS and FMS sufferers, the sympathetic nervous system will have been placed under stress for many years before the onset of the signs and symptoms. This stress may be of a physical nature due to postural strain or an old injury, or it may be emotional stress, or environmental, such as pollution, or due to stress on the immune system due to infection or allergy (see Figure 3).

The sympathetic nerves spread out from the thoracic spine to all parts of the body. The hypothalamus, just above the brain stem, acts as an integrator for autonomic functions, receiving regulatory input from other regions of the brain, especially the limbic system which involves emotion, motivation, learning and memory (see Figure 1). Significantly, the hypothalamus also controls all the hormones of the body.

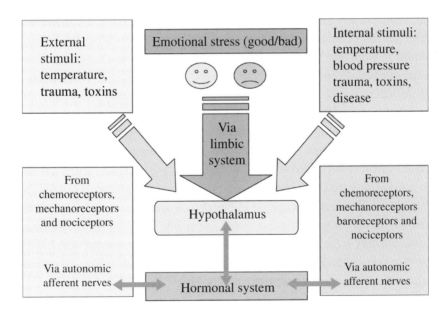

Fig. 3 Long-term build-up of internal and external stress.

Fact 5: Biofeedback

The hypothalamus controls hormones by a process called biofeedback. This mechanism can be explained with the following example. If the sugar levels in the body are too low, it may be due to a rise in the hormone insulin, which is produced in the pancreas, which lies in the upper right side of the abdomen beneath the liver. Insulin, like other hormones, is a large protein molecule that travels through the blood and stimulates the breakdown of sugar. It passes from the blood into the hypothalamus, which will calculate if more or less insulin production is required and, accordingly, send a message to the pancreas to make the necessary adjustments.

The region of the hypothalamus is one of a few sections of the brain that allow the transfer of large molecules into the brain from the blood (known as circumventricular organs). In all other parts of the brain there is a filter known as the blood–brain barrier (BBB) that separates the blood from the cerebral interstitial fluid and which was first hypothesised in 1906[28]. In the circumventricular organs there are natural gaps in the BBB.

The BBB contains tight junctions that prevent toxins and other harmful material entering the brain's cells from the blood. However, protein transport molecules that can cross the BBB can carry these huge protein molecules, enabling the biofeedback mechanism to work and allowing the transfer of hormones into the brain. The unit of molecular size is the Dalton and water molecules, which are only 18 Daltons, are small enough to naturally pass through the BBB via channels within membrane proteins known as aquaporin. Due to the tight junctions in the BBB, the transport of larger molecules is limited through the endothelial cells between the blood and the brain's tissue. The same arrangement is present in the blood–cerebrospinal fluid barrier, which restricts the circulation of macromolecules between the blood and cerebrospinal fluid. Evidence in the past decades suggests that these barriers are also subject to toxic damage from neurotoxic chemicals circulating in blood. The ageing process and some disease states render barriers more vulnerable to damage arising inside and outside the barriers. Hormones are very large protein molecules, and the hormone insulin, which we know has receptor sites on the hypothalamus, is 5808 Daltons, which is huge compared with the water molecule and yet it is able to enter the brain[29, 30].

Unfortunately in many disease states, further gaps in the BBB plus dysfunctional protein transporters mean that large toxic molecules can invade the brain and wreak havoc on the normal functioning of the central nervous system[31, 32, 33, 34, 35, 36, 37], and, as we will see later in this book, in ME/CFS it has now been proven that many immune cells that are pro-inflammatory do just this[38].

Fact 6: What goes wrong

The central nervous system, composed of the brain and the spinal cord, is the only region in the body that for hundreds of years was believed to have no true lymphatic system. Since we now know the lymphatics exist to drain large molecules, what can the central nervous system do if attacked by large toxins? It has now been demonstrated that the cerebrospinal fluid (see Fact 1) drains toxins along minute gaps next to blood vessels, called **paravascular spaces** and these transport the toxins into fluid in spaces within the arterial walls known as **perivascular spaces** (also known as Virchow-Robin spaces), and then onto the lymphatic system outside the head through perforations in the skull. We also now know that, as well as through the cranial perforations, drainage occurs from the perivascular pathways into newly discovered true lymphatic vessels in the outer layer of the meninges, the membranes surrounding the brain[21]. The lymphatic vessels found in the head and around the spine take the toxins away via the thoracic duct and right lymphatic duct (see Figure 2) into the blood and the liver where they are broken down[39].

This drainage mechanism has now been filmed, with the largest amount draining through a bony plate situated above the nose (known as the cribriform plate, see Fig. 4)[3, 12, 14, 15]. The toxins then drain into lymphatic vessels in the tissue around the nasal sinuses. There is further drainage down similar channels next to blood vessels supplying other cranial nerves, especially the optic, auditory and trigeminal nerves

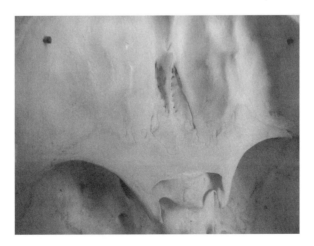

Fig. 4 Superior view of the cribriform plate with observed perforations.

in the eye, ear and cheek respectively, and also down the spinal cord outwards to pockets of lymphatic vessels running alongside the spine[4, 5, 7]. It has been shown that perivascular spaces enlarge in patients with cognitive problems[40], and this can be seen on a scan taken of the brain of one of my patients (see Figure 5). The radiological report on the scan stated 'the hyperintensity in the parahippocampal gyrus was most probably an enlarged Virchow-Robin space'.

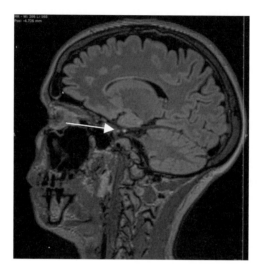

Fig. 5 Hyperintensity (marked by white arrow) in the parahippocampal gyrus

Fact 7: Build-up of toxins

In ME/CFS, I believe it is these drainage pathways, both in the head and the spine, that are not working sufficiently, leading to a build-up of toxins within the central nervous system. The reasons for drainage problems can vary from patient to patient. It may be trauma to the head from an accident; it may be hereditary or due to a problem at birth. The spine may become out of alignment – especially in very active teenagers – which can lead to a disturbance in the normal drainage (see Figure 6). If the spine and brain are both affected, the increased toxicity will disturb hypothalamic function and thus will further affect sympathetic control of the central lymphatic vessels. This in turn pumps more toxins back into the tissues and the brain via the aforementioned perivascular and paravascular spaces, which further affects hypothalamic and sympathetic control. With this, a vicious circle (see Figure 7) has started[41, 42, 43].

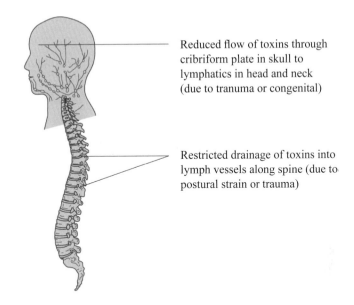

Reduced flow of toxins through cribriform plate in skull to lymphatics in head and neck (due to tranuma or congenital)

Restricted drainage of toxins into lymph vessels along spine (due to postural strain or trauma)

Fig. 6 Restricted drainage of toxins from the central nervous system.

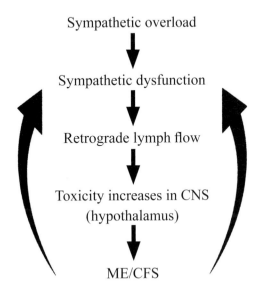

Sympathetic overload

Sympathetic dysfunction

Retrograde lymph flow

Toxicity increases in CNS (hypothalamus)

ME/CFS

Fig. 7 The downward spiral into ME/CFS.

Conclusion

ME/CFS is very much a biomechanical disorder with clear and diagnosable physical signs, including disturbed spinal posture, varicose enlarged lymph vessels and specific tender points related to sympathetic nerve disturbance and backflow of lymphatic fluid. The fluid drainage from the brain to the lymphatics moves in a rhythm that can be palpated using cranial osteopathic techniques. A trained practitioner can feel a disturbance of the cranial rhythm in ME/CFS sufferers[43, 44].

The Perrin Technique helps drain the toxins away from the central nervous system and incorporates manual techniques that stimulate the healthy flow of lymphatic and cerebrospinal fluid and improve spinal mechanics. This in turn reduces the toxic overload to the central nervous system which subsequently reduces the strain on the sympathetic nervous system, which ultimately aids a return to good health.

Chapter 2

ME/CFS: What it is

Life is not what it's supposed to be. It's what it is.
The way you cope with it is what makes the difference.
Virginia Satir (1916–1988) American author and therapist

Case: Heather's story

I was 19 years old and living a very active life when I suddenly got ill. I was working part-time as a cleaner and doing a lot of voluntary work which involved a considerable amount of walking. I always enjoyed walking, had had a dog since I was 10 years old and lived in a beautiful but very hilly area, so thought nothing of walking up and down hills most days.

Suddenly, I needed to rest in the middle of the day, just to get through the day; then just resting wasn't enough, and I went from this very active lifestyle to crawling up the stairs on my hands and knees and barely being able to dress myself and get downstairs to the sofa, where I then needed to lie to 'recover' from the effort of getting dressed. I knew I wasn't well... but what was wrong?

I was actually quite fortunate in one way, in that I got a diagnosis quite quickly. Having heard other people's stories later on, I realise that just getting the diagnosis itself can be a very frustrating journey, let alone working out how to get better.

This was towards the end of 1995, so 'yuppie flu' was in all the news at this time. My local General Practice got a new doctor who had just completed a study of this 'yuppie flu', and so he diagnosed me with chronic fatigue syndrome, or ME. So, I did get a diagnosis, but no real way to treat it, or how to deal with it. The only advice given was to gradually increase activity to try to get back to my former state. I remember timing myself hoovering, and then having to rest on the settee to recover, so I don't think this advice really worked!

Gradually you learn how to live with it; I had to give up work, both the cleaning and the voluntary work. At 19 years old, I was suddenly at home a lot and in bed a lot! Time passed, I met and married my husband and I moved. We got a home in the area he grew up in, as he had work there. I was able to stay at home, and just care for the house in between resting a lot.

It was now early 1999 and in the local church we both attended was another young couple; they had been married a year longer than us, and were a couple of years older. She had also been diagnosed with ME. In reading everything she could about it, she had discovered what was then a very 'new' treatment, which had had some success, but was still so new it was not really recognised by the mainstream medical profession. She showed me an article about Mr Raymond Perrin, an osteopath from Manchester. He had treated a patient who was a cyclist. He had advised the cyclist that he could help him with his lower back injuries etc, sustained from years of cycling, but he could not help him with his ME. However, after some time, the cyclist said he felt like the treatment was working on his ME, and he was getting better. This beginning led to Mr Perrin doing more research on ME, and in particular the lymphatic system. He had developed a treatment which did indeed seem to have some success on various patients. I must admit that, on hearing about this initially, I was somewhat sceptical as

I didn't believe in so-called 'miracle cures'. However, our friends were enthusiastic, and my husband wanted to see if I could improve my health, even by a small amount, so we agreed to go together one day, the four of us (both couples). We drove over to Manchester to what is now The Perrin Clinic.

We met Mr Perrin, who took over an hour to do an initial diagnosis and explain the treatment. At that first session he gave me a score of 3 out of 10 (on a scale of 1 to 10, 10 being good health) and told me if I followed his treatment, I could get better, and it could take approximately two to three years.

So, I settled into a pattern of treatment. I initially went to Mr Perrin's every six weeks, and in between visited another osteopath, whom Mr Perrin had trained. This osteopath was in Leeds, so it was much easier to get to for weekly treatment, as obviously travelling at that point was very exhausting. Gradually, very slowly at first, I started to see improvement. Appointments went from weekly to fortnightly, and check-ups with Mr Perrin went from every six weeks to every three months.

The summer of 2002 came; I was gradually feeling better and starting to build up my stamina and my immune system. My husband was by then working delivering papers. I would go and meet him later in the day, towards lunchtime, and walk round all afternoon delivering newspapers (using a paper trolley – I could not carry a bag). At first I only managed an hour or so, then I would sit in the car for a while, then do a little more; all that summer I slowly increased my stamina.

We then asked Mr Perrin whether he felt it would be advisable for me to try working. He said I should look for part-time work only and VERY slowly increase the hours, seeing how I went first. I was by this time now going for 6-monthly check ups with Mr Perrin.

So, I then got the first job I had had since I was 19. Obviously, I did not go back to cleaning work! I found an evening job in a call centre, starting on 15 hours a week, Monday, Wednesday, Friday evenings, 4–9pm. This was a good place to start for me. After years of ME, getting up in the mornings was still very hard work. It took me years to overcome that, so an evening job was ideal for my circumstances at the time. In those first few months I had to work on building up my immune system. I vividly remember working with vitamin C, echinacea and cough sweets lined up on my desk, as I got sore throat after sore throat when I first went back to work. Very slowly I increased my hours; I did the 15 hours for eight months, and then went to 20 hours and so on. My last check up with Mr Perrin was sometime in 2003, when he gave me 9.5 out of 10. He said I would never be a 10, as I would always have a residual weakness towards ME.

Time passed, as it does, my health was reasonably okay and I gradually increased my hours at work, until I was doing 32 hours a week, something I would never have thought possible years before.

Then in 2012 I started to have panic attacks and anxiety, something I had never had before, and this resulted in another diagnosis in 2013.

Mid-2015 and I definitely felt unwell again, by this time I was clearly intolerant to various foods but was struggling to pin down which foods and solve the issues. I was now having IBS-like symptoms and had put on weight, and generally felt unwell. Towards the end of 2015, I was again struggling to manage a full workload, and was back to doing a lot more resting, and less activity, though I somehow still held onto my job.

A lot of things then happened in quick succession. I was made redundant from the same job I had now held from 2002 to 2015. I was getting no real answers about the IBS-like symptoms, the weight gain and general fatigue. I still felt at this point that it was not the ME that had come back, as it 'felt different' from the last time, perhaps because I was focusing on the food issues this time round, which was definitely a different problem from the first time I got ill. That time I was 19 and had no issues at all with food. Then in late 2015, when I was still looking for work, my husband said, 'Why don't we go back to Mr Perrin and just get a check up. We can rule out if the ME has come back, and that might help then see if there was some other issue, which the GP or hospital could help with?'

So, in February 2016 I got an appointment with Mr Perrin. He did a check up for me and said that yes, unfortunately the ME was back. Not quite as badly as the first-time round; this time he gave me 5 out of 10. He also explained why I had more food intolerances, and how going gluten free could help the ME.

In the time since I had last seen him, he had gained his doctorate and was now Dr Perrin, and had had some of his research published and his theories proved. There were also a LOT more success stories now for The Perrin Clinic. Dr Perrin now explained that going gluten free would help my body recover better from the ME, as it was spending time breaking down the gluten being consumed and could instead use its limited energy to help repair itself.

I explained to Dr Perrin about the search for work, and how I did need to work this time round. He said I MUST get a part-time job only, preferably 20 hours or less. (This was his opinion about my work from a health point of view.) The very same week I saw Dr Perrin and learnt the ME had returned, I was offered a part-time job, exactly 20 hours! This job was Monday to Fridays 10 am to 2 pm, more call-centre work, for a different company this time. On really bad days, I made it to work for the four hours, came home and crawled back into bed.

So, a lot of things happened in early 2016. I found out my ME had come back, I got a new job and I went gluten free. I was now back to having regular appointments with Dr Perrin, and treatment from another physiotherapist, who had trained with Dr Perrin, in between times. In 2017, I was making slow progress, and I only increased to 6 out of 10 that year. Dr Perrin explained that working part-time this time round, during recovery, was slowing my progress. In keeping up the treatment, I would recover, but more slowly. I went mostly dairy free in 2017; using lactose-free products eliminated some of the IBS-like symptoms, but not all.

In 2018, as well as keeping up my treatment with Dr Perrin, I decided to do *Slimming World*. (I am not recommending any diets or treatments, just telling my story and what worked for me). My weight loss was VERY slow, partly because due to the ME and my stamina; my main exercise was only walking. But after some tough initial times, getting used to the new way of eating, I noticed something unexpected. My panic attacks and anxiety dramatically decreased (very noticeably so), and my IBS-like symptoms all but disappeared. Clearly for me, reducing processed foods and sugar helped both these things. I now cook from scratch and enjoy mostly fresh, unprocessed foods, a personal choice that works for me.

The last check-up I had with Dr Perrin was January 2019, when he gave me an 8 out of 10. I continue to make good progress and have been happy to be feeling noticeably better since mid-2018.

The years of on-and-off illness have left their mark. I find it hard to differentiate between 'normal' tiredness and the ME feeling, and I still even now have to rest on certain days at certain times. But I will always be grateful to Dr Perrin for getting me well enough to work for 13 years, and to enjoy at least most things a normal 20 to 30-year-old should be able to do. After being ill from such a young age, it was precious to me, to have better health in my 20s and 30s. Thank you.

Heather Kaye, Leeds, Yorkshire, UK
Patient of Dr Perrin and Sylveen Monaghan, Chartered Physiotherapist and Licensed Perrin Technique Practitioner.

Chronic fatigue syndrome affects the communication between the internal organs and the musculoskeletal components of the body. This organ of communication is known as the **sympathetic nervous system**, which may be likened to a transmission station in a power station.

In our homes and at work, we use electricity for lighting, for cooking, refrigerating and freezing, for electrical appliances, and for music centres, TVs and computers. The electrical energy required is produced by power stations and is monitored by controllers in transmission stations, which channel the amount of electricity through to us, the consumers.

If we were all suddenly to use substantially more electricity, simultaneously, the transmission station would allow more electricity to flow, signalling to the power stations to produce more energy. This occurs, for example, at half-time during major international televised sporting events, when everybody turns on the kettle at the same time to make a cup of tea.

If something were to go wrong with the operator, or the equipment in the transmission station were to develop a fault, the power required to cope with the increased demand would be insufficient. This would eventually lead to a power cut and blackout. Alternatively, if a situation were to arise when too much electricity passed into the household's supply, an overload or power surge could damage the appliances in use at that time.

In the body, the muscles are the principal 'electrical appliances', utilising most of the energy produced. The power station of the body is the gastro-intestinal system, together with the respiratory system, which consumes fuel in the form of food and utilises oxygen to produce the energy.

The sympathetic nervous system is the transmission station, which connects the visceral 'power station' of the body to the musculoskeletal 'appliance'.

Blackout

When we are active, the sympathetic nervous system stimulates an increase of energy production and a release of stored energy. If this is not accomplished, the result is that the muscles will not receive the nutrients normally obtained from the blood, and the natural function of the muscles, nerves and joints will break down. There will be a power cut in our body and we will suffer fatigue.

This is precisely what occurs in patients suffering from ME/CFS. The body demands more energy, especially when under any form of stress, mental or physical. However, the mechanism normally operated to transform the stored energy into a usable form is not functioning, and thus the patient's body simply stops working effectively.

It is therefore not surprising that ME/CFS is a profoundly debilitating disorder and requires as much rest as possible to reverse the process by minimising the amount of stress on the body. The power station analogy explains why some sufferers seem to display signs of too much sympathetic activity, such as palpitations and excessive sweating, as well as reduced sympathetic activity, such as fatigue and low blood pressure. The fault with the 'transmission station' could lead to the body working in overdrive as well as the power cut scenario, and sometimes in the same patient at the same time. Reducing the demand on the sympathetic nervous system helps the patient on to the road to a full recovery.

As stated in the introductory chapter, scientists from Rochester University, in New York State, have discovered that there is drainage of toxins from the brain into the lymphatic system, which supports my original hypothesis that ME/CFS is due to a dysfunction and backflow in the neuro-lymphatic pathway. The scientists at Rochester University further explored what was happening to this pathway when the drainage was unable to occur in their genetically engineered laboratory mice. They discovered that in these mice, the main areas of toxic build-up in the brain were the thalamus and the basal ganglia.

The thalamus is a small structure located just above the brain stem between the cerebral cortex and the mid-brain and has many influences on both. Its main function is to relay motor and sensory signals to the cerebral cortex. It also contains nuclei in its lateral-posterior section that increase pain and temperature sensation[1].

The thalamus also plays an important part in regulating sleep, and since it is an important part of the limbic system in the brain, also helps control emotional functions.

Therefore, patients with a dysfunctional thalamus, besides suffering from widespread pain, will also complain of mood swings and difficulty moving, reading, talking and processing information. They become less alert and suffer from sleep disturbances, often complaining of vivid dreams. The thalamus contains NMDA (*N*-methyl-D-aspartate) receptors which are severely affected by alcohol, and therefore in ME/CFS and FMS patients, alcohol is definitely a No! No!

Studies have indeed shown overactive NMDA receptors in both ME/CFS[2] and fibromyalgia[3] patients. Activation of NMDA receptors causes the release of the neurochemical, neuropeptide P ('substance P'), that actually enhances painful stimuli around the body[4]. Therefore, a toxic overload in this section of the brain accounts for some of the major symptoms of ME/CFS and fibromyalgia.

ME/CFS also affects another part of the limbic system, the basal ganglia, which together with the thalamus, are also a major junction box between the frontal parts of the brain, which is where thoughts and decisions take place, and other regions of the brain, including the activity centres which are situated in the back of the brain. This turns every action into a chore and creates difficulty in reasoning, making decisions, and other everyday activities, such as reading, writing, talking, walking and even sitting up. In some severe cases, it completely prevents the patient from conducting a normal life.

All nerves use chemicals known as 'neurotransmitters' to pass signals from one nerve to the next. The main neurotransmitter in the brain is the protein glutamate. However, certain specific nuclei in the basal ganglia produce the neurotransmitter gamma-aminobutyric acid (also known as GABA), which is a pain suppressant, centrally dampening pain. Therefore, if this activity is reduced by toxins, it will lead to the increasing generalised pain that plagues both ME/CFS and fibromyalgia patients who also find that any painful stimuli are enhanced. Indeed, over the years, I have had some patients who have had brain scans that reveal structural and functional problems in the thalamus and basal ganglion. It is no surprise that the basal ganglia have been suspected by many other neuroscientists of being involved in ME/CFS[5].

The target of some treatment strategies, such as the Gupta programme, are talk therapy methods that aim to improve the function of the amygdala, part of the basal ganglia (see Chapter 5). Occasionally, brain scans of ME/CFS patients reveal problems in the basal ganglia. Just recently one of my patients, a 64-year-old woman, had problems with balance as well as other severe symptoms of the illness that she had suffered for many years. A CT scan revealed, and I quote from the reporting radiographer's report: 'Several foci or hypodensity within the basal ganglia bilaterally, most likely representing established perforator vessel infarctions, or Virchow-Robin spaces as a differential'.

In other words, there were obvious radiological signs of fluid drainage disturbance in this region. An 'infarction' being an obstruction of blood supply and the Virchow-Robin spaces that may be a factor refer to the perivascular spaces in the brain that surround some cerebral blood vessels, which we now know should drain toxins away via cerebrospinal fluid. It would be interesting to know how many other ME/CFS patients would show similar abnormalities if they had the same scans.

Brain fog

One of the most common symptoms of ME/CFS and fibromyalgia is described by many patients as 'brain fog' or, as I like to call it, 'muzziness'. Their ability to think properly about anything is usually disturbed. Scientists have examined the cognitive symptoms of ME/CFS for many years and have come to the conclusion that it is partly due to altered blood flow to parts of the brain as sympathetic nervous dysfunction leads to patients often complaining of neurally mediated hypotension (low blood pressure) leading to 'orthostatic intolerance' – inability to keep standing. This is coupled with disturbed neurotransmission within the brain[6].

The main parts of the brain affected by neuro-lymphatic drainage problems are the frontal and pre-frontal lobes concerned with thought, plus, as we have said earlier, the basal ganglia and thalamus, which are concerned with emotion and relay messages from the frontal region to the rest of the brain. This leads to the brain fog that some patients find the worst of all the symptoms, especially if prior to their illness they had a job that required major cognitive skills. This, due to the connection with the limbic system, makes them even more depressed.

ME/CFS: 'The Black Hole of medicine'

ME/CFS has been given more names than any other disease, and yet there is still no universally accepted way of positively diagnosing it, and therefore, treatment remains controversial and, by many schools of thought, unscientific. Because the disease is such an enigma, with so many problems affecting the patients and countless different ideas being bandied about, it is often diagnosed without practitioners following the basic and essential procedure in clinical medicine – namely, that of properly examining their patients before making a diagnosis or providing treatment. As it is often diagnosed when other, more common conditions have been excluded, it has been called 'The Black Hole of medicine'[7].

I once had the pleasure of hearing a Stanford Professor of Medicine, Dr Abraham Verghese, at an international ME/CFS conference in California who made the most profound statement: 'The Doctor's round … has become square'. In other words, instead of physically examining the patient, as in days gone by, most physicians are busy looking at a screen for pathological tests etc, In most cases, they should be looking at and listening to the patient to work out what is really going on. As a trained osteopath, I listen to, observe and palpate all patients before any diagnosis is made. Sometimes pathological tests and computers are needed to confirm the diagnosis, but one should always carry out a physical examination first.

Many patients who suffer from ME/CFS are left untreated, with the physician hoping that the patient will spontaneously recover, learn to live with the problem, or change doctors. Despite the fact that the World Health Organization (WHO) has recognised myalgic encephalomyelitis (ME) as a neurological disease since at least 1969, when it published the 8th edition of *The International Statistical Classification of Diseases and Related Health Problems* (ICD-8), and despite thousands of scientific papers being published which demonstrate that ME/CFS is a real physical disease, with many different pathological findings, there are still many GPs who refuse to believe in a physical source of the symptoms and refer their patients to a psychiatrist. Meanwhile, the WHO continues to classify ME/CFS as a disease of the nervous system (ICD-10 G93.3).

Diagnosis of many conditions employs techniques such as MRI (magnetic resonance imaging), using computer-enhanced prints of the body. Electron microscopy shows each cell of the body in greater detail than ever before. Endless numbers of viruses have been identified, and yet, there are still some common ailments that continue to baffle medical scientists, including ME/CFS and fibromyalgia; slowly, however, more and more members of the scientific and medical community are beginning to understand these diseases.

The naming of the disease

Fibromyalgia or fibromyalgia syndrome (FMS) has not suffered as much from an identity crisis as has ME/CFS. FMS is now accepted worldwide as a rheumatological disease affecting the musculo-skeletal system and causing widespread pain.

This acceptance is completely different to the way the medical and scientific camps have viewed the disorder known to many as ME or chronic fatigue syndrome (or post-viral fatigue syndrome, or post-infectious disease syndrome, or chronic Epstein-Barr syndrome, etc etc). In the United States it used to be commonly referred to as chronic fatigue and immune dysfunction syndrome (CFIDS). It has been known by so many names that eminent American specialist Dr David Bell referred to it as the 'disease of a thousand names' in his seminal work[8].

Most diseases are classified according to the type of change that takes place in the cells of the body – e.g. chronic lymphocytic leukaemia. Some diseases are categorised according to causative factors – e.g. caused by *Mycobacterium tuberculosis* or COVID-19. The problem with chronic fatigue syndrome (ME/CFS) is that it does not fit into any particular category. ME/CFS is so diverse in its signs and symptoms that no specific disease classification fits the bill. Thus, we have the term 'myalgic encephalomyelitis': myalgic refers to pain in muscles and encephalomyelitis relates to the possible effect on the brain and spinal cord. This term may suggest that there is inflammation of the central nervous tissue. However, with ME/CFS, inflammation of the spinal cord is not always present.

Although many in the medical profession now recognise the category ME/CFS and realise that there is something physically wrong with the patient, they do not know how to diagnose nor how to treat it.

Most of my patients who suffer from this condition have been to neurologists, undergone brain scans, X-rays, blood tests and many other exhaustive examinations, all of which have yielded inconclusive evidence that there is anything wrong at all. This may lead to the patient being told to get on with life as best as possible and to try and forget about it. The usual advice given to sufferers is to rest until the body sorts itself out, or worse, to gradually increase activity, which mostly causes the patient's symptoms to quickly deteriorate. Sadly, in many cases patients end up forgotten by their health-care providers as they spend months and often years bed-ridden in darkened rooms in silence with little communication with the outside world, which can hardly be called 'living'. Many ME/CFS and fibromyalgia patients just exist, waiting for the miracle cure that never comes.

Even more depressing is that often the patients' own family and friends do not give the patient the support they need. Even in cases where the patient does have a loving and caring family and group of friends, there is a lack of understanding regarding both ME/CFS and fibromyalgia. This lack of understanding is compounded by the media, which often belittles these diseases as just 'in the mind' and suggests that these patients are actually not that ill.

How many 'get well' cards are ever received by ME/CFS or fibromyalgia patients? …Usually none!

Defining ME/CFS

Chronic fatigue syndrome (CFS) or myalgic encephalomyelitis (ME), as it has been known in the UK since an outbreak in 1955 at London's Royal Free Hospital, was first identified by consultant physician in infectious diseases, Dr Melvyn Ramsay[9]. It is a clinically accepted condition now referred to in Great Britain as ME/CFS. As the suffix '-itis' means inflammation of some kind, some health professionals now use the term 'myalgic encephalomyelopathy', signifying a disease state within the head and the spine but not necessarily accompanied by inflammation.

The defining symptom of ME/CFS is post-exertion malaise, but there are many other symptoms, the most common being:
- generalised abnormal muscle fatigue that occurs after relatively mild activity
- difficulty getting to sleep
- sleep disturbance which includes insomnia but sometimes too much sleep (hypersomnia)
- vivid dreams and sometimes very weird ones
- headaches
- problems with short-term memory
- difficulty reading
- cognitive dysfunction
- 'muzziness' in the head/'brain fog'
- frequent rashes on the face, back and/or chest
- dry skin
- frequent spots on the face, back and chest
- panic attacks
- breathlessness
- palpitations
- anxiety and depression (not primary but secondary to the disease)
- increased sensitivity to light and sound
- tinnitus (continuous buzzing or ringing in the ears)
- over-sensitivity to smells
- food sensitivities or allergies
- back pain
- shoulder pain
- neck pain

- generalised muscle pain (myalgia)
- frequent sore throats
- irritable bowel
- bad breath
- frequent fungi and yeast infections
- nausea
- dry eyes
- profuse sweating
- irritable bladder
- numbness
- pins and needles (paraesthesia)
- cold extremities
- pre-menstrual syndrome.

The name chronic fatigue syndrome is used by most medical practitioners around the world, although most patients I meet prefer the term ME (myalgic encephalomyelitis/ myalgic encephalomyelopathy) as this implies a disease state and is much more than just fatigue. However, the term ME by itself is not widely used except in the UK, Norway and Canada and can lead to confusion and may substantially undermine the progress that has been made by many scientists' original research into CFS.

The joint term ME/CFS was agreed upon by the UK's independent working group in its report to the Chief Medical Officer, Sir Liam Donaldson, published on 11 January 2002[10] into the condition, so I have used it in my work, but there is still much debate over the most suitable name. Patient groups in the UK prefer the term ME, whereas on my travels I have learnt that some countries have never heard of ME, but they do know of CFS.

ME/CFS, according to Dr Keiji Fukuda and his colleagues[11] at the Centers for Disease Control and Prevention (CDC) in Atlanta, USA, was defined in 1994 as the presence of the following:

- clinically evaluated, unexplained persistent or relapsing chronic fatigue that is of new or definite onset (has not been lifelong)
- is not the result of ongoing exertion
- is not substantially alleviated by rest
- results in substantial reduction in previous levels of occupational, educational, social, or personal activities.

In addition, the co-occurrence of four or more of the following signs and symptoms must exist, all of which must have persisted or recurred during six or more consecutive months of illness and must not have predated the fatigue:

- self-reported impairment in short-term memory or concentration severe enough to cause substantial reduction in previous levels of occupational, educational, social, or personal activities
- sore throat
- tender cervical or axillary lymph nodes
- muscle pain
- multi-joint pain without joint swelling or redness
- headaches of a new type, pattern, or severity
- un-refreshing sleep
- malaise lasting more than 24 hours following exertion.

Another frequently used but highly controversial set of diagnostic criteria developed by Dr Michael Sharpe and colleagues in 1991 and used by some practitioners in the UK, is the Oxford criteria[12], which is similar to CDC's definition (stated above) but differs in the number of signs and symptoms needed to confirm the diagnosis and, most significantly will still diagnose ME/CFS in patients who are known to suffer from psychiatric disorders, such as depression or anxiety states.

In 2007, Canadian physician Dr Bruce M Carruthers and colleagues published a new working case definition of ME/CFS[13]. It was the first set of criteria for the diagnosis of ME/CFS rather than the less specific CFS. This clinical case definition has been updated to what is now known as the International Consensus Criteria (ICC), which is gradually being accepted around the world, and states that, in order to be diagnosed with ME/CFS, the patient:

- must become symptomatically ill after exertion
- must have signs and symptoms, other than fatigue, such as neurological, neurocognitive, neuroendocrine, immune manifestations and signs of autonomic disturbance.

The history of ME/CFS

The nineteenth century

Many terms have been given to ME/CFS-type disorders, and some of these may actually be different names for the same disease. As early as 1871, Union Army doctor Dr Jacob Mendez Da Costa described a fatigue disorder that affected about 300 soldiers during the American Civil War[14]. The soldiers had all been in active service for some while.

The signs and symptoms listed were as follows:
- abdominal problems, including diarrhoea and frequent indigestion
- palpitations, usually induced by exertion
- chest pain
- shortness of breath, again aggravated by exertion
- rapid pulse
- headache and dizziness
- disturbed sleep
- excessive perspiration.

Dr Da Costa noted that when the soldiers' signs and symptoms had eased, and after they had returned to duty, their performance on the battlefield was of low standard and that they were unable to keep up with their healthy comrades. Dr Da Costa suggested that the cause of the problem was due to physical over-exertion and physical stress of the body, leading to an 'irritation of the heart'. He proposed that the condition was sustained due to an imbalance in the nerve supply to the heart, which includes sympathetic nerves. It became known as 'Da Costa's syndrome', also called 'irritable heart disease' or 'soldier's heart' and had already been recognised in the Crimean War (1853–1856). The famous 'Lady with The Lamp', Florence Nightingale, was ill for most of her life after working as an army nurse in the Crimea. Many believe she was suffering from ME/CFS.

It is something of a coincidence that, as well as Dr Da Costa, another physician practising during the American Civil War has been a major influence on my theories – Dr Andrew Taylor Still. Shortly after serving in the Union Army, Dr Still founded the mechanical treatment of the body that he termed 'osteopathy' (see Figures 8 and 9).

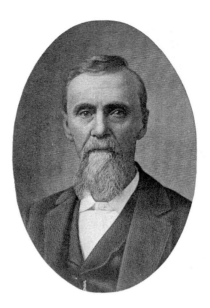

Fig. 8 Dr Andrew Taylor Still (founder of osteopathy) (1828–1917).

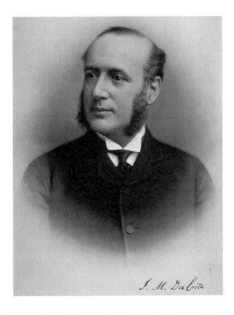

Fig. 9 Dr Jacob Mendes Da Costa (1833–1900).

Clinical scientist and cardiologist Sir Thomas Lewis (1881–1945), the pioneer of the electrocardiograph, wrote a paper in 1920 noting similar cases during the First World War, which he labelled 'effort syndrome', also known as 'neurocirculatory asthenia'. Lewis concluded that an infection was at the root of the problem[15].

The twentieth century

Since Lewis, a number of physicians, neurologists, cardiologists and others have searched for the cause, constantly redefining this mysterious disorder. An outbreak was identified by physician Dr Melvyn Ramsay in 1955 at London's Royal Free Hospital, as I mentioned before[9]. After many doctors, nurses and patients were struck by a mysterious virus, there was one group that did not recover but continued to suffer from lethargy and a range of signs and symptoms now known to be associated with ME/CFS. The group you would expect to be most severely affected by a virus were obviously the patients; however, the sufferers of what came to be called myalgic encephalomyelitis or 'Royal Free disease' were mostly nurses. In the 1950s, nurses often had to lift heavy loads and were in a very demanding job, mentally as well as physically, placing significant strain on the spine. This is also true of many ME/CFS sufferers.

Eminent psychiatrists have pointed to a possible psychological source of the disease[16]. Indeed, many viewed 'soldier's heart' and 'neuro-circulatory asthenia' as forms of what was later termed 'shell-shock' and 'battle-fatigue' and is now known as post-traumatic stress disorder – PTSD.

Even though Da Costa originally linked the condition to fevers, diarrhoea, physical overload and injuries to the body causing a neurological problem, and Lewis thought the cause was an infection aggravated by physical exertion, it is a travesty that the condition they actually described has been reclassified by many as psychiatric in origin.

From the label 'yuppy flu' of the 1980s to the dismissive attitudes of some practitioners, many patients feel isolated and depressed as a result of ignorance. The inability of most of the healthcare profession to legitimise this illness has been shown to aggravate psychiatric problems in patients. Sufferers have been labelled as unmotivated and school- or work-phobic, although many of my patients are well-motivated, high-achieving type 'A' personalities[17].

The twenty-first century

Research findings continue to lay the blame of ME/CFS on the patient's inability to cope with daily problems, fear of physical activity[18], altered perception of the sufferer[19] or worse, the result of parental attitude such as maternal overprotection in childhood[20]. It remains a condition that attracts controversy since many of the signs and symptoms are non-specific and are common to many other illnesses, including psychiatric disorders. Atypical depression, which is a common feature of the disease, has been viewed as a sickness behaviour seen in many chronic illnesses. ME/CFS continues to be an enigma that confounds medical research. Apart from the strain of suffering from a severely debilitating illness, much emotional stress emerges from the refusal of others to accept the validity of the illness, leading to strained relationships at home, work and school, and with members of the social services and medical profession.

There is light at the end of the tunnel, as has been shown in the international consensus criteria (ICC) for medical practitioners, which were formulated by a group of 26 leading doctors and scientists from all around the world with a wealth of knowledge and many years of clinical experience treating the disease. The editors of the ICC (which were based on the widely used Canadian criteria) were Bruce M Carruthers from Vancouver, Canada, and Marjorie I Van de Sande[21].

I had the great honour to meet the late Dr Carruthers a few times at international conferences and I still remember one of his lectures when he said with ME/CFS we have to look at the 'dis-ease' of the patient and treat the whole person rather than try and kill the virus or bacteria possibly causing the disease. This holistic approach was advocated by someone who was probably one of the most experienced orthodox medical physicians in the world trying his best to treat ME/CFS. So, for any physician reading this book, I urge you to follow his advice… treat the dis-ease and not the disease!

More recently, in 2014, a report from the Institute of Medicine of the US National Academy of Sciences, based on a review of more than 9000 published articles, concluded that ME/CFS is a 'biologically based illness'. Since post-exertion malaise is the main common feature in ME/CFS, a new name for the disease has been proposed by the Institute of Medicine: 'systemic exertion intolerance disease' (SEID)[22].

In fact, during the initial consultation with any new patient, I will always ask how they are after exertion, not just exercise (which is often mistaken for exertion). Exertion involves pushing yourself beyond what you consider normal healthy activity.

Unlike some psychiatric illnesses that are helped by exertion, ME/CFS patients will sometimes or always worsen following exertion and sometimes the post-exertion symptoms take up to three days to surface. This has been found to happen in a study by a leading ME/CFS expert, Dr Lily Chu at Stanford University, California. The patient may feel well after exertion for the first couple of days but by the end of the third day their symptoms will have deteriorated.

The fact that some exercises do not seem to affect many patients at the time has been confirmed in another comprehensive study in California. Even after exertion the study showed the cardiopulmonary system seemed to be functioning well in many patients with ME/CFS[23]. The cardiopulmonary exertion test and retest procedure that has been developed by this Californian team is used by some insurance companies and legal teams in the USA to show that, although the patient does not have initial physiological signs of malaise after exertion, a day later a re-test shows a completely different picture, with a post-exertional malaise and impaired recovery due to muscular, cardiovascular, pulmonary or autonomic dysfunction[24, 25].

The patient profile

ME/CFS sufferers tend to be highly motivated individuals who were very active before the illness struck them down. They find it highly depressing being inactive. The depressed feelings and attitude of ME/CFS patients is commonly mistaken for clinical depression. Clinically depressed patients feel better when involved in increased activity, which, unfortunately, aggravates the symptoms of ME/CFS. ME/CFS patients feel miserable, not due to a psychiatric disorder, but from profound frustration.

Case: Miss D

This is a typical example of a ME/CFS patient. This young (age 20), trendy drama student lived life to the full, except at exam times. She presented at my clinic complaining of frequent headaches, drowsiness and lethargy, plus abdominal pain. Her GP had initially suspected that she was suffering from appendicitis. He had then investigated a possible kidney infection. Eventually, a consultant diagnosed that she was undergoing 'some form of stress-related disorder'.

On examination, I detected the familiar restricted dorsal spine, with associated tension within the surrounding musculature. The postural problem was mostly related to the position she adopted whilst studying. She also had certain personal problems at that time which contributed to her overall stress.

The treatment helped relieve all her symptoms in only seven sessions. These were spread out over the year, since she visited my practice during college holidays. To restore proper mobility to the thoracic spine was relatively easy. The patient was quite young, and the mechanical difficulty in the back had only been a recent development. Mobility exercises were prescribed, and she managed to finish her course without ME/CFS giving her any further cause for concern.

Case: Miss P

Another student I saw over a decade ago was an 18-year-old schoolgirl who, for three months prior to the commencement of my treatment, had spent all day in bed. She had fallen ill suddenly in early spring, during the build-up to her A Level exams through which she was hoping to enter a university after the summer recess. She was a grade 'A' student who was expected to achieve just reward for the hard work and effort she had put into many years of study. Instead, she could hardly move out of her bedroom, she could not concentrate or read any book, never mind the school textbooks. Besides the severe fatigue, she suffered from pain in her shoulders, arms and legs, headaches and dizziness.

This girl had been diagnosed as suffering from ME by a specialist who advised her to live as restful and healthy an existence as possible, and the disease would eventually burn itself out.

Her mother and father heard about the results that I was achieving with ME/CFS patients, and thus brought her for a consultation. She was virtually carried in by her parents who seemed to be desperate and looked as though they had little hope in an osteopath being able to help. Quite frankly, her condition was very serious, and she was obviously severely affected by the ME/CFS.

Once I had examined her, I found mechanical problems common to all my ME/CFS patients. They were surprised by my enthusiasm in treating their daughter, and that I was so positive that I could help her.

With an intensive course of treatment, the same girl, at the end of the summer, had restarted her A-level coursework and subsequently gained three As in her exams. She then studied English at university for three more years and gained a first-class honours degree. After a successful career as a PA for a leading actress and film director, she is now happily married with a family and, most importantly, perfectly healthy.

Professional sportsmen, or those people who are keen on sporting events, usually start participating in their discipline at an early age. These competitive individuals are more likely to suffer from developmental disorders commonly associated with overtaxing growing bones and joints.

One such disorder is osteochondrosis in the spine, known as 'Scheuermann's disease'. It is also referred to as 'osteochondritis' as it is an inflammatory disorder of the bone and cartilage which often affects an active, growing spine, and is a frequent cause of backache in adolescents. The disorder usually leaves a slight, permanent deformity in the spine, especially in the thoracic area, with an associated restriction of the affected region. This stiffened area may be asymptomatic for the rest of the person's life, but it may also lead to other mechanical problems of the back. This condition could eventually cause the permanent irritation of the surrounding sympathetic nerves and also affect the lymphatic drainage from the spine, and thus be a further reason for the high incidence of ME/CFS in active and sporty men and women.

The cost of ME/CFS

The UK government's independent working group's report into chronic fatigue syndrome/myalgic encephalomyelitis in January 2002[10] estimated that a general practice with 10,000 patients was likely to have between 30 and 40 ME/CFS sufferers. Prognosis of this complex disorder was recognised as very variable. The economic impact on individuals in the form of informal care and lost employment is devastating. Statistical analysis carried out in 2003 by the Survey and Statistical Research Centre at the UK's Sheffield Hallam University revealed that ME/CFS annually costs the UK government around £3.5 billion in benefits payments, caring and loss of taxation[26].

The rest of the world does not fare any better. An American study in 2004 by Cynthia Bierl and colleagues at the National Center for Infectious Diseases in Atlanta, found that 2.2 million American adults between the ages of 18 and 69 years suffered from CFS-like illness[27]. On a global scale, the impact of ME/CFS on society in both human and economic terms is of great magnitude. As you will understand after reading this book, following the Covid-19 pandemic there will almost certainly be a huge rise in ME/CFS among the survivors, which will place a further financial strain on the world's health services.

Research into ME/CFS

Although many relatively small research projects have been carried out, financed mainly by private charitable trusts and pharmaceutical firms, the main sponsors of medical research have tended to shy away from financing any major studies investigating ME/CFS. As demonstrated from present socio-economic research, there is clearly no evidence to justify this lack of interest compared with the research funding for other global diseases, such as AIDs[28].

Some breakthroughs have been made which may mean objective clinical tests become available to assess the severity of ME/CFS – such as the head-up tilt test using a haemodynamic instability score, which measures the change of flow and pressure of blood when the patient is placed on a tilt table, turning them upside down and then upright. ME/CFS patients take longer for their blood pressure to be increased when changing from horizontal to upright and thus many feel initially faint. This phenomenon, known as neurally mediated hypotension (see earlier – page 32) is due to disturbed sympathetic nerve activity which then fails to monitor changes of position and make the correct adjustment in the cardiovascular system[29]. Yet there are still no universally accepted investigative tests for this condition that have been validated in scientific studies. From the diagnostic viewpoint, there has been little movement in classifying the disease in over a decade, although the recent Canadian/ICC initiative to standardise the diagnostic criteria may help[13].

The symptoms of ME/CFS typically become apparent following a common viral infection, although many other causative factors have been suggested.

- Vaccinations against cholera, tetanus, typhoid and influenza have been associated with the onset of ME/CFS[30].
- Organophosphate pesticides have been suggested as an aetiological (initiating) factor, as have other environmental toxins[31, 32, 33, 34].
- Patients with ME/CFS have been shown to have greater chemical sensitivity than healthy controls[35, 36, 37].
- It has been observed that the psychological disturbances in ME/CFS occur secondary to, or share a common pathophysiology with, immunological dysfunction[38].

Important research[39] is investigating common viral gene expressions found in ME/CFS, which will help with earlier diagnosis, and perhaps some patients identified with the viral signature will soon have a treatment to help rid their body of the offending microbe. However, in many cases there appears to be no apparent cause triggering the condition[40]. Diagnosis of ME/CFS can be made only after all other medical and psychiatric causes of chronic fatiguing illnesses have been excluded.

Red blood cell structure has been studied in various diseases and has shown that the most common aberrant shape of a red blood cell in ME/CFS patients is a flattened disc, with up to 80% of cells having this abnormal shape[41, 42]. Some red blood cells in patients with ME/CFS have also been found in clusters rather than individual cells. This clustering, known as agglutination, is seen due to the presence of antibodies in some ME/CFS and FMS patients who also have chronic infections as well as sympathetic nervous system disturbance leading to clumping as the blood flow slows. These aberrations may lead to loss of fluidity and flexibility of the cell wall, resulting in reduced access of these cells to the deep capillary beds, thereby reducing oxygen supply to tissues and exacerbating any fatigue.

Decreased concentrations of essential fatty acids in red cell membranes of ME/

CFS patients are also thought to be causing the malformation of the red blood cells. In fact, research at London's Hammersmith Hospital in 2003 by Professor Basant Puri revealed a deficiency in fatty acids, which are important for the healthy maintenance of all cell membranes[43]. Puri and his colleagues discovered that a combination of eicosapentaenoic acid (EPA), an omega-3 essential fatty acid, together with unprocessed and unrefined virgin evening primrose oil (an omega-6 essential fatty acid), was the best supplement. In the body, EPA naturally converts to another fatty acid, docosahexaenoic acid (DHA). DHA then combines with a brain chemical, choline, to form a bond that strengthens and even repairs damaged brain cell walls. However, Puri has discovered that if DHA is taken as a supplement, as in many fish oil preparations, it inhibits some of the health effects of EPA, such as an antiviral property. Thus, any omega-3 supplement, to begin with, should contain only EPA and not DHA. I usually recommend that for the first three months at least, EPA only, and then I recommend a product with both EPA and DHA as a maintenance dose.

The amount of EPA and DHA long-chain omega-3 fatty acids within the red blood cells can be expressed as a weight percentage of total fatty acids. This is known as the omega-3 index. If this index is low, it can lead to many health problems including diseases affecting the cardiovascular and especially the nervous systems. Maintaining a high omega-3 index has been shown to help reduce inflammation and oxidative stress in the body. Patients can have a blood test from some private clinics and some nutritional support companies to see if the omega-3 index is high enough and, if not, use supplements to raise this index[44].

As will be shown extensively in this book, there is much evidence to indicate that the central nervous system is profoundly involved in the process leading to ME/CFS. There have been scientific studies for many years focusing on the high levels of toxicity found in ME/CFS patients caused by an array of toxins, such as organic solvents and heavy metals such as mercury, which have a detrimental effect on nerve transmission in the brain and throughout the body[45, 46, 47, 48].

Fibromyalgia

Fibromyalgia, also known as fibromyalgia syndrome (FMS), was first observed by Dr William Balfour in 1824, who described 'tender points', which were then examined in detail by French physician Francois Valliex in 1841. It was referred to as 'fibrositis' in the *British Medical Journal* in 1904 by British neurologist, Sir William

Gowers. However, the term wrongly implied that the pain and discomfort were due to inflammation[49]. The more correct term fibromyalgia has been used since 1976.

It is viewed by many as a form of ME/CFS, but with severe widespread pain in all four quadrants of the body being the principal symptom.

From 1990 until 2010, the American College of Rheumatology (ACR) classified fibromyalgia based on the existence of 11 of 18 tender points on the body known as the fibromyalgia trigger points.

There were nine tender muscular points on both sides of the body:

1. The suboccipital muscles where the upper neck joins the skull.
2. The lower neck muscles.
3. The trapezii muscles where the shoulder joins the neck.
4. The supraspinatus muscle at the back of the shoulder covering the upper part of the shoulder blade.
5. The muscle over the front of the second rib below the collar bone.
6. The tendons attached to the lateral epicondyle, the bony prominence on the outside of the elbow.
7. The gluteii muscles in the upper outer part of the buttocks.
8. The tendons attached to the back of the greater trochanter (the bony prominence at the top of the hip).
9. The tendons attached to the inside of the knee.

However, the problem with these tender points was that some doctors pressed too hard and virtually all patients were diagnosed as having fibromyalgia, while some doctors pressing too little, with hardly any diagnosis consequently being made. Also, many patients were being pressed in the wrong places, and so in 2010 the ACR developed new criteria for the diagnosis of fibromyalgia.

According to the present information from the ACR, fibromyalgia is a neurologic chronic health condition that causes pain in all four quadrants of the body if one divided the body into segments, as shown in Figure 10, plus other symptoms listed below.

Other symptoms of fibromyalgia that patients most often have are:
- tenderness to touch or pressure affecting muscles and sometimes joints or even the skin
- severe fatigue
- sleep problems (waking up unrefreshed)
- problems with memory or thinking clearly.

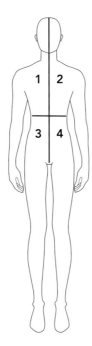

Fig. 10 The main feature of fibromyalgia is pain in the four quadrants of the body.

Some patients may also have:

- depression or anxiety
- migraine or tension headaches
- digestive problems: irritable bowel syndrome (commonly called IBS) or gastro-oesophageal reflux disease (often referred to as GERD)
- irritable or overactive bladder
- pelvic pain
- tempero-mandibular disorder – often called TMJ – a set of symptoms including face or jaw pain, jaw clicking, and ringing in the ears.

The 12-point symptom questionnaire known as the 'symptom severity scale' which has the unfortunate initials SS, and was developed by the ACR in 2010, has many of the symptoms contained in the Perrin fatigue questionnaire (PFQ) for ME/CFS. This questionnaire was developed by myself and fellow scientists and used in the 1990s for the clinical research projects that were carried out at the University of Salford and are still used today by many practitioners around the world (see Appendix, page 420).

The SS scale assesses three main features of the disease: fatigue, unrefreshed sleep and cognitive symptoms, scoring the level of severity over the past week using the following scale:

  0 = no problem

  1 = slight or mild problems, generally mild or intermittent

  2 = moderate: considerable problems, often present and/or at a moderate level

  3 = severe: pervasive, continuous, life-disturbing problems.

This score is added to the severity score (0–3) of physical symptoms in general, which may include any of the 41 symptoms listed below:

muscle pain	pain in upper	loss/change in taste
irritable bowel	abdomen	seizures
syndrome	nausea, nervousness	dry eyes
fatigue/tiredness	chest pain	shortness of breath
thinking or	blurred vision	loss of appetite
remembering	fever	rash
problems	diarrhoea	sun sensitivity
muscle weakness	dry mouth	hearing difficulties
headache	itching	easy bruising
pain/cramps in	wheezing	hair loss
abdomen	Raynauld's	frequent urination
numbness/tingling	hives/welts	painful urination and
dizziness, insomnia	ringing in the ears	bladder spasms
depression	vomiting, heartburn	
constipation	oral ulcers	

Therefore, the final score of the SS scale is between 0 and 12.

Patients are assessed by the SS scale and the widespread pain index (WPI), which divides the body into 19 regions and scores how many regions are reported as painful (see Figure 11).

A patient satisfies diagnostic criteria for fibromyalgia if the following three conditions are met:

1. Widespread pain index (WPI) ≥7 and symptom severity (SS) ≥5 or WPI 3–6 and SS ≥9.

2. Symptoms have been present at a similar level for at least three months.

3. The patient does not have a disorder that would otherwise explain the pain[50].

To answer the following questions, patients should take into consideration
- how you felt during the **past week**
- while taking your current therapies and treatments, and
- excluding your pain or symptoms from other known illnesses such as arthritis, lupus, Sjögren's etc.

Check each area you have felt pain in over the past week

Shoulder girdle, left	☐
Shoulder girdle, right	☐
Upper arm, left	☐
Upper arm, right	☐
Lower arm, left	☐
Lower arm, right	☐
Hip (buttock), left	☐
Hip (buttock), right	☐
Upper leg, left	☐
Upper leg, right	☐
Lower leg, left	☐
Lower leg, right	☐
Jaw left	☐
Jaw right	☐
Chest	☐
Abdomen	☐
Neck	☐
Upper back	☐
Lower back	☐
None of these areas	☐

Determining your Widespread Pain Index (WPI)

Count up the number of areas checked and enter your Widespread Pain Index score here _____ .

Fig. 11 The widespread pain index (WPI):
New clinical fibromyalgia diagnostic criteria – Part 1.

The last condition of not having any other disorder that would explain the pain is a tricky one as you can have two conditions at the same time. This presents the same dilemma as ME/CFS being diagnosed by exclusion. The criteria do not account for people having another disorder at the same time (known as comorbidity) which unfortunately can happen and does so quite often, especially with ME/CFS, which also leads to general muscle pain (myalgia). As you can see, the symptoms of FMS are very similar to those of ME/CFS and this is why I feel they are on the same spectrum of the disease process, with FMS being diagnosed when there is widespread severe pain in all parts of the body, not just aching muscles or minor discomfort. For years, FMS was considered a rheumatologic disorder; however, the immune system has been shown to be important in the pathological process of this disease[51]. There is much evidence to show that FMS, like ME/CFS, also arises from disturbed connections between the central autonomic nervous system, the hormonal system and the immune system[52, 53].

Case: Bev's story

I was 49 years old when I was diagnosed with an aggressive form of breast cancer. Up to that point I had been very fit and healthy, going to the gym three or four times a week, often doing classes back to back.

I had a left mastectomy, all the lymph nodes removed from my left armpit as the cancer had spread there, and surgery to use the latissimus dorsi muscle from my back to create a new breast. This was followed by six cycles of chemotherapy. After allowing myself time to recover from the treatment I returned to the gym but instead of feeling energised my energy levels continued to deteriorate. I had severe fatigue which was unrelenting. I then started to get pain all over my body, right down to my feet.

I bought extra-soft towels as my skin felt so sensitive to touch. I struggled to walk; normal daily activities became impossible; I couldn't chop vegetables or cut up meat. I struggled to shower and found washing my hair impossible. All my teeth were painful; I had pain on my face which made eating difficult as I could barely open my mouth. I went to see my dentist, who did a full mouth x-ray and told me there was nothing wrong.

I suffered from terrible brain fog, had no concentration, couldn't follow conversations, and didn't have the energy to talk. My life changed beyond recognition. My GP did numerous blood tests, which all came back clear. I had scans to ensure the cancer hadn't returned. Eventually she, along with another GP I had seen for a second opinion, diagnosed fibromyalgia. My GP prescribed amitriptyline, which didn't alleviate any of my symptoms and I gained weight. She took me off that and referred me to a rheumatologist who prescribed gabapentin. Nothing changed apart from the fact I felt even more like a zombie.

I went to see Dr Perrin hoping he could help. He had treated my daughter, Olivia, who had made a full recovery from severe ME. Following a physical examination and assessment he diagnosed me with ME/fibromyalgia. Listening to him explain the science behind the Perrin Technique made so much sense and for the first time I felt that my illness was finally understood. His research shows that in some patients with ME the toxins, which aren't draining from the brain due to dysfunction of the lymphatic drainage system, affect the pain receptors in the brain, resulting in the symptoms of fibromyalgia.

Dr Perrin explained to me that the damage to my lymphatic system, together with the high toxicity of the chemotherapy, had triggered the illness. What may have exacerbated my symptoms is the fact that one of the main drainage points of the lymph system is near the lefthand side of the breast area, which was where all of my surgery was. I started the Perrin Technique straightaway, initially having weekly treatments at the Perrin Clinic in Prestwich. I did the self-treatment regime at home every day, with the help of my daughter, as well as following the pacing advice from Dr Perrin. After three months I was pain free and my energy levels had improved dramatically. It was unbelievable. I realise that three months is a relatively short period of time to see such huge changes but we caught it early. As Dr Perrin says 'early diagnosis improves patient outcomes'. That was six years ago. I will not make a complete recovery due to the extensive damage to my lymphatic system, but I have a good quality of life and am pain free.

I continue to have a treatment at the Clinic every four weeks, and do the self-treatment at home about three times a week as a maintenance programme. I pace myself using Dr Perrin's 50% rule – that is, to only do half of what you are capable of doing without the onset of symptoms. That was a learning curve and on occasions, when I hadn't quite got it right, I started to feel the slow return of symptoms, which serves as a stark warning to not overdo things and keep up with the treatment.

With the Perrin Technique I am able to have a social life, go on holiday, go shopping and generally enjoy my days. It really has changed my life.

Postscript: On 9 September 2020 I tested positive for Covid-19. I felt very unwell but did the self-treatment regime [chapter 10] every day. My symptoms began to improve and after only a couple of weeks I was back feeling great. Soon after that my daughters, who usually do my massage for me, were away for 12 days and during that time I neglected to do the massage myself. Some of the Covid symptoms returned. However, within a week or so of doing the massage I felt back to my usual self. I believe without doubt that the Perrin Technique helped my recovery from Covid-19.

Bev McDonald, Lancashire, UK

Authors note:
I have included this story as it aptly illustrates a few interesting points:
1. A patient can be diagnosed with fibromyalgia and have both FMS and ME/CFS.
2. Trauma to the lymphatics from surgery, especially to the breast, can lead to dire consequences and trigger the onset of ME/CFS and FMS (see Chapter 6).
3. Predisposition to ME/CFS can run in families, even if the triggering factor is different (see Bev's daughter Olivia's story at the beginning of Chapter 1).

Chapter 3

The role of the sympathetic nervous system in disease

I advocate for a totally new view of the role of the patient:
patient as engaged partner, not passive recipient.
Richard Davies (Dave) de Bronkart Jr (1950–)
author, international speaker and blogger

Case: Penny's story

In 2009, life took a turn I could never have envisaged.

Prior to this, I had enjoyed a very active and interesting life flying around the world working for British Airways as cabin crew and then, later, on the ground at Manchester which was more conducive to family life. My husband and I were doing up a house together, we enjoyed long walks in the countryside, and I cycled whenever I got the chance. I enjoyed meeting friends, going out for dinner and learning to play the piano. Busy, busy, just like any other family.

In 2004, when my youngest daughter started school, I retrained as a teaching assistant and took a job in a small primary school in Wilmslow, Cheshire. I had truly found my vocation, working with children who had special educational needs. Being in the 'viral pool', as we affectionately called it, had its challenges – lots of runny noses etc. I think you get the picture! I built up resistance like the other staff. After all, I had worked in 'tin tubes' with recycled air and in an air-conditioned airport!

In December 2009, I caught a nasty virus and was in bed for two weeks. Following this, I had several infections, mainly chest, sinusitis and bugs a plenty. This pattern continued on and off, but in December 2012, I had the flu and spent 10 days on sick leave. With the usual guilt in tow, I went back to work too early. I felt very weak and as a result was back in bed again within two weeks of my return. However, this time things spiralled. By January 2013, I was in hospital with suspected viral meningitis.

From this point onwards, my pre-2009 good health never returned. It was Easter before I managed to go back to work on my original hours, but it was a massive struggle and took every ounce of energy I could muster just to get there. The fatigue was crippling. I had gone from a robust individual to one who now picked up every illness that was circulating.

When I fell asleep in a lesson (the teacher wasn't that boring!) I knew I couldn't carry on like this. My GP was very compassionate but had not seen anyone with such prolonged and debilitating symptoms of fatigue, muscle pain/twitching, sleep disturbance, nausea, racing heart, joint pain, memory problems, brain fog etc as I was now presenting. With such an endless list of ailments, I started to sound like a mad woman. Who would even believe me? When I did sleep, I woke up still feeling drained. I was continually off work when my legs refused to 'work' and I was unable to get out of bed. During these episodes, my husband had to take over, which included him carrying me to the bathroom. I was so weak I was unable to reach and lift up a glass of water. The most terrifying part was the not knowing if or when each 'episode' would end. That really played with my head. 'Will this be the one that leaves me bedridden for years?' I used to think. This, of course did not help my cause as it resulted in even more stress, but I'm only human.

I am not going to lie. There were times when I felt that no life at all was a better option than the one I was trying to live. My emotional wellbeing was taking a battering. I felt angry. After all, I had tried to be a kind and good person. I didn't drink or smoke. Why had this happened to me? Looking back, I was mourning the loss of my old, active life and the freedom of choice it gave me. I would and will never, ever take that for granted again.

My first of many consultations was with a haematologist who found nothing amiss. Next was a rheumatologist who said I should take antidepressants and suggested it was psychological. Very helpful! To cut a very long story short, I saw an endocrinologist, had a brain scan to look at the pituitary gland, endless blood tests and finally ended up at Liverpool Hospital for Infectious Disease where I was diagnosed with ME/CFS. It was now June 30th, 2014. I was overwhelmed with relief. Bizarre isn't it, to be told you have a chronic illness and feel such an emotion? At last it had a name and I was, above all, believed. If I had a pound for every person who had told me that 'they got tired too' I would be very rich indeed. I could only try and describe to them that ME/CFS is like having the worst flu you have ever encountered coupled with the worst jetlag.

From diagnosis, the search began for help. I tried lots of complementary therapies which helped short-term with the pain, but didn't last. I now think the benefit lay in the relaxing and calming effect on my central nervous system. I reduced my working hours, tried CBT, mindful relaxation, took advice from a clinic in London, changed my diet and took supplements. I tried to do yoga and Pilates. The exercises proved to be too difficult as my muscles wouldn't cooperate, and it was too exhausting. Having seen a very knowledgeable endocrinologist at Salford Royal, I knuckled down to a strict pacing regime. I was still in a 'boom and bust' cycle and it was extremely difficult to manage. When was too much too much? Sadly, I only found out when it was too late, and I ended up in bed.

I limped on over the months, trying to get the balance right, micromanaging and assessing everything I did on a daily basis in order not to overdo it, but the episodes kept coming. If I picked up a cold it would be devastating. An ear infection saw me off work for several weeks. Some days, I was having difficulty verbally retrieving everyday vocabulary. Words often just didn't look right. My memory was deteriorating. At one low point, I entered my classroom and realised I couldn't remember the name of the teacher I had worked with for years. I had to excuse myself to the loo whilst I racked my brains. I thought I was going mad.

Feeling more and more isolated, I stopped trying to explain the illness to people and no longer read everything I could find on the internet. Other than my immediate family, I felt nobody understood how desperate I was starting to feel. By this point I no longer engaged socially. I felt I had literally exhausted every avenue, and this was now going to be my life.

In the Spring of 2018, my husband came home from his usual golf match and told me about a conversation he had had with a man he had been paired up with. Both his wife and daughter had ME and had visited Dr Perrin in Prestwich. They had been successfully treated and were much improved. What did I have to lose?

I saw Dr Perrin in April 2018. He confirmed I had ME and gave me a score of 4.5. out of 10 – 10 being fit and well. He explained that people with ME often think they are healthier than they really are. I had been quite proud of my now, well-established pacing regime but Raymond said I was still in boom and bust and should give up work. I was upset. I felt I had sacrificed so much in life already. To give up my job completely would leave me with no sense of purpose whatsoever. We compromised and I cut my work back to nine hours a week.

Thank goodness my bosses were so understanding and supportive throughout.

I began treatment soon after with Collette, at the Village Osteopaths in Timperley, as it was closer to get to. I had prepared myself for feeling worse before feeling better, but it wasn't too bad within that first three months; I just got a bit spotty, had a bout of sinusitis and some weight gain from doing half of what I felt I could (as instructed).

At 12 weeks, I was reassessed, and Colette gave me a new score of 6. I was delighted to say the least. I cried all the way back to the car where my husband was waiting to drive me home as usual. He looked worried until I told him they were tears of joy! I had not felt such a sense of hope in years.

At the end of October I took my first holiday in nine years. Nigel and I went to a wedding in Maryland. He sorted everything out and made plans A, B and C depending on energy levels and covered every eventuality. Other than a couple of dips where I had to rest up, we had the most wonderful time. I now feel anything is possible.

I have had what I would describe as 'mini episodes' where I definitely have identified stress to be the cause (bereavement). Overall, these haven't been as prolonged as they used to be, and I think I am more 'accepting' of them. I think fighting this illness feeds it but that's easier said than done when you are so debilitated.

When you feel you have tried everything to get better, but to no avail, it can be very daunting to commit to something new. That fear of disappointment is a hard one to overcome.

This is not a quick fix or magic bullet. It requires total commitment; sometimes when you least feel like it. In my experience, the improvement is very gradual and almost natural. You aren't aware you can do more physically until you look back and reflect. I am still pacing and being careful. I have the support of my husband, family and close friends without which I could not have survived this disease.

At the end of my treatment, if I can do 80% of what I used to prior to the onset of ME, I will be very happy indeed. If I can get back on a bicycle, I will be ecstatic. I'll even settle for an electric one!

The future already looks brighter. I have even taken up the piano again. That's only good news for me of course. I pity those around me having to listen! After all, this treatment can't fix everything.

Update in August 2020: Following regular 12-week reviews through the summer of 2019 and a lot of hard work, I continued to gradually improve. By December 2019 I was 8/9 out of 10 and hadn't had a flare up for four months. This is the point where I felt I was at a plateau but to be honest, I was happy to settle for that. Sadly, life is a rollercoaster (cue song!) and in January 2020 I became extremely poorly. I had the worst episode since my diagnosis and couldn't move out of bed for eight weeks and was very weak for several after that. I will never know if I had Covid -19 but Collette pointed out that my immune response may not have been typical of others with the disease (I didn't present with the cough etc.) I was devastated both mentally and physically. Obviously, I was unable to go for treatment during lockdown but I have now returned to the practice and feel I am back to where I was when reviewed in December 2019. My energy levels are much improved and I have been able to do some gardening for the first time in years so who knows, I may be even stronger than I think!

Penny Naden, Cheshire, UK
Patient of Collette Nelstrop (B Ost) Registered Osteopath and Licensed Perrin Technique Practitioner

Note from the author: Penny's story is similar to that of many recovering patients with a resurgence of symptoms following an infection of Covid-19. In the UK, some Perrin Technique practitioners, such as Penny's osteopath, have been on lock-down during the height of the pandemic. However, some clinics like mine remained open for emergency and urgent cases. If there is a relapse following an infection or other stress factors, it is important to intervene as soon as possible for a better chance of a quick recovery. Fortunately, in this case, the delay in receiving the necessary treatment was not too damaging.

RP September 2020

Many terms have been given to ME/CFS-type disorders, as we saw in the previous chapter, and these may be different names for the same disease. As mentioned in the previous chapter, Dr Jacob Mendez Da Costa wrote in 1871 about Da Costa's syndrome in the *American Journal of Medical Science*, a paper[1] suggesting that the cause of the problem was physical over-exertion and stress of the body, leading to an irritation of the heart. He proposed that the condition was sustained due to an imbalance in the autonomic nerve supply to the heart. However, there is a major difference between Da Costa's beliefs and mine. He and his colleagues believed the problem led to a psychiatric condition which is now known as post-traumatic stress disorder (PTSD), whilst I believe the illness is a physical one, namely ME/CFS.

PTSD has also been linked with fibromyalgia syndrome by many physicians. Häuser and colleagues concluded that PTSD was a potential risk factor for fibromyalgia syndrome (FMS) and vice versa. FMS and PTSD are common comorbid conditions because they are frequently associated with previous traumatic experience[2].

This is different to a much rarer condition known as post-traumatic fibromyalgia, which is a very severe form of fibromyalgia that occurs as a result of a traumatic injury, usually to the neck, such a whiplash injury sustained in a car crash, and remains very difficult to treat (see Chapter 10)[3].

The autonomic nervous system

The autonomic nervous system controls the automatic functions of the body. It is divided into two sections, the sympathetic and parasympathetic. One of the main functions of the sympathetic nerves is the control of the walls of the arteries, which supply blood to most parts of the body. The heart (and heartbeat) is predominantly stimulated by the sympathetic nerves aided by the parasympathetic vagus nerve. It is interesting to note that when the sympathetic nerves supplying the heart are over-active, the heart rate can increase to over 200 beats per minute, whereas the average normal adult heart rate is 50–100 beats per minute (bpm).

The sympathetic nervous system has its entire origin within the spinal cord. Along with the other part of the autonomic system, the parasympathetic nerves, as well as the hormones of the endocrine system, the sympathetic nerves are responsible for tuning visceral, circulatory and metabolic activity to muscular demand. The overall control centre of the autonomic nerves lies in the brain. However, the performance of the sympathetic system can be greatly affected by mechanical and postural strain to the middle section of the spine, from the first thoracic vertebra to the second lumbar segment.

Neurotransmitters

Research in the 1930s by Dale and Gaddum[4] and Feldberg and Gaddum[5] revealed that the transport of nerve impulses across synapses involved the release of chemicals, now known as neurotransmitters. There are two types of neurotransmitter involved in the autonomic control of the viscera:

1. The cholinergic neurotransmitters, which use the chemical acetylcholine.
2. The adrenergic neurotransmitters, which use noradrenaline (known as norepinephrine in the USA).

One of the main transmitter substances in the sympathetic nervous system is noradrenaline. This is formed in the adrenal glands and in a small organ in the brain stem known as the locus coeruleus, which is under the direct influence of the hypothalamus (see Figure 1, Chapter 1).

Research by Xie and fellow scientists at Rochester University, New York, published in 2013, showed that the hypothalamus–locus coeruleus axis is a vital area in the brain for healthy neuro-lymphatic drainage[6].

I first drew Figure 1 (see Chapter 1) in 2004 for my doctoral thesis, to show the importance of these two regions in the pathological mechanism leading to ME/CFS. I knew that, since noradrenaline is so important in the functioning of the sympathetic nervous system, this axis must be disturbed in neuro-lymphatic disorders. This is exactly what Xie and his colleagues discovered with their ground-breaking work, showing why we all need restorative delta-wave sleep (see below), as the neuro-lymphatic drainage system occurs mostly during this sleep phase.

Recent studies on human sleep have discovered a pumping mechanism in the brain, hitherto unknown, that is produced during … you guessed it … delta-wave sleep. The research team was led by Professor Nina Fultz at the Department of Biomedical Engineering at Boston University in the USA[7].

The researchers used MRI scanners to examine 13 healthy young people whilst they slept, and found that every 20 seconds a wave of cerebrospinal fluid (CSF) flows into the brain, replacing a large flow of blood that is stimulated by delta-waves during deep restorative sleep. This extra pumping action of CSF leads to an increase in pressure within the ventricular system and is most probably the mechanism that improves neuro-lymphatic drainage during delta-wave sleep as described in the research by Xie and colleagues on mice. Further research is necessary on humans, but I would be very surprised if this new pumping mechanism induced by delta-waves was not found to be under the influence of the hypothalamus and the sympathetic nerves.

One of the most common symptoms of ME/CFS is unrefreshing sleep. The reason for this is that ME/CFS patients have too high a level of non-restorative alpha-wave sleep.

There are five stages of sleep: 1–4 (non-REM sleep) and REM (rapid eye movement) sleep. During these stages neurological activity within the brain changes. These stages progress cyclically from 1 to 4 through to REM, then begin again with stage 1. A complete sleep cycle takes an average of 90 to 110 minutes, with each stage lasting between five and 15 minutes.

- Stage 1 is light sleep where you drift in and out of sleep and can be awakened easily.
- In stage 2, eye movement stops and brain waves become slower, with only an occasional burst of rapid brain waves.
- In stage 3, extremely slow brain waves, called delta-waves, are interspersed with smaller, faster waves. This is deep sleep. It is during this stage that a person may experience sleepwalking, night terrors, talking during one's sleep, and bedwetting.
- In stage 4, deep sleep continues as the brain produces mostly delta-waves.
- During REM (rapid eye movement) sleep, brain waves mimic activity during the waking state. The eyes remain closed but move rapidly from side-to-side, which is often due to brain activity that occurs during dreams. During this phase the rest of the body is immobilised.

Brainwaves

In the brain we have around one hundred billion nerve cells (neurones) that are constantly in communication with each other through trillions of connections known as synapses. Brainwaves are produced by synchronised electrical pulses from different areas of neurons communicating with each other.

Brainwaves can be detected using sensors placed on the scalp. They are divided into bandwidths which each have different functions. Slower brainwaves, such as delta-waves, make us feel tired, slow, sluggish, or dreamy. The higher frequencies can create a hyper-alert state, which some call 'wired and fired'. In practice, things are far more complex, and brainwaves reflect different aspects when they occur in different locations in the brain.

Brainwave speed is measured in Hertz (cycles per second) and they are divided into bands delineating them as slow, moderate, or fast.

The waves are as follows, starting with the slowest:
- Delta-waves = 0.5–3 Hz; they occur during deep sleep.
- Theta-waves = 4–7 Hz; they are present during deep meditation and dreaming.
- Alpha-waves = 8–13 Hz; they appear during visualisation and meditation.
- Beta-waves = 14–40 Hz; they are present during wakefulness and REM sleep.
- Gamma-waves = more than 40 Hz; as with Beta waves, they occur spontaneously during wakefulness and REM sleep.

Most patients with ME/CFS complain that they don't get enough sleep and that they when they do, they still feel exhausted. The problem for them is that though they may often have plenty of sleep, it isn't the restorative kind as it is consists of a high proportion of alpha-waves. This is known as alpha-wave intrusion and was shown in a study published in 2007[8].

It has further been demonstrated by researchers at Stanford University that ME/CFS patients have fewer delta-waves during the night, but too many during the day[9].

The drainage of the brain and spinal cord occurs more during waking hours in ME/CFS and FMS, making those patients feel ill and shattered during the daytime. However, during the night in ME/CFS and FMS, the hypothalamus–locus coeruleus axis switches on, leading to the 'wired and fired' state, affecting the patient's ability to fall asleep.

Not only does the type of sleep affect neuro-lymphatic drainage, but it is the position a person adopts during sleep that is also vitally important. A side-lying posture during sleep aids neuro-lymphatic drainage as well as being the best position for the spine in general[10]. Often, I am asked 'which side is best?'. Regarding neuro-lymphatic drainage, I don't think it matters that much and I would advise you to start with lying on the side you feel most comfortable on. However, the left side is believed to be the better for improving venous return to the heart and also has been shown to reduce gastric reflux and heartburn[11].

To maintain a balanced spine in bed, as well as lying on your side, I recommend a small pillow, such as a scatter cushion, placed between your knees throughout the night (see Chapter 10).

Further investigation has found that the hormone adrenaline (epinephrine) acts on two receptors at the target organ. These receptors are called alpha and beta receptors. When an alpha receptor is stimulated, it causes constriction of the blood vessels. Vasodilation occurs if the beta receptors are excited. Thus, adrenaline can produce an increase and decrease of blood flow. The neurotransmitter noradrenaline, on the other hand, predominantly acts on alpha receptors, leading to vasoconstriction.

More research has discovered a further division of the receptors of the neurochemical transmitters: alpha-1 and alpha-2 plus beta-1 and beta-2. The transfer of messages to the types of four receptor is blocked by different chemical antagonists – for example, the antagonist drug prazosin blocks only alpha-1 receptors. Stimulation of the alpha-1 receptors leads to constriction of the blood vessels, thus prazosin, by blocking this effect, aids vasodilation, thus reducing overall blood pressure. This is because the larger the diameter of the vessels, the less the resistance against the flow of blood. This selectivity makes prazosin useful in treating hypertension (high blood pressure).

The autonomic nervous system maintains an important function in regulating the body's inner environment. This process, known as homeostasis, is clearly demonstrated when there is a break in the spinal cord above the first thoracic vertebra following a major trauma. The lesion of the cord at this level would cut off the whole thoracic-lumbar sympathetic outflow from higher control. After such an accident, tilting the patient from supine (lying down) to an upright position has been shown to lead to:

• decrease in blood pressure
• increase in the rate of the pulse
• loss of consciousness.

These effects occur since there is no compensatory control of the blood vessels to adjust to the change of position.

At the same time, the skin blood vessels do not adapt to any change of body temperature, so there is no vasodilation or sweating. If cold, there is no shivering of the muscles controlled by nerves below the spinal lesion. It is important to note that the lower the damage to the cord, the smaller the disturbance of autonomic control.

Sympathetic nerve fibres reach the blood vessels via two distinct paths:

1. Directly, from the sympathetic chain to the plexuses around the aorta controlling the vessels in the abdomen, thorax, skull and upper parts of the arms and legs.
2. Via peripheral nerves to the forearms, hands, lower legs and feet. Surgeons often help circulatory problems by an operation known as a 'sympathectomy' (destruction of a portion of the sympathetic nervous system in the thoracic or the lumbar spine. The results of this form of surgery include widespread and lasting dilation of the arterial supply in the limbs, especially in the skin.

If the signs and symptoms of ME/CFS are due to a dysfunction of the sympathetic nervous system, a sympathectomy is obviously not the desired treatment: although the peripheral circulation may improve, cutting off the sympathetic control would have unwanted side-effects. This is also the case with some medications, such as beta blockers, which are regularly prescribed for cardiovascular signs and symptoms, such as palpitations and high blood pressure.

A very low dose of the beta blocker propranolol has been shown to reduce overall pain and some other symptoms in FMS, but higher doses could have the opposite effect by over-stimulating the sympathetic nervous system[12]. Low dose (one fifth to one tenth of normal) propranolol blocks sensory receptor activity without activating the adrenergic receptors that constrict the blood vessels.

There are also alpha and beta cholinergic receptors (i.e. stimulated by the neurotransmitter acetylcholine) on both the muscle sensory neurons that signal fatigue and others that signal muscle pain; there are also some on circulating immune cells. These receptors are blocked at lower doses (one tenth of the usual dose) than is necessary to block alpha and beta receptors on vascular smooth muscle.

This means that extremely low doses of propranolol can block the sensory receptors, reducing the total signal to the sympathetic nervous system, allowing the normal sympathetic reflexes to be re-established. However, the regularly prescribed levels of beta blockers for patients with hypertension will exacerbate the fatigue and should be avoided if possible. (Consult your GP/family doctor for possible alternatives.)

The sympathetic nervous system

The role of the sympathetic nervous system is to co-ordinate the functioning of the viscera (the internal organs), via messages and impulses from the musculo-skeletal system, thus allowing the healthy existence of the whole body.

The concept of the primary machinery of the body being the neuromuscular-skeletal system, with the internal organs being secondary and supportive, is a fundamental principle of osteopathic philosophy. When one observes a fellow human, it is the make-up of the person that is apparent – their build, and shape and how they utilise their structural assets is what is most important. In everyday existence, it is the muscles, tendons, ligaments, joints, skin and bones, together with the nerves supplying these structures (the somatic nerves), that form the 'primary machinery of life' as it was described by one of the past luminaries of the osteopathic and chiropractic world, physiologist Irvin M Korr (1909–2004) in his studies on the autonomic nervous system[13, 14, 15, 16, 17].

Since Korr's research there have been new discoveries concerning sympathetic nerves that further help explain many of the symptoms of ME/CFS. In Bidiford, Maine, USA there is a wonderful osteopathic college which was host to my first workshop teaching American osteopathic physicians, UNECOM (University of New England College of Osteopathic Medicine). Among the first American doctors of osteopathy to train in the Perrin Technique was a neurologist who, after the course, told me that my work had managed to combine the neurology and neuroscience she had learnt with the basic osteopathic principles.

At UNECOM there is an anatomy lab run by arguably the world's leading anatomist involved in the autonomic nervous system, Professor Frank Willard.

A few thousand miles away from Professor Willard at Kiel University there is German neurophysiologist, Professor Wilfred Jänig. Thanks to Willard's and Jänig's in-depth knowledge and ground-breaking discoveries we now know that the sympathetic nervous system has a major influence on the sensory component concerned with many more messages entering the spinal cord and brain compared with the signals being sent out to different organs as originally thought at the time of Korr's seminal work. The sympathetic nerves are very narrow fibres compared with the much larger sensory nerves. Sympathetic nerves, because of their frailty, are found lying along blood vessels in the deeper tissues. However, when they travel to the surface, they can be found lying along somatic nerves – that is, the nerves involved in the voluntary control of the body. Connectors between sensory nerves that send pain signals to our brain, known as peripheral somatic nociceptive afferent fibres, and sympathetic nerves have been observed in many pathological mechanisms to affect nociceptive (pain) pathways and vice versa.

Noradrenaline, one of the main neurotransmitters of the sympathetic nervous system as explained earlier, acts directly on these sensory nerves. It also stimulates the release of chemicals that excite these sensory nerves, such as prostaglandins. Noradrenaline release may have local effects on blood flow, resulting in skin-enhancing activity.

Different nerve fibres join each other at points known as synapses. In the autonomic nervous system, a large number of nerves join each other in separate bundles of synapses. These bundles of nervous tissue are situated throughout the body and are known as ganglia (singular: ganglion). The nerves between the spinal cord and the ganglia are known as preganglionic fibres, and the nerves between the ganglia and the target organ are called postganglionic fibres. One preganglionic fibre may synapse with many postganglionic nerves, thus increasing the overall area in the body affected by one impulse from the spine.

The sympathetic ganglia mostly lie at the side of the middle section of the spinal cord in two parallel chains. There are other sympathetic ganglia that lie in front of the main artery in the abdomen, the aorta. Some form large bundles of nerve fibres, each known as a plexus – for example, the solar plexus found in the upper central part of the abdomen.

The role of the ephapses

One fact about neurotransmission that most practitioners in the medical world find truly amazing when I give my lectures is that, as well as nerves connected chemically via synapses, sympathetic and sensory fibres which lie close together in the surface tissues are coupled electrically by lesser known 'ephapses' resulting in 'cross talk' which was originally shown in the 1950s[18], but has been examined in detail more recently by Jänig.

Most people have heard of synapses where neurotransmitters travel from one nerve to another, continuing messages along the neural pathway. However, very few in the scientific or medical world know anything about ephapses which cross over at the main long body of the nerve (known as the axon).

As the peripheral sympathetic nerves become overstimulated in ME/CFS, they begin to send messages over to their neighbouring sensory nerve leading to sympathetic-induced pain, tingling or burning. Sometimes it is just a 'trickling' sensation, with patients describing the feeling like running water just beneath the skin. It can also cause itching or a creeping sensation, with sometimes numbness and occasionally pins-and-needles in one area of the body, or just the arms and legs. However, in some distressing cases, the whole body can be affected.

When one understands that the ephapses can transfer signals from sympathetic nerves to the sensory (afferent somatic) nerves, and vice versa, then one can understand why many symptoms do not follow the normal patterns in ME/CFS and FMS, which confuses clinicians the world over. For example, many ME/CFS and FMS patients may have pain or sensitivity in their feet which normally would relate to a possible problem affecting the nerves that come from the lower lumbar region of the spine, but these often appear normal on further examination. However, investigation of the upper lumbar region (at about the waistline) of the spine will often reveal problems as these segments are where the bottom of the sympathetic chains leave the spinal cord. The sympathetic chains, or sympathetic trunks, are paired bundles of nerve fibres that run down both sides of the spine, passing to and from the central nervous system via the thoracic and upper lumbar spine. This is why treatment to the lower thoracic spine and upper lumbar region in ME/CFS and FMS often helps foot pain (see Figure 12).

It may be that sympathetic nerves also act the same way on motor fibres near the surface, leading to the twitching and even muscle spasms that affect many patients, but at the time of writing this new edition no evidence of motor ephapses has yet been found.

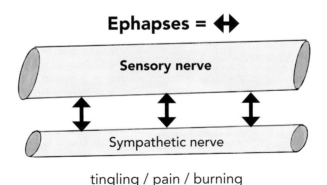

Fig. 12 Ephapses: cross fibre stimulation of parallel nerves.

Fibromyalgia vs ME/CFS

Since 2010, the American College of Rheumatology has classified fibromyalgia as a syndrome with many similar symptoms to ME/CFS and with widespread pain in all four quadrants of the body.

There is an argument and evidence to show that ME/CFS and fibromyalgia are genetically different diseases. However, although they obviously present differently, my view is that both illnesses are due to the backflow of neurotoxins in the neuro-lymphatic system, leading to many common symptoms and epidemiological characteristics, such as both conditions affecting more women than men and being found more in previously highly motivated and active people. Most importantly, the same five physical signs that I have discovered in patients with ME/CFS, also exist in fibromyalgia. However, when the main symptom is fatigue with post-exertion malaise, it is most likely to be ME/CFS, and when the main complaint is severe widespread pain, then I feel fibromyalgia (FMS) may be a more correct diagnosis. Often in clinic, due to the difficulty in determining what the predominant symptom is, I will diagnose 'ME/CFS with FMS'.

The reason for the different emphasis of symptoms in ME/CFS and FMS, I believe, is the amount of toxicity affecting areas of the brain that control pain perception. This theory is supported by the work of USA fibromyalgia expert Dr Robert Bennett, who has been involved in fibromyalgia research since 1979 and has published countless original studies in this field. He explains that in fibromyalgia, specialised receptors called NMDA receptors are stimulated by large levels of the neurotransmitter glutamate. Activation of these receptors, together with the abnormal levels of substance P (see page 30), greatly enhances the intensity of the pain signal transmitted.

These alterations in the nerve pathways involved in the transmission of pain lead to a state of hypersensitisation, where pain is felt at a much lower threshold, referred to as 'central sensitisation'. As mentioned previously in Chapter 2, toxins can affect the production and action of neurochemicals such as GABA as well as substance P. These neurotransmitters are affected in fibromyalgia as well as ME/CFS, but more so in the former.

How the sympathetic nervous system responds to stimuli

Rapid adjustments in accordance with levels of exertion and posture are orchestrated largely by the sympathetic nerves. The parasympathetic system makes long-term adjustments to maintain and replenish stores of nutrients and fuel, which have been utilised under the direction of the sympathetic system. In other words, both sections of the autonomic nervous system work in conjunction with each other. From this viewpoint, illness results from the inconsistency between demands of the neuromuscular-skeletal system (the primary machinery) and the ability to maintain adequate provision for the normal functioning of all of the body's systems. Thus, a patient requires rest when ill, reducing demands until this disparity has been corrected.

Conventional medicine places an emphasis on the demands made by the internal organs: however, by virtue of their mass and their rapidly changing metabolic rate, the muscles are the main consumers of the body's energy supply. The energy production in cells takes place in a structure known as a mitochondrion. Muscle cells contain large numbers of mitochondria to produce the energy needed to move about.

Disease within the body can be divided into four categories depending on the different systems affected:

1. Damage to the neuromuscular-skeletal system commonly due to trauma, postural problems or over-use.
2. Visceral disorders due to physical or operational defects in one or more of the internal organs; these are often due to infection or other disorders affecting the immune system, such as autoimmune diseases.
3. Emotional or psychosomatic disorders.
4. Communicative disorders, which occur when there is impaired communication between the musculoskeletal system and the internal organs. This happens when either the nervous or vascular channels are either incomplete or interrupted.

ME/CFS and FMS are primarily forms of this fourth category of disease origin, with the other three often being predisposing factors to differing degrees in each individual case.

The parasympathetic nervous system

The parasympathetic ganglia are mainly situated in the various organs which they supply. Their postganglionic fibres innervate all the internal organs and the eye. The uppermost fibres in the head supply the lachrymal glands of the eye, which produce tears, and the salivary glands. A major parasympathetic nerve from the head is the vagus, which supplies the organs of the neck, thorax, abdomen, pelvis and genitalia.

The sympathetic postganglionic fibres supply all the organs innervated by the parasympathetic nerves, although the distribution to different parts of the organ may vary. The blood supply to the body is almost entirely under the control of the sympathetic nervous system, except the vasculature of the pelvic organs and genitalia, which is under parasympathetic regulation.

The sympathetic influence over arterial pressure and peripheral blood resistance affects cardiac output, and many other metabolic processes. The parasympathetic vagus nerve modifies the rhythm of the heart, but the sympathetic nerves regulate the entire cardiovascular system, in accordance with what is going on in the body as a whole.

The differences between the sympathetic and parasympathetic nervous systems

The sympathetic nervous system differs from the parasympathetic in the following ways:

1. The parasympathetic nerve supply is almost entirely visceral, exerting most of its control over the internal organs. The sympathetic nerves, however, regulate functioning of the skin, bones, ligaments, tendons and parts of the somatic nervous system, plus the skeletal muscle as well as the organs.
2. The parasympathetic nerves are more specific, with individual nerves supplying a specific target organ. The sympathetic effects are more widespread due to a fanning out of the nerves to all the tissues.
3. The blood supply of the genitalia is primarily controlled by the parasympathetic nervous system whereas the sympathetic nerves control the circulation throughout the rest of the body. Erectile dysfunction is, however, sometimes seen in ME/CFS[8] and fibromyalgia, due to the central autonomic dysfunction leading to parasympathetic disturbance. Reduced sexual activity is a common problem in both ME/CFS and FMS, although more often due to lack of libido, pain or just plain exhaustion.
4. The parasympathetic system is not directly affected by the requirements of the body, but the sympathetic nerves are influenced and controlled by the demands of the other bodily systems.

It has always been assumed that the parasympathetic nervous system has an overall calming effect on the body and dampens overexcited nerves, and, until recently, was never thought to be a major factor in the disease process unlike the sympathetic nerves. However, due to new findings, especially through the work of Dr Stephen Porges and the 'polyvagal theory', we now know different. Dr Porges has discovered that there are not just two components to the autonomic nervous system, but in fact the main parasympathetic pathway is divided into two sections, front (ventral) and back (dorsal). The ventral vagus is a signalling system for motion, emotion and communication which forms our social engagement system... this is the vagus nerve that is well known.

Although the dorsal vagus is a more recent discovery, it is a remnant of our primitive ancestry and is advanced in reptiles and possums, which use it when they play dead as a defence mechanism. It is the immobilisation system which is our passive defence system and, if overstimulated, can lead to pathological mechanisms that cause symptoms such as bradycardia (extremely slow heart rate) and sleep apnoea, when some sufferers stop breathing for a dangerously long time in their sleep. The vagus nerve can be affected biomechanically by problems in the suboccipital region at the very top of the neck, and so this is an important region to examine in ME/CFS and FMS patients, and also to concentrate on when attempting to improve spinal movement and stability to balance the overall autonomic control (see Chapter 10).

Pain, numbness and muscle spasm in ME/CFS

As explained earlier, an intimate relationship exists between part of the somatic nervous system and the sympathetic nerves. The somatic motor nerves, which stimulate skeletal muscle contraction, contain fibres that lie alongside the fibres of the sympathetic nerves as they leave the spinal cord. The sympathetic fibres connect with the motor nerves as they travel down to the tissues being supplied.

As explained above, the sympathetic sensory nerves are excited by painful states in the internal organs. The reduction of blood flow when there is a spasm in the organ leads to a chemical irritation, stimulating the preganglionic sympathetic nerves in the spinal cord. This leads to physiological changes within the target organs – dilation of blood vessels resulting in increased circulation, for example. The neighbouring motor neurones are excited, prompting a sustained muscular contraction – for example, muscle spasm and pain in the right shoulder in cases of gall bladder inflammation.

This is a classic example of what is known as 'referred pain', in which pain is felt at one site of the body although its cause lies within another part of the body.

Case: Mr G

An elderly man visited my practice, complaining of an ache in the right shoulder. He informed me that all he needed was a 'good rub' on the offending joint. I took his full medical history and carried out an examination, as is usual practice, before treatment. As I went through his symptoms in more detail, it emerged that the shoulder pain worsened after eating fatty or fried foods. When I examined the region of the gall bladder in the upper right section of the abdomen, underneath the ninth rib, I noted that pressure caused the patient severe pain. This positive test, known as Murphy's sign, confirmed my suspicions, and I promptly sent the patient to hospital. The following day he had successful surgery on his gall bladder, to remove a large stone. The shoulder pain disappeared soon after his operation.

This case demonstrates how the sympathetic nerves' connections with the somatic nervous system co-exist and can lead to many varied referred symptoms.

Stimulation of the sympathetic nervous system

If the sympathetic system is stimulated, it causes the following effects[20, 21]:
1. On muscles: The force of muscle contraction is increased and there appears to be a delay in the onset of fatigue in over-stimulated muscles.
2. There is an increase in excitability of sensory mechanisms.
3. The bone marrow, which is very rich in sympathetic nerve supply, is stimulated to produce lymphocytes to help the immune system fight disease.
4. The endocrine system, which is under the influence of the sympathetic nerves, is stimulated to release hormones from glands such as the thyroid, adrenals and other organs, such as the pancreas.

It therefore follows that if there is an impairment in sympathetic control, the opposite effects may occur, thus reducing muscle contraction, increasing fatigue, reducing sensation and lowering resistance to disease.

Sympathetic stimulation only modifies the inherent physiology rather than introducing new qualities, so that each tissue responds in its own particular way. This is why ME/CFS can affect different patients in such a variety of ways. Some sympathetic paths may be functioning correctly, others may be overactive or underactive, while in severe cases they may be severely blocked. The common factor is that with any form of ME/CFS there is a general disorder, or dysfunction, of the sympathetic nervous system as a whole, causing widespread signs and symptoms of ill health within the body. Some of the signs and symptoms are due to an over-activity of the sympathetic nerves, other effects relate to a reduction of sympathetic activity.

It is interesting that Sir Thomas Lewis observed in the 1930s that the patients with 'effort syndrome', as he called it, displayed a characteristic drooping posture, which he attributed to the fatigue and depression[22]. The concept that the bad posture might be related to the root cause of the disorder in the first place, rather than the result, evaded him. The mechanical strain that a kyphotic, or bowed, upper spine, places upon the sympathetic nervous system is immense and, over a period of time, can directly lead to the patient developing ME/CFS. This is why so many people who develop ME/CFS are in occupations placing postural strain on the thoracic spine, such as nursing, teaching and studying.

Genetics research

A chronic sympathetic nerve irritation may stem from a postural problem of the thoracic and upper lumbar spine. Although bad posture may be brought about by unhealthy habits – for example, slouching in soft chairs – the shape of the back may also be determined by genetic factors. This also goes for the shape of the cranium which may genetically predispose an individual to many problems and lead to neurolymphatic drainage disturbance in the early years and structural problems, such as cleft lip and/or palate. Hereditary disorders can also lead to soft tissue abnormalities such as tongue tie. As in all areas of medicine, gene studies have a major role to play in improving our future understanding of aetiological mechanisms that may pre-dispose patients with ME/CFS and FMS.

A gene is a sequence of DNA which encodes molecules in your cells to have different functions. The transmission of genes to one's children is the basis of the inheritance of what are known as 'phenotype traits' (e.g. eye colour). These genes make up different DNA sequences called 'genotypes', which, along with environmental and developmental factors, determine what the observable characteristics of its structure and function will be. These, as well as the susceptibility to disease, are known as the phenotypes.

Single nucleotide polymorphisms, frequently called SNPs (pronounced 'snips'), are the most common type of genetic variation among people. Each SNP represents a difference in a single DNA building block, called a nucleotide.

There are about 10 million SNPs in the human genome. Scientists often use SNPs as biological markers to locate genes that are associated with different diseases and genes that may predict a person's susceptibility to environmental toxins and risk of disease, and to check for susceptibility to an inherited disease.

Major research into SNPs associated with ME/CFS is taking place in many research labs across the world. One of the leading centres for genetic research into ME/CFS, fibromyalgia and other neuro-immune disorders is the Institute of Neuro-immune Medicine at NOVA Southeastern University College of Osteopathic Medicine in Fort Lauderdale, Florida. In 2016, I had the honour of being one of the first scientists to give a lecture to Professor Nancy Klimas and her research team at their new $200m centre. At this centre, they are examining many different SNPs that may provide evidence of problems in metabolic pathways in ME/CFS, such as MAO, MTHFR and MTHFD, which are involved in the methylation cycle, a major process in most cell functions, especially in the brain and nervous system plus energy production in the mitochondria.

Variant genotypes associated with muscle metabolism and physical endurance have been discovered in Gulf War veterans that made them much more likely to develop ME/CFS[23]. Clinically, one can see a genetic pattern in the family history data where there is more than one family member with ME/CFS and fibromyalgia. It is thought that 15% of ME/CFS is familial and I have seen patients where more than four members of the same family are affected. There have been recorded cases of occurrences of the disorder in three generations. Research has shown evidence of a heritable predisposition to ME/CFS[24]. Genetic susceptibility is now considered to influence the aetiology of fibromyalgia and is often also seen in family clusters[25].

The genetic coding can lead to susceptibility for disease but, just as the colour of one's eyes and hair are hereditary, so can stiffness and curvature of the spine and developmental problems in the cranium run in families. Structural anomalies of cranial bones have been linked to genetic mutation as have spinal deformities[26, 27]. A virus may strike at those in the unfortunate family who possess the same mechanical problem of the spine, affecting the drainage of the post-viral inflammatory toxins.

Genetic researchers are looking at the possibility that one malfunctioning gene could be at the heart of a group of comorbidities commonly seen together – namely, EDS, POTS and fibromyalgia (see Chapter 6).

ME/CFS, although a neuroimmune disorder with many differing aetiologies (causes and triggers), may actually target genetically predisposed individuals[28]. Environmental and genetic factors will alter the rate of chemical metabolism[29] and may predispose the person to the development of multiple chemical sensitivity. The prognosis of diseases such as ME/CFS will depend on the many factors affecting the body's capability to eliminate toxins.

In fact, as I am finishing the editing of this book, a new UK study into how genetic factors may predispose people to ME/CFS has just been announced (June 2020), after receiving £3.2m of funding from the Medical Research Council and National Institute for Health Research.

The DecodeME project will collect DNA samples from 20,000 ME/CFS patients. The hope is that the study will aid the development of diagnostic tests and targeted treatments by pinpointing tiny differences in a person's DNA that may affect their risk of developing ME/CFS and reveal the underlying causes of the condition.

The trouble is that this research will probably find a huge number of subgroups due to the huge variety of biological mechanisms that can lead to ME/CFS and therefore it will be almost impossible to develop a successful treatment that works universally, unless you look at the common biophysical problems affecting the neuro-lymphatics and address these first.

A recent scientific review by Gerwain Morris and colleagues into the cause of ME/CFS has highlighted a wide range of biological abnormalities, most notably in the neuroendocrine, autonomic, neurological, bioenergetic, redox and immunological domains referred to in this book. It has also been seen that toxins and environmental changes can affect the variation in immune response genes that play a major part in determining the development of damage-associated molecular patterns (DAMPs). The DAMPs involved in the pathogenesis of ME/CFS activate innate immune machineries which promote certain inflammatory changes occasionally associated with adaptive autoimmune processes.

According to the authors of a paper which included leading ME/CFS specialist Professor Basant Puri of Imperial College London[30], these specific molecular patterns seen in ME/CFS could change an acute pathogenic infection into a state of escalating chronic systemic inflammation, which in turn can give rise to many of the reported symptoms and biological abnormalities.

How viruses affect nerves

As mentioned earlier in this chapter, Sir Thomas Lewis surmised that the disorder was due to an infection. An infection is defined as the invasion of tissues by living micro-organisms. Disease is produced by their subsequent multiplication. Bacteria and viruses are the most common type of pathogenic (disease producing) organisms in man. It is a widely held belief that a virus is the underlying cause of ME/CFS. Many practitioners still refer to the illness as 'post-viral fatigue syndrome'. They believe a virus was initially present in the body and has now been eradicated, but that it has left its mark, causing the disorder. A virus would be the most plausible explanation when dealing with certain recorded outbreaks of ME/CFS, where the incidence has almost reached epidemic proportions – for example, as previously mentioned, at the Royal Free Hospital, London in 1955[31].

A virus is the smallest micro-organism known, measuring only nanometres in length (one meter = one billion nanometres). Viruses sometimes are known to attack specific parts of the nervous system. A well-known viral infection, shingles, affects sensory nerves due to the virus *varicella zoster*. With shingles there is an initial infection by the varicella virus, usually in childhood, causing chicken pox. The child recovers but the virus lies dormant for many years in the root of a sensory nerve as it leaves the spinal cord. Eventually, the virus may reactivate in the form of shingles. This is an example of a latent virus infection.

There are also slow-acting viral infections, such as scrapie which affects the nerves, albeit in sheep. Severe damage to the animal's nervous system results after an incubation period of many years. There is a rare nervous disease, similar to scrapie, which is found in some tribes of New Guinea, known as kuru. This disorder shows that chronic disease of the nervous system can be of viral origin in humans as well as animals.

Another viral infection that involves the central nervous system is polio (poliomyelitis). The infection occurs after the virus has entered the body via the mouth (in food or drink). It then attacks specific cells in part of the spinal cord. There is a tendency for the polio virus to affect the lumbar region, in the lower section of the cord, more than the dorsal or cervical areas.

This demonstrates that viruses are capable of targeting precise regions of the spine and concentrating their effect on particular nerve cells. This may be precisely what occurs with ME/CFS, with the unknown virus attacking the thoracic and upper lumbar areas, acting on the sympathetic nerves or ganglia as well as the brain itself.

Severe acute respiratory disease (SARS) was a corona A virus that in 2003 killed over 40 Canadians after travelling from Hong Kong to Toronto. It was a deadly virus with almost a 20% fatality rate. However, it didn't spread as quickly and did not affect as many people as the Covid-19 causing the pandemic of 2020.

Post mortems found that the SARS coronavirus had crossed the blood-brain barrier (BBB) via the olfactory pathway and ended up in the hypothalamus – that is, the pathway of the virus in severe cases followed the same pathway of neurotoxins as seen in ME/CFS patients. Not surprisingly, many of the survivors of SARS in Toronto ended up with ME/CFS[32].

At the time of writing, the world is in the grip of the Covid-19 pandemic so I do not know exactly how the future is going to pan out. However, I fear that via the same pathological pathways as with SARS, there will be a huge upsurge in the numbers of ME/CFS and FMS patients in the years following Covid-19. In relation to this, I can report in November 2020 that a team of researchers from Charité – Universitätsmedizin Berlin have produced the first electron microscope images of intact coronavirus particles inside the olfactory mucosa, showing that the main entry of SARS-CoV-2 into the brain is via the olfactory nerve pathway. They also suggest that migration of SARS-CoV-2 across the blood–brain barrier (BBB) is a valid possibility as they found immunoreactivity to SARS-CoV S protein in leptomeningeal endothelial cells (that is, cells in the region between the pia and arachnoid layers of the membranes of the brain containing cerebrospinal fluid), which happens to be a main pathway in the neuro-lymphatic drainage[32a].

In the 1980s, ME/CFS epidemics broke out in a number of American towns, where the blood tests showed that the patients had been infected with the Epstein-Barr virus[33, 34, 35], the herpes virus that causes glandular fever ('mono' in the US). This led many US doctors to refer to the disease as chronic Epstein-Barr virus syndrome. However, the signs and symptoms were different from glandular fever, and the patients seemed to be suffering from different viruses at the same time.

Researchers have concentrated on other viruses – namely polio, Coxsackie's and cytomegalovirus (CMV), a recently discovered herpes, HHV-6[36, 37], but none has shown up exclusively in every patient with ME/CFS. I believe the long-term irritation of the brain, hormonal system, and ultimately the sympathetic nervous system, leads to a disorder in the normal functioning of the blood plus lymph circulation, and visceral activity, which directly affects the immune system. This results in the body as a whole being susceptible to viral infections of more than one type.

Infectious diseases usually focus on weak areas in the victim's body. If a virus is to blame for ME/CFS, then a long-term irritation of the sympathetic nerves could lead to a weakness in the system, which may render it prone to a viral infection.

Viruses or other infectious agents are normally dealt with by the immune system and the different antibodies that attack the offending pathogen. The body knows what cells to attack by virtue of signalling molecules that attach to the virus, bacteria or fungus, or whatever has invaded the body. The signalling molecules are large proteins known as cytokines. Being large molecules means that they need to be drained away by the lymphatics after the infection has been dealt with. If the drainage doesn't occur efficiently, or there is a backflow of lymph, then there will be a build-up of cytokines. This is exactly what has been discovered in ME/CFS and this explains why the symptoms are often seen in a post-viral stage, although, as you will learn from reading this book, the problems that cause ME/CFS and fibromyalgia to develop are pre-viral and may even begin at birth, and in some cases may be genetic as discussed above.

Pre-viral or post-viral?

My hypothesis does not rule out the possibility of viruses and indeed any infections being involved in the pathology of ME/CFS. However, as I have already stated, the condition is pre-viral rather than post-viral. The sympathetic nervous system's dysfunction leads to a reduction in the body's immune system. This in turn results in the entire body becoming susceptible to infections of more than one type. This explains why research into viral causes has been going on for some years, with many different viruses being suspected of playing a part in the establishment of the disease.

I believe that Lewis wrongly concluded that the poor posture he observed was a result of the fatigued and depressed state of the body and not part of the cause. Viral infections are often the trigger for ME/CFS and are a result of a disturbed immune system, but never the creator of the disease. This is why in the very early stages of the disorder, only a mechanical and postural-based examination can detect the development of ME/CFS and FMS before the sympathetic nervous system breaks down. In other words, the severe symptoms of ME/CFS and FMS can even be preventable if treated and managed properly in the early stages.

If disturbance of the sympathetic nervous system is allowed to take place unhindered, the ultimate result is the manifestation of the many signs and symptoms and complications that we now associate with ME/CFS and FMS.

The Greek playwright Euripides (c. 480–406 BC) said that 'the best and safest thing is to keep a balance in your life, acknowledge the great powers around us and in us. If you can do that and live that way you are really a wise man'. The autonomic nervous system, and primarily its component the sympathetic nervous system, provides the balance in the homeostatic mechanism. If this balance is not maintained, the overall nervous system is compromised, leading to disturbed biochemistry and cell structure damage, which in turn affects the immune system, leading to the body spiralling further out of balance.

Chapter 4

The causes of ME/CFS

The knowledge of anything, since all things have causes, is not acquired or complete unless it is known by its causes.

Avicenna (c. 980–1037 AD)
Persian philosopher, astronomer and physician

Case: Jeff's story

I met Ray Perrin back in the late 1990s to discuss his planned research trial of ME patients and we talked about my health issues and background. He was unsure given that I was aged 52 that he could achieve any success but was willing to give me a try.

He was the first person to explain about why I had back pain and other physical issues as well as the ME, and the effect these had on my health.

As part of the trial, he explained, I was to have no treatments other than the Perrin Technique so that if there was any change, then it must be down to what he was doing in terms of massage and manipulation. He also explained everything he wanted me to do as part of the process on a daily basis, also to attend for treatment weekly with him.

Also, he wanted me to attend various tests to set base lines and check on progress.

Well, within months a number of the symptoms had gone; these included a sensitivity to light and loud noise and a change in the food I could absorb without suffering. As time has gone on, my quality of life has vastly improved, from those terrible times when most of my days were spent mostly at home eating bland food in a quiet environment with only occasional trips out.

I was also able to return to work, only part-time but I then continued to work for another nine years, rather than – as the occupational health doctor had predicted – never working again at all.

My energy levels improved, not dramatically but slowly and surely; my need to sleep diminished and I was better able to socialise with others.

Over the years, with less and less treatment from Ray and Gail Sumner, my health in terms of my ME has got better and better, and at present – 20 years on – as far as I am aware I am having no side effects from the ME, despite the fact I no longer have treatment or do any massage for it.

Please remember that in the beginning Ray had made no promises that I would see any improvements in my condition at all, so all the better for how much better my quality of life has become

I have managed to do a whole range of things with my life, such as go on an African safari on my own with no assistance, visit Disneyworld in the middle of summer when the temperature was in the nineties, travel the world mainly on my own and, more recently, I am planning a cruise to Norway for a couple of weeks.

Without Ray's treatment I do worry where I would be now; possibly my mobility would have been very poor. I would have been on strong painkillers and spending much of my time alone at home with no quality of life.

Again, many thanks for all your time and effort in treating me and giving me back some quality of life.

Jeff Glasser, Bolton, UK
Patient of Dr Perrin and Gail Sumner, Chartered Physiotherapist and Licensed Perrin Technique Practitioner

Considerable controversy surrounds the cause or causes of ME/CFS. This chapter looks at the following possibilities:
- immunological
- inflammatory
- viral
- hormonal imbalance
- depression
- allergy and sensitivity
- oxidative stress
- hyperventilation syndrome.

Immunological disorder

Many people believe that ME/CFS is an immune disorder[1, 2, 3, 4] that enables viruses, which are normally controlled within the body, to go rampant and start to attack healthy body tissue in a similar way to AIDS, but usually without fatal consequences.

Many symptoms associated with ME/CFS, such as enlarged lymph glands, fever, gut symptoms, recurrent infections and pharyngitis, appear to indicate an immunological disorder. Indeed, as noted in the previous chapter, the onset of the disease often appears to follow a viral infection.

The body has an innate immune system that defends non-specifically against attack from any source. It also has a defence mechanism that is more specific to the type of infection. This specific immune response utilises cells known as lymphocytes. The body provides two basic forms of immune response: humoral (in the body fluid) and cellular (cell-mediated). Both forms are coordinated by the cells of the immune system and their mediators. B lymphocytes are responsible for humoral immunity and T lymphocytes are responsible for cell-mediated immunity.

Humoral immunity

Humoral immunity is a specific defence mechanism that involves the production of antibodies, distributed in the blood, lymph and interstitial fluid, which attack foreign antigens throughout the body. Humoral immunity is the major defence mechanism against bacterial infections and utilises circulating antibodies that are produced by specialised B-cells, supported by other cells called T-helper cells (Th cells) which are an important component of the immune system as far as the pathogenesis of ME/CFS is concerned.

T-helper cells circulate through the blood and lymph nodes for many years and are important in facilitating activities of other cells in immune reactions that destroy invading organisms. T-helper cells can be separated mainly into two categories:

- Th1 cells are mainly involved in cell-mediated immunity, as described below, which leads to activation of T lymphocytes within specific cells.
- Th2 cells stimulate B-cell activity.

The balance between Th1 and Th2 cells is very important for a healthy immune system. In many disease states there is a dominance of one or the other. For example, Th1-mediated diseases include multiple sclerosis, Crohn's disease of the bowel and lupus (SLE). Diseases that are Th2-mediated include asthma and allergic rhinitis. With ME/CFS there is often a disturbed Th1/Th2 balance with both Th1 and Th2 dominance possible. This is because ME/CFS affects the central control mechanisms within the brain via the sympathetic nervous system that influences immune regulation.

After recognising foreign material, B-cells multiply rapidly and produce antibodies comprised of large protein molecules known as immunoglobulins. These proteins are produced in large numbers and are usually specific to the infective or foreign agent. The antibodies form complexes with the foreign material and these complexes are then destroyed by other cells, such as macrophages (see below).

Activated B-cells differentiate into plasma cells, which are specialised to synthesise and secrete 1 to 2 trillion immunoglobulins found in the healthy adult.

The immunoglobulins are divided into different categories, such as IgG and IgM, depending on the type of infection and whether the infection is acute or chronic. IgM levels are usually high in short-term infections, whereas IgG levels are raised in long-lasting infections. If there is a long-term co-infection, such as Lyme disease, then the IgG for the bacterium *Borrelia burgdorferi* will usually be high. Sometimes the immunoglobulin levels are found to be lower than normal, which could indicate an exhaustion of the immune system leading to a susceptibility for some patients with ME/CFS to pick up any infection going.

Cellular (cell-mediated) immunity

Cellular immunity involves a variety of T-cells that are responsible for protection against viruses, cancers and some disease-causing bacteria, such as tuberculosis. T-helper (Th) cells assist cytotoxic T lymphocytes (Tc), which actively destroy abnormal cells in disease and malignancies.

A further group of lymphocytes are natural killer (NK) cells, which are part of the body's innate immune system and play an important part in surveying the body for any anomalies and counteracting viral infections and cancer.

Patients with ME/CFS initially have an overactive immune system producing far too many lymphocytes. Certain enzymes, which help drive the immune reaction, such as RNaseL, have been shown to be overactive[5, 6, 7]. This leads to an interesting phenomenon experienced by most ME/CFS patients, at least in the early stages of the disease. Their families and friends may suffer from the occasional cold and bout of flu, but ME/CFS patients will just feel groggy and weak with a worsening of their usual symptoms but without full-blown cold or flu symptoms. This is because the viruses in their upper respiratory tract are already being blasted by far too many lymphocytes, and, consequently, the usual viral symptoms, which are due to the normal immune response, do not occur.

After a while this situation may reverse and the immune system may become severely depressed, with the patient suffering from constant recurrent infections, with depleted immunoglobulin levels as mentioned above.

The complex interactions between all the B- and T-cells require cytokines, which are large protein signalling molecules. There are many types of cytokine, which are subdivided into smaller groups (e.g. interleukins and interferons). During an infection, both T- and B-cells multiply rapidly, with cell numbers returning to normal levels after the antigen has been defeated. However, some memory cells remain so that a second infection is more rapidly combated. Cytokines can produce nasty side effects, such as sickness and lethargy, as many cancer patients know too well with the infamous side-effects of chemotherapy. Chemotherapy often involves the injection of large amounts of interleukins and/or interferons which target the cancer cells. Once they have attached to the cancer cell, they signal to the body's immune system to destroy the malignancy. However, with the large amounts of cytokines involved in some chemotherapy treatments, they will also attach to healthy cells, which then are attacked by antibodies, leading to hair loss, nausea, lethargy etc. Being large protein molecules, excess cytokine activity requires the lymphatic system to drain the surplus away, otherwise the consequences will be dire.

With ME/CFS, when there is a reversal of lymphatic drainage back up to the central nervous system through the neuro-lymphatic system, one would expect a high concentration of cytokines in the cerebrospinal fluid in the brain and the spinal cord, which has been shown in previous studies[8, 9]. There are several specialised regions of the brain's ventricular system, termed circumventricular organs (see Figure 13), which interact closely with the reservoirs of cerebrospinal fluid contained in the ventricles. In these regions some of the tight junctions between the endothelial cells are missing, allowing the entry of macromolecules into the brain and therefore, the passage of hormones. These zones, for example the area 'postrema' in the fourth ventricle, are chemical-sensitive regions that may react with toxins, sending messages to other parts of the brain, especially the hypothalamus. The 'subfornical organ' is another area active in many bodily processes, including cardiovascular regulation, and preserving water and salt balance and maintaining energy through the control and release of hormones, especially angiotensin and vasopressin.

The most important circumventricular zones without a complete BBB are the 'median eminence' of the hypothalamus and the pituitary gland.

The median eminence, which is part of the hypophyseal portal system connecting the hypothalamus with the pituitary gland, sends chemicals that inhibit or stimulate the release of hormones from the pituitary gland, which is so important in hormonal control, together with the hypothalamus. Most hormones are controlled via the hypothalamic-pituitary axes. In the medical model of stress, the hypothalamic–pituitary–adrenal (HPA) axis is always mentioned due to the role of adrenaline (epinephrine) and noradrenaline (norepinephrine) produced in the adrenal glands.

Toxins entering the region of discontinuous tight junctions at the pituitary gland can cause havoc with hormonal control, as they do in ME/CFS and FMS. So many

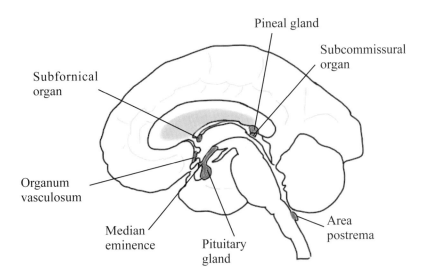

Fig. 13 The natural gaps in the blood–brain barrier (BBB).

patients have problems with their adrenaline and noradrenaline levels. One axis even more commonly found disturbed in ME/CFS and FMS is the hypothalamic–pituitary–thyroid (HPT) axis, with many patients having too low and some too high levels of thyroxine.

Another significant circumventricular organ is the pineal gland, which is important in maintaining the circadian rhythms in the body, the 24-hour biological rhythms that regulate our sleep and awake cycles, in addition to many other important physiological processes discussed in more detail later in this chapter.

Also important is the *organ vasculosum* (vascular organ) of the cup-shaped *lamina terminalis* found at the front end of the third ventricle projecting into the hypothalamus. In inflammatory and infective disorders, cytokines such as interleukin-1 have been shown to pass through the *lamina terminalis* into the hypothalamus, raising the body's temperature and causing a fever. The permeability at both the *organ vasculosum* and the median eminence facilitates the brain's ability to monitor hormone levels in the blood but equally makes the hypothalamus one of the most permeable regions of the BBB and one of the regions in the brain most prone to suffer toxic damage.

So, when toxins pass through these gaps in the BBB, hormonal, sleep, temperature and general metabolic dysfunction occur.

Research findings have demonstrated cytokine involvement in the patho-physiological mechanisms found in ME/CFS[10, 11], especially the hormone leptin which is a cytokine that attaches to the fatty cells of the central nervous system and has an effect on the brain's control of satiety and hunger, appetite and loss of appetite, and which has been found to fluctuate almost identically with the severity of the patient's symptoms[12]. It is interesting that this hormone is much more prevalent in women and is probably one of the reasons why ME/CFS occurs more in the female population.

Recent evidence from studies in the USA has revealed as many as 17 cytokines in the brain of ME/CFS patients, which were found to correlate with the severity of the disease. Of these 17, 13 were pro-inflammatory, which Stanford University's research showed was likely to contribute to many of the symptoms experienced by patients whilst also establishing a strong immune system component of the disease[13].

However, if the brain is overloaded with pro-inflammatory activity, then one would expect this to create a fever in all patients, but although some patients with ME/CFS and FMS do have symptoms of a fever with high temperature or shivering with chills and feeling clammy all the time, and have signs of chronic inflammation, many others don't. The answer to this conundrum is that it all depends on which neurotoxins affect which part of the brain and even which part of the hypothalamus, but first we have to explore the exact mechanism in our brain that can cause fever to occur.

The inflammatory response

Inflammation is a complex response to localised injury and trauma and, although it is usually an acute response, there are a number of well-known chronic inflammatory diseases, such as rheumatoid arthritis and sinusitis. The inflammatory response involves cytokines together with other classes of large molecular inflammatory modulators, known as prostaglandins. In recent years, researchers have found that prostaglandins cross into the brain and bind to a specific kind of receptor, called EP3, to cause fever.

Research has shown that EP3 receptors are found in a tiny region in the hypothalamus, the size of a pin head, known as the 'median preoptic nucleus', that is crucial in causing fever[14].

The median preoptic nucleus is found behind the eyes, where the optic nerves cross paths as they enter the brain. If the toxic drainage along the perivascular space in the optic nerve pathway is affected, then it could lead to a build-up of pro-inflammatory cytokines and prostaglandins around this nucleus, and in these patients will lead to feverish symptoms in ME/CFS. In other patients, where different regions of neuro-lymphatic drainage are affected, or if there are different neurotoxins involved, such as heavy metals, then the symptoms will be different, without noticeable symptoms of fever.

Inflammation and the gut

The controversy about the MMR (measles, mumps and rubella) vaccine being associated with the development of autism involved the identification of grossly inflamed tissue in the lower part of the small intestine in autistic children who had previously been vaccinated[15].

Inflammation of this part of the gut is common among ME/CFS patients and many have been diagnosed with irritable bowel syndrome or inflammatory bowel disease and specifically Crohn's disease. Allergic reactions to food containing gluten are common. The best known condition involving such a reaction is coeliac disease in which the structure of the small bowel is destroyed, with a flattening of the deeply folded villi of the gut wall, and diminished capacity to properly absorb many key nutrients from food. Generally, ME/CFS patients do not test positive for coeliac disease, but many become sensitive to a variety of chemicals and foodstuffs, especially gluten.

When digestion is impaired, the larger peptide fragments that make up proteins in food are not broken down. Among these are opioid peptides derived from two principal sources, casein in milk (the casomorphins) and gliadin in gluten (the gliadomorphins), which occur in wheat and other cereal crops, such as rye and barley. Opioids are peptides that have been found to possess morphine-like activity and are known to be naturally occurring in important transmitter molecules, particularly in the gut, brain and immune system.

When the gut wall has increased permeability, these opioid peptides, which would normally be kept inside the gut, are absorbed and act both locally in the gut and in other organs, particularly the brain. The same factors that render the gut permeable appear to increase the permeability of the BBB and allow access of these compounds to the brain.

Depending on the concentration of opioids in the gut, as well as the permeability of the gut wall and BBB, the overall level of these compounds in the bloodstream and the brain may be unstable and give rise to variable expressions of symptoms and dysfunction. Opioids play a significant part in the immune response through receptors found on cells of the immune system. Generally, they suppress the immune response and increase susceptibility to infection. The gut and the brain communicate via messenger molecules generated by the immune response.

The gut and brain also communicate neurologically. The enteric nervous system (ENS), which is an elaborate nervous system controlling the whole gut, is connected to the central nervous system (CNS) through innervation by the autonomic nervous system, often referred to the gut–brain axis. The ENS has been referred to as 'the second brain'.

The gut has an intricate immune system network controlled by the ENS that produces a number of neurotransmitters, such as serotonin, acetylcholine and substance P. These have been shown to play a part in the communication between the gut and the brain and vice versa, and influence the activity of the gastrointestinal microbiota. It is now known that the gut's communication to the brain is as important as the messages from the brain to the gut[16, 17].

Messages between the brain and the rest of the body are modified by a regulatory action of the gut microbiota on the BBB converting from hormones into neurotransmitters in the brain affecting control of the entire nervous system[18].

Lymphocytes involved in the immune response in the gut lead to the secretion of small amounts of hormones that are thought to play a local part in regulating inflammation in the gut. Due to the processes mentioned above, it is also possible that the release of hormones in the gut is influenced by stress and that problems affecting the gut and the brain may be a result of disrupted communications in the neuroimmune network.

It is now known that the microbiome helps produce around 70% of the neurotransmitters used in the brain. Unbelievably, over 90% of serotonin is produced in the gut. Serotonin is essential for feelings of wellbeing and is often the neurochemical targeted by antidepressants. Disruption of the gut microbiome can lead to an imbalance of serotonin and melatonin; melatonin is an essential component of the circadian rhythm, the 24-hour biological rhythm that regulates our sleep and wake cycles, in addition to many other important physiological processes.

In addition to the pineal gland in the brain, the gut is known also to produce melatonin. The microbiome has its own separate rhythm but is connected with the circadian rhythm; these two need to be in sync with each other, otherwise the person may be hungry and want to eat at all the wrong times for their body clock, something which is very common in ME/CFS and fibromyalgia[19, 20].

The role of the microbiome in neuro-immunology can explain why probiotics are so important following a short course of antibiotics and imperative if one is prescribed long-term antibiotics for chronic bacterial illnesses such as Lyme disease. Many patients with ME/CFS and FMS have a history of repeated infections in their younger life, such as tonsilitis, requiring large amounts of antibiotics which would also reduce the quantity of good bacteria. The gut-brain axis can equally be disturbed due to an excess of bacteria in the gut seen in the condition, small intestinal bacterial overgrowth (SIBO), which also causes chronic diarrhoea, weight loss and malabsorption and is becoming more commonly identified.

The link between ME/CFS and other diseases

Sometimes the process that leads to ME/CFS may be linked to other even more serious illnesses. A subset of ME/CFS-free breast cancer patients complained of a level of symptoms almost identical to ME/CFS sufferers, such as fatigue, sleep disruption and loss of concentration[21]. A previous link had been made between non-Hodgkin's lymphoma and ME/CFS after a 1988 epidemiological investigation into a cluster of ME/CFS sufferers in North Carolina[22].

The symptoms and signs of ME/CFS are very similar to Addison's disease (primary adrenal insufficiency – that is, failure of the adrenal glands). However, corticosteroid replacement, where there are no physical signs of adrenal failure, is clearly not warranted, and usually exacerbates ME/CFS signs and symptoms. Drugs containing adrenaline (epinephrine) usually worsen ME/CFS symptoms. This is commonly seen when ME/CFS and fibromyalgia patients need local anaesthetics – for instance, when visiting the dentist. It is therefore important always to insist on a non–adrenaline-based anaesthetic. The only physical sign of adrenal dysfunction I have observed in ME/CFS patients is one usually attributed to *high* levels of cortisol – namely striae gravida (stretch marks), seen in Cushing's syndrome.

However, the striae occasionally seen on the thighs and breast tissue of ME/CFS patients are most probably due to damage of collagenous fibres attached to surface lymphatic capillaries. This will happen when there is a major backflow of lymph and is nothing to do with the adrenals. In some patients, however, there will be a disturbance of the adrenals due to the dysfunctional hypothalamus which controls all the hormonal system, as discussed in more detail later in this chapter.

The immune system has been shown to exert numerous effects on the hypothalamus and thus the autonomic nervous system. Immune activation is associated with increased firing rates of hypothalamic neurones. It is known that activated immune cells can cross the BBB and release cytokines and other immune mediators into the central nervous system. Central and peripheral release of cytokines affects a range of behaviours, including feeding, sleeping, drinking, levels of activity and mood, presumably by their action on receptor sites in the limbic system, the emotional control centre in the brain. Infections have an effect on the limbic system, which also plays a major part in regulating memory and learning and is directly involved in hypothalamic and autonomic function. Dysfunction of the limbic system in the brain leads to many of the symptoms associated with this illness and thus ME/CFS patients are very sensitive to both physical and psychological stress[23].

Functional changes in limbic areas have been demonstrated in ME/CFS using SPECT scans (single photon emission computerised tomography)[24]. The limbic system controls emotions and dream states and it is significant that patients with ME/CFS often complain of mood swings and weird or extremely vivid dreams, nightmares or, in some cases, hallucinations.

The basal ganglia and thalamus form a major part of the limbic system and, as shown in 2012 in ground-breaking research at Rochester University[25], when the 'glymphatic' drainage of the brain through the paravascular spaces was stopped there was a build-up of large protein molecules around the basal ganglia and thalamus.

The viral trigger

Some viruses have been implicated as possible causal factors in ME/CFS. As noted in the previous chapter, a class of virus, known as enteroviruses – such as the Coxsackie B group – are believed to be particularly important in triggering ME/CFS[26]. Polio is also caused by an enterovirus, leading sometimes to what is known as post-polio syndrome, yet another name for a group suffering with ME/CFS. Treatment approaches over recent years have focused on antiviral medications. However, most antiviral treatments have very unpleasant side effects and should be used with caution.

The antiviral drug acyclovir has undergone vigorous tests[27] to analyse its efficacy in treating ME/CFS. Acyclovir has been successful against the Epstein-Barr virus, but double blind trials have shown it to have no greater effect on ME/CFS than a placebo[28]. Most patients on the acyclovir drug trials reported that any improvement was short-lived, and their symptoms returned soon after the treatment was completed.

There is no doubt that in many cases the full blown symptoms of ME/CFS do start after a virus but it is important to understand that we are dealing with an illness that builds up for many years and is only triggered by a virus and that the virus has usually been destroyed before the major symptoms begin in the post-viral stage due to the build-up of pro-inflammatory toxins.

Hormonal imbalance

As explained earlier, the hypothalamus is the main region of the brain that controls and receives messages from the sympathetic nervous system and becomes dysfunctional in ME/CFS. The hypothalamus also controls the release of the body's hormones, thus hypothalamic dysfunction in ME/CFS may affect the entire endocrine (hormone) system. Therefore, one might find excesses or deficiencies in many hormonal levels in patients with the disease. Both raised[29] and reduced[30] levels of a precursor of the major sex hormones – serum dehydroepiandrosterone (DHEA-S) – secreted from the adrenal glands, have been found in ME/CFS sufferers. As with many hormones, both high and low levels of melatonin, produced by the pineal gland, have been reported in a sample of patients with ME/CFS. Melatonin levels are found to be high when daytime drowsiness and excessive sleep are reported[31]. However, when insomnia is a major symptom, supplements of melatonin usually prove to be beneficial[32].

All organisms, even bacteria, as we have mentioned earlier in this chapter, possess internal 24-hour cycles termed circadian rhythms, which provide a means of anticipating changes in night and day. In humans this occurs through a process known as 'entrainment', which continues to reset and maintain synchronicity with the biological 24-hour clock. This process is under the control of our good friend the hypothalamus.

In the retina at the back of the eye, there are three basic types of photoreceptors (cells sensitive to light). There are rods and cones which are involved in image formation and there are the photosensitive retinal ganglion cells (pRCGs) which, when stimulated, send information to the hypothalamus. Receptors in the hypothalamus send messages directly to the pineal gland, located behind the third ventricle of the brain, which produces and secretes the hormone melatonin in the human body.

Therefore, when the hypothalamus is disturbed with ME/CFS and FMS, circadian rhythm regulation is disturbed. Some patient's internal body clocks are so dysfunctional that they remain awake for most of the night and sleep most of the day. This is also partly due to problems with the hypothalamic–locus-coeruleus axis mentioned in Chapter 3.

Insulin-like growth factor (IGF-1), the main mediator of growth hormone effects, has been found to be reduced in ME/CFS sufferers. Growth hormone has been used to treat ME/CFS patients, showing a significant improvement in symptoms after six months in the experimental group compared with the control group of patients treated with a placebo[33]. However, the improvement proved short lived after medication was discontinued.

One of the main reasons why ME/CFS affects women much more than men is the influence that oestrogen and progesterone, the female sex hormones, have on many women. To quote Christiane Northup MD, author of *The Wisdom of Menopause*: 'Women can be, and many are, greatly affected by hormone fluctuations. Sometimes it gets to the point of feeling totally overwhelmed – as if for a time they have lost control of their life'.

It is no surprise then that in a 2016 report from the Centers for Disease Control and Prevention (CDC), based on results from three US population-based studies, ME/CFS was found to be three to four times more common in women than in men and that the highest prevalence of the illness was in persons aged 40–50 years, affecting over a million people in the USA[34].

Fibromyalgia has also been found to be much more prevalent in women, with some studies showing a 9:1 ratio of women sufferers to men[35]; it also affects many peri-menopausal women for the same reason as does ME/CFS[36].

Depression

The secondary feelings of depression and anxiety in ME/CFS are different to primary psychiatric conditions. Many patients with ME/CFS cannot tolerate the effects of antidepressants, such as fluoxetine, thus dropout rates from studies of antidepressant therapy in ME/CFS exceed those of patients with depression[37, 38]. Signs and symptoms of depression in ME/CFS may occasionally be sufficiently severe to require antidepressant therapy; however, the patients in these cases may have two distinct disorders: (a) ME/CFS and (b) clinical depression. Patients are allowed to have more than one thing wrong with them at a time, but mostly the symptoms are secondary to having such a depressing disorder as ME/CFS – what I term TPOS (thoroughly p*****d off syndrome) or TFUS (thoroughly fed up syndrome) if your great aunt Nellie is around.

However, antidepressant drugs have been used for symptomatic relief in many non-psychiatric illnesses, such as Parkinson's disease, multiple sclerosis and hypothyroidism. In the same way, antidepressants can sometimes reduce the signs and symptoms of ME/CFS; however, symptomatic improvement occurs at much lower doses and more rapidly than in depression. Many patients with ME/CFS who find it difficult to relax when trying to fall asleep are regularly advised to take 10 to 25 mg of amitriptyline one hour before retiring to bed. This is significantly less than the normal dose of the mild tricyclic antidepressant, which when prescribed for anxiety/depression can be up to 75 mg twice a day. When the patient suffers badly from anxiety/depression, a low dose of a selective serotonin reuptake inhibitor (SSRI) type antidepressant, such as sertraline hydrochloride, has been shown to help but should be taken with caution.

Clinically, as mentioned in Chapter 3, since we know the noradrenaline levels in the brain are affected by CSF/ME, the class of antidepressant that also affect noradrenaline levels – known as SNRIs (such as duloxetine) – seem to help more with some patients, and should be considered by the doctor if the patient is also suffering from major depression or anxiety. The drug should be taken first thing in the morning as it will stimulate the release of noradrenaline during the day via the hypothalamic–locus-coeruleus axis, which, as stated in Chapter 3, is a vital area in the brain for the regulation of healthy neuro-lymphatic drainage.

In other words, if you can stimulate the release of noradrenaline during the day, the brain will hopefully revert to the normal healthy cycle of drainage at night during deep restorative sleep. In the morning you will then feel more awake and refreshed, and during the day, the drainage of toxins from the brain will be reduced due to the increase in noradrenaline improving your drive and vitality during the day.

Allergy and sensitivity

Some ME/CFS patients, with high levels of sensitivity bordering on allergy, have been treated by Miller neutralisation. The Miller technique involves provocation of the skin followed by the administration of a neutralisation 'vaccine' of individual allergens. It acts by stimulating the body to produce higher levels of detoxification enzymes, thus helping the body cope with the allergen[39].

Enzyme-potentiated desensitisation (EPD) is another anti-allergy treatment that has benefited many ME/CFS patients by actively adding enzymes to enhance the desensitising effect. It is applied to a scratch on the skin or by intradermal injection[40].

Oxidative stress

Oxidative stress has been acknowledged as a common feature in many disease processes, including ME/CFS. Oxidative stress may induce many of the symptoms of ME/CFS.

In an atom, small negatively charged electrons spin around the central nucleus, akin to planets orbiting the sun. Some atoms have electrons on their outer rings that are shared with other atoms. A group of atoms join to form a larger molecule. A free radical is a molecule with an atom that has lost one of these shared electrons from their outer ring. This will make it highly unstable and it will damage healthy tissue by trying to obtain another electron from an adjacent molecule. The movement of electrons between chemical species is known as 'reduction' for the electron acceptor and 'oxidation' for the electron donor. Reduction and oxidation always go together and are referred to as 'redox reactions'. Free radicals create problems with healthy redox reactions and can therefore lead to what is known as oxidative stress and, subsequently, many disease processes.

Oxygen reacts with free radicals to form peroxidised radicals, which further damage healthy molecules. Oxidative stress increases free radical production, leading to further cell damage and worsening toxicity. External factors, such as environmental pollutants and radiation, can lead to major free radical production. Overall, the synthesis of the free radical nitric oxide is increased in ME/CFS and may be induced by inflammatory cytokines[41]. The neurotoxic effect is further aggravated by amplified sensitivity due to increased nitric oxide stimulation of the neurotransmitter glutamate[42].

Antioxidants restore free radicals to healthy molecules. Antioxidants such as vitamin C have been shown to be major combatants in fighting disease ever since the 1950s when Harman[43] discovered the role of free radicals. The rationale for vitamin C infusion in ME/CFS rests on the traditional use of megadose vitamin C infusion treatments in autoimmune disease, allergy and a range of other conditions[44].

I always advise caution when taking any supplements, even vitamin C, as there is a risk of developing kidney stones if the vitamin C intake is too high, so a safe dose that I recommend is up to 500 mg every day. Vitamin C aids calcium absorption, and too much calcium over a long period can lead to kidney stones. Swedish researchers carried out a large study on 23,000 Swedes over an 11-year period and those who reported taking vitamin C supplements were twice as likely to have kidney stones[45].

Interestingly, this has only been proven to happen in men[46] but I still feel that both men and women should be cautious about overloading vitamin intake and only receive a vitamin infusion from medically-trained practitioners who can correctly evaluate and reduce any health risks to each individual patient.

Remember that too much of anything, even the good stuff, requires the body to work harder to remove the excess chemicals, whether they be inflammatory toxins, environmental pollutants or vitamins. So even an excess of vitamin C will lead to more strain on the lymphatics to remove the molecules that are not required. This obviously is not what we wish to achieve so I stress with ME/CFS and fibromyalgia, always err on the side of caution, even with vitamins and other supplements.

Hyperventilation syndrome

Hyperventilation syndrome is a collection of many symptoms similar to ME/CFS and FMS that is caused by long-term breathing that is too fast and too heavy. This upsets the balance of oxygen and carbon dioxide in the body. Since the symptoms are so similar, many doctors believe that many cases of ME/CFS and FMS are actually hyperventilation syndrome. I feel that sometimes the conditions overlap and some of my patients have hyperventilation syndrome as well as ME/CFS and FMS, but they have very different pathophysiology and patients with this syndrome require much more treatment than just correcting their breathing pattern.

Hyperventilation causes a reduction in carbon dioxide by exhaling more than you inhale, creating more alkaline blood. This leads to a narrowing of the blood vessels and reduces the blood to the brain, leading to cognitive problems and light headedness. The ratio of oxygen to carbon dioxide in the blood is important for the amount of oxygen released to the tissues. Danish physiologist Christian Bohr discovered that without carbon dioxide, oxygen is bound to the haemoglobin in the blood and not released[47]. Consequently, in hyperventilation the lack of carbon dioxide leads to too little useable oxygen.

Therefore, although an increase in oxygen intake is useful in ME/CFS, too much oxygen without carbon dioxide may be detrimental. So, if one has access to an oxygen tank it is best to use it sparingly, for up to one hour spread over a 24-hour period and using a rebreather mask that allows the intake of carbon dioxide as well as pure oxygen is preferable.

In cases of hyperventilation, the Buteyko method has been helpful to some of my patients. It is a therapy using specific breathing exercises developed by

Ukrainian doctor Konstantin Pavlovich Buteyko in the 1950s and focuses on nasal breathing, breath holding and relaxation methods.

However, although in cases of hyperventilation syndrome this method might work, one should be very cautious with ME/CFS and FMS. Many patients I have seen, and it is usually the severe bedridden cases, have too little carbon dioxide in their blood (known as hypocapnia) and may improve with rebreather masks and doing Buteyko breathing, but there are many who may just have low oxygen and too much carbon dioxide in their blood (hypercapnia), causing an increase in carbonic acid levels (acidosis). In such cases, the last thing patients need is more carbon dioxide and they will respond more to just a normal oxygen mask or machines that increase the amount of oxygen in the room. Many patients benefit from using an oxygen concentrator, which is a device that concentrates the oxygen from the air by selectively removing the nitrogen.

The problem of using oxygen as a therapy is that, if one just breathes in oxygen, the increased levels in the blood may exacerbate the oxidative stress mentioned above, which won't help at all. It is, as always with ME/CFS and FMS, complicated, and every patient is different so, unless one has access to specialist clinics with labs that can monitor blood oxygen and carbon dioxide balance, one has to be cautious with any breathing therapy.

Chapter 5

Treatments for ME/CFS and FMS other than the Perrin Technique

Though the doctors treated him, let his blood, and gave
him medications to drink, he nevertheless recovered.

Leo Tolstoy (1828–1910) Russian author

Case: Gail's story

In the year 2000 I was a fit and healthy 24-year-old and my life was great. I had been on my first long-haul holiday to the Caribbean, moved out from my parents into a rented house and just got promoted at work doing a job that I loved as a physiotherapist within the NHS. My weekends were filled going out with my friends, I played hockey for one team and sometimes two teams on Saturdays, and I went to the gym four nights per week. And then it happened... I woke up on October 6th 2000 and I could barely move; every muscle and joint in my body ached so much I could barely lift my limbs or my head. I felt dizzy, I sweated profusely at night but was freezing cold, I couldn't think clearly, my glands were swollen, my heart pounded, my head hurt and I was utterly exhausted... It felt like I had run a marathon, coupled with the worst hangover I had ever had, on top of having completely debilitating flu.

My initial thought was that I must have the flu and it would pass, but after several weeks I felt worse. I struggled to stand; just sitting up was a real effort, and talking was proving difficult as I couldn't think quickly enough to find the words. Just having a conversation would leave me exhausted. I was told I had a virus and it would pass; then I was told I had vertigo, but the medicine made no difference. I was then referred to ENT but told everything was fine. Meanwhile my occupational health doctor told me there was nothing wrong with me, but I wasn't getting any better; in fact I was getting worse.

My head pains were now constant, my limbs felt like lead and the pains throughout my body made it painful just to lie in bed. My exhaustion was so great that after being unable to shower for weeks, I had a shower and had to crawl back to my bed. People visited whilst I was in bed and I didn't have the energy to talk, yet I would lie in bed completely exhausted but unable to sleep. I tried to go out with my mother and my 88-year-old nan and had to swap with her and sit in her wheelchair. I had more in common with my nan than anyone else, because I too had a body that was willing and wanting to do things but would fail me.

I felt as though my life was falling apart. I was unable to work, I was unable to socialise, let alone do any sport, which had always been a huge part of my life. I didn't know who I was anymore as all of the things that I had defined myself by had gone. I was no longer the person I had been. It was as if someone had drained my battery and left just a shell, a shell that was exhausted and wracked with pain.

Months passed and one of the GPs in my practice said in a nonchalant manner that I might have ME/CFS and if it was that, there was nothing they could do. I was devastated. Nevertheless, I was referred to a neurologist and sent for a CT head scan. At this stage I had tried to resume duties at work and was desperate for any diagnosis, no matter how serious, as I wanted something that could be done. Yet again I was told that the CT scan was normal, but the neurologist recommended a drug and discharged me. I tried the drug, but it didn't help; I felt lost again. To add to matters, my occupational health doctor said that I had to change my attitude and see a psychologist or therapist to change my perspective and that I was depressed. He also said that ME/CFS did not exist when he did his training therefore it did not exist today.

Regarding my occupational health doctor, my preferred GP asked what I would do to get better. I said that I would do anything, I was desperate to do anything! Thankfully she didn't believe I was depressed and believed something was physically wrong, saying that she would do everything she could to help, but didn't know what to do. At least somebody believed me.

I experienced such stigma surrounding ME/CFS. I walked into work one day and overheard a member of staff saying, 'Well I get tired too. You just have to push through', then silence as I walked into the room. People often said that I just needed to push through, keep going and try harder, but the more I tried the worse I became, and after trying to return to work I finally had to resign from the job which I loved in May 2002 – ironically, the same day that ME/CFS was officially recognised by the World Health Organization.

At this stage I could barely function after pushing myself so much, and completely crashed. I became housebound and, for periods, bedbound. The only reason that forced me to get out of bed, when I could, was to see Tango, the dog that lived with me. I realised at this point that any recovery was going to be down to me.

I found an amazing private doctor called Dr Andrew Wright, who conducted private tests to look at my individual biochemistry. He advised on various treatments to help my body make energy at a cellular level. I spent hours looking at other therapies and treatments, and recovery became my new job and focus. Alongside Dr Wright's treatment I tried numerous other therapies and for periods made some improvements, but then my health deteriorated again.

I came across an article that mentioned research which had been conducted at Salford University by an osteopath called Raymond Perrin, looking at the Perrin Technique for ME/CFS treatment. I contacted a local osteopath and they said they could do the Perrin Technique, so I went for treatment. I later saw Dr Perrin speak at a local ME/CFS group meeting and realised that I was not receiving the Perrin Technique treatment at all! I then booked into his clinic and was assessed by Raymond Perrin himself. It was a relief to meet somebody who not only did a thorough history but did a physical assessment to confirm the diagnosis too. I was treated by himself and one of his practitioners, Melissa, who were both wonderful, knowledgeable, and very supportive. I felt unwell to start with: my exhaustion, headaches and muscle pains got worse, as did my night sweats, and my sleep was still terrible and this went on for some time.

At the same time, I consulted with a nutritional therapist who specialised in ME/CFS, had tests done, made significant changes to my diet and took specific supplements. Alongside this I also started therapy to help with the stress of having a chronic health condition and to work through the characteristics and thought processes that could be adding further stress. As well as doing the Perrin home treatment of drainage, stretches and spinal compresses, I also started to do breathing exercises lying down, every day; then I started to do gentle stretches while sitting. This progressed on to meditation, relaxation programmes, sleep audio programmes, progressive breathing exercises and yoga, which I did without fail every day.

Finally, improvements came! First, they were very gradual, and I barely noticed them unless I looked back to what I had been able to do six months earlier, but then they became more noticeable. I remember being able to drive for the first time into town and meet a friend for lunch. I remember forgetting something and running up the stairs to get it, actually running! I started to be able to plan things in advance and be able to attend. Months passed and, with the help of Raymond Perrin and Melissa, my confidence grew. So much so that Raymond asked me if I would consider working at the clinic in the future. Pre ME/CFS, my aspirations had been to work in the field of sport but having been through what I had for the previous seven years my aspirations had changed. So, in April 2007 I started to work at the Perrin Clinic and also set up my own practice, focusing on ME/CFS treatment using the Perrin Technique.

I have not looked back since. Twelve years on I still work at the Perrin Clinic, alongside Dr Perrin and an amazing team of dedicated practitioners and staff. I now work full time, manage my own clinic, have gone on to study for a PGDip in nutrition and have even had the privilege of being involved in Dr Perrin's research study published in the *BMJ* in 2017. I meet amazing patients every day who still face the same challenges and battles that I did 19 years ago, and I am in awe of them and want to do everything that I can to help.

In addition, I have also been able to return to the things that I love, spending time with my family and friends, travelling the world, joining a hockey team and even doing a 10 km run and four sprint triathlons for ME/CFS charities. I now live life to the full, but with a greater appreciation of being able to do things after not being able to. I will be eternally grateful to Dr Perrin, Elaine, Colin, Melissa and all of the wonderful team at the Perrin Clinic and the huge impact they had in turning my life around. They truly are life changers and I cannot thank them enough for what they did for me and the world of ME/CFS.

Gail Sumner
Physiotherapist and Licensed Perrin Technique Practitioner, Bolton, Lancashire, UK

No one can be certain of the best possible treatment for ME/CFS until the cause is established and accepted. However, the one common feature of all the treatments for the condition is the removal of stress-producing factors. We know that stress is damaging to the body in some way or another, whether it is through physical exertion, emotional trauma or too much yeast, too little magnesium or a viral infection (see below).

A build-up of stress in the body eventually reaches a point at which the slightest overload causes a complete collapse. This is similar to a child building a tower of wooden blocks, one on top of another. Sooner or later, one too many will cause the whole stack to become unbalanced and collapse.

The accumulation of any stress in the body can be due to many causes, but by treating each individual stress factor separately, rather than the problem as a whole, the pressure on the body may be reduced, but will not be totally alleviated.

Current therapies used to treat ME/CFS are based on differing opinions as to the cause of the disorder. I described these possible causes in Chapter 4, including:

- immunological factors
- inflammation
- viral infection
- hormonal imbalance
- depression
- allergy and sensitivity
- oxidative stress.

One has to treat all the causative factors together in order to reverse the whole process; therefore, in this chapter I will consider:

- diet
- supplements
- immunological therapies
- adaptogens
- exercise
- antidepressants
- talking therapies
- acupuncture
- ozone therapy
- Alexander technique
- neural therapy
- electrotherapy.

Diet

In the wild, when animals are poisoned, they naturally seek out waterholes. With ME/CFS one should drink around 2 litres of fluids, such as mineral or filtered water, every day. This helps with detoxification, but care should be taken not to drink too much, thereby diluting sodium and other essential minerals to dangerously low levels.

Simple, sensible dietetic practices should also be followed, such as avoiding foods with too many additives, artificial flavourings and colourings and rejecting junk food whenever possible.

However, for those of you reading this book who believe a healthy diet full of fruit and vegetables improves health, then you better look up the work of author and investigative food journalist Joanna Blythman who has revealed over the years that most of the food we buy at the supermarket contains toxic additives: plastic-like toxic wax coatings on citrus fruits, herbicides such as chlorpropham used on potatoes, chlorine on ready-to-eat salads and all manner of chemical enhancements that are poisonous[1]. Fortunately, some countries have banned the use of these chemicals, but they are still used by some farmers around the world so continue to enter the food chain.

Organic food and home-grown fruit and veg are much healthier but unfortunately, due to global pollution of the environment, there are toxins in everything we eat and drink and so no foodstuff is totally healthy nowadays, only healthier.

Over the years I have found many ME/CFS patients have benefited from certain nutritional advice given by experts in the field. Having attended many conferences and discussed hundreds of cases with colleagues who are trained nutritionists or nutritional scientists, I have found that many symptoms of ME/CFS and related conditions are helped by certain nutritional support and I will endeavour to summarise the nutritional advice that has benefited patients for their particular condition. However, as everybody in this field of medicine knows, every ME/CFS patient is different, and nothing is truer when trying to satisfy the patient's nutritional needs and avoid any sensitivities and/or intolerances.

For those of you who wish to know the very basics regarding dietetic advice for ME/CFS and FMS and don't want more detail or can't cope with too much information, I generally recommend the following:

1.   Drink around 2 litres of water a day.
2.   Avoid alcohol like the plague.

3.   Reduce stimulants such as caffeine.
4.   Reduce dairy (milk) products.
5.   Reduce gluten-based products.
6.   Reduce yeast, which also means reducing sugar that feeds yeast.
7.   Eat regular meals with as many plant-based foods as possible but aim to have as much variety as possible in the foods and food types you can eat.

In other words, do not have the same food or food types (including even fruit and veg) meal after meal, day after day… variety is the spice of life. And, unless allergic to dairy, gluten or yeast … cheat occasionally with a little treat. (This is to occasionally stimulate the production of the enzymes that break down these foods. Total avoidance of particular foods or food types leads to a depletion of the body's natural enzymes and eventually can lead to total allergies.)

Elimination and avoidance diets

Many ME/CFS patients suffer from food intolerances. Diets, including low-carbohydrate, gluten-free and yeast-free, have all been proposed. However, nutritionists Morris and Stare of Harvard Medical School[2] found that there is no clinical scientific evidence to substantiate claims about the efficacy of various dietary approaches in the treatment of ME/CFS.

However, many patients with ME/CFS suffer with irritable bowel syndrome (IBS) and certain foods known as FODMAPs can lead to an increase of IBS symptoms. 'FODMAP' stands for a group of poorly-absorbed sugars found in some fruit and vegetables, milk and wheat – namely, fermentable oligosaccharides, disaccharides, monosaccharides and polyols. High FODMAP foods include, for example, common dietary items like apples, milk, broccoli, leeks, garlic, onions, peas, dried beans, bread, breakfast cereals, biscuits, barley, beer and fruit juices.

The process of drawing fluid into the bowel and the fermentation of FODMAPs by bacteria is one of the causes of the symptoms experienced by people with IBS. Reducing the intake of high FODMAP foods can help reduce symptoms of IBS.

However, not all FODMAP food may be bad for the individual and one should try and reintroduce some of the FODMAPs after a four to eight week restriction diet. It has been shown that some FODMAPs have pre-biotic qualities that are important in maintaining the good bacteria of the gut, so it isn't a good idea to go on a total FODMAP exclusion diet for too long.

These, and other specific dietary plans, should always be under the strict supervision of a dietitian or nutritionist. Patients often ask what the difference is between the two, to which I answer: one instructs you which foods you can't eat... and the other tells you which foods you can! Joking aside, a dietitian usually has more university-based nutritional training, but over the years I have known of numerous extremely knowledgeable nutritionists who have spent many years training and are more than capable of giving the best nutritional advice. Without stepping on both professions' toes, I will endeavour to impart my advice on what patients with ME/CFS need to know from a nutritional viewpoint.

However, as I keep reiterating, no two ME/CFS patients are the same and as such they all have different dietary requirements. After years of dealing with thousands of patients and consulting with experts in nutrition, I have learnt that no one diet is the universal answer for ME/CFS or FMS. Some patients respond badly to some diets, other patients swear by regimes such as the Paleolithic (Paleo) diet (also known as the Stone Age diet) which contains food that in ancient times was obtained by hunting and gathering rather than farming methods of the last few thousand years. A Paleo diet therefore includes foods such as meats, fish, fruits, vegetables, nuts and seeds but no dairy, grain or processed food . Other patients are devoted followers of the ketogenic diet, which is low carb, high fibre and fat. And some combine the two i.e. paleo AND ketogenic PK diet[3]. It is always a case of trial and error until you find what best suits you.

Anti-candida diets

Infection with the yeast *Candida albicans* has been cited as a cause of ME/CFS and can lead to chronic candidiasis hypersensitivity syndrome (CCHS)[4]. Candida has also been shown to be a major cause of oesophagitis, leading to severe 'heartburn' which is a common symptom in ME/CFS.

The recommended treatment for candida infections is usually oral antifungals nystatin or ketoconazole, together with strict diets that prevent the development of further candida overgrowth by excluding many foods[5]. However, in his 1989 research, Renfro and co-workers noted that the 'yeast connection' is frequently a self-diagnosed condition on the basis of having typical symptoms and a history of frequent yeast infections and multiple courses of antibiotics.

Diets aimed at eliminating *Candida albicans* overgrowth are based on avoiding the foods on which candida thrives – for example, sugar. However, there is little scientific evidence that such regimes do control candida overgrowth.

The use of some antifungal agents such as ketoconazole and itraconazole, in some patients has also resulted in hepatitis[5, 6], with many patients showing no improvements in ME/CFS symptoms. (Nystatin stays within the gut so is much safer but will not act on any fungal infection elsewhere in the body.) I have also seen many patients who have had extensive tests that revealed no abnormal levels of candida in their body, although they definitely suffered from ME/CFS.

I do advise patients to reduce sugar intake as this will reduce the production of yeast and does help many female patients who have frequent bouts of oral and vaginal thrush. Anti-candida creams have helped reduce rashes I have seen on some of my ME/CFS patients which may be due to yeast expelled through the skin when the lymphatics are not working properly. However, it is important to remember that it is always best to check with your doctor if the rash doesn't clear up quickly or worsens and spreads.

Dietary advice for ME/CFS

The usual dietetic advice that works best for most ME/CFS sufferers is that the patient should eat healthy, regular meals, and vary the types of food. Eating the same food types again and again may stimulate the continual release of particular enzymes and overload the body, thus a rotation diet should be followed with plenty of variety[7, 8, 9].

In the years that I have been treating ME/CFS and FMS, some of the weakest, most emaciated and immobile patients I have seen are those that have been following strict avoidance diets, often for many years. They usually start by being slightly intolerant of certain foods and within some months of avoiding those may become completely intolerant of many. As time goes on, more allergies seem to develop, with the body's immune system going into 'free fall' mode, and the patient rapidly descending into a form of total allergic syndrome where almost every food, perfume or deodorant causes adverse reactions[10]. My advice is that in the early stages, if any food sensitivity has been discovered, do not abstain totally for more than a month and, occasionally cheat, eating a little of that substance. The exception to this rule would be if the patient was proved to be allergic, such as in the case of coeliac disease when one is allergic to gluten.

Why do these intolerances and allergies exist in patients with ME/CFS and FMS?

It all goes back to the lymphatic system. As stated earlier in the book, we need the lymphatics to cope with draining an excess of larger molecules. One of the common symptoms of ME/CFS and FMS is irritable bowel syndrome (IBS) which takes the form (usually) of loose bowels and/or constipation, bloating and pain in any part of the abdomen. This is due to the dysfunction of the sympathetic nerves controlling the smooth muscles of the bowel wall. The irritable bowel in ME/CFS and FMS usually occurs together with gut dysbiosis.

Gut dysbiosis is the term used for an imbalance of the flora in the gut, with normally dominating healthy bacteria in the gastrointestinal tract overtaken by harmful bacteria, viruses and fungi, including candida. The beneficial microbial colonies aid healthy digestion and also help protect the body from pathogens. However, the good bacteria can be overtaken by the bad and upset the fine healthy balance of the microbiota.

Microbial colonies excrete waste by-products and the excess waste, especially larger molecules, require a healthy lymphatic system. When there is also a leaky gut, these waste products from the harmful microbes, plus yeast, gluten and the milk protein casein (which are all large molecules and need to drain via the lymphatics), will overburden the lymphatic system, which, if the person has ME/CFS or FMS, is pumping the fluid in the wrong direction.

So, one can understand why too much sugar, wheat and other gluten-based foods plus dairy foods should be reduced with ME/CFS and FMS, especially if the patient suffers from IBS. The lymphatic fluid around the bowel, which is known as chyle, absorbs fat and is thus creamy white in colour, unlike the clear colourless lymphatic fluid in the rest of the body, and so excess fat in the diet when there is a reversal of normal lymphatic flow, as in ME/CFS and FMS, does not drain away in the chyle but may remain congested in the gut. This resultant build-up of fat becomes a collecting depot for further neurotoxins.

The way the cells in our body react to disease relies on what is known as the 'gene expression' of a cell. As many scientists keep on saying, 'it's all in the genes'. We now know that the expression of genes can change and often does due to external influence, such as increased toxins. This is known as epigenetics.

The genes of all the microbes in our bodies are known collectively as the human microbiome. There are 10 times more bacterial cells than human cells in our body and these bacterial cells contain 5 to 8 million genes compared with ours which number about 20,000. A healthy diet is required to improve the health of all the microbiome to fight disease, especially in conditions that affect the whole body, such as ME/CFS and fibromyalgia.

Dr Romain Bouziat and colleagues at the University of Chicago, in collaboration with scientists at Pittsburg University, recently showed that a type of virus stimulates a TH1 immunity reaction against gluten[11]. Dr Peter Green, director of the Celiac Center at New York-Presbyterian/Columbia University Medical Center commented:

'This study demonstrates the mechanism of how a viral infection can cause a switch in the immune system that results in the development of food intolerance', noting that further study might show that other organisms, such as bacteria, do the same. Dr Gerard Mullin, director of the Celiac Disease Clinic at Johns Hopkins School of Medicine in an interview with NBC News said: 'We have more viruses in our gut than bacteria and we know very little about what they do at this point'.

So, in theory, viruses and bacteria can lead to many intolerances and switch on genes that wrongly cause our body to recognise regular foods as harmful, leading to autoimmune reactions and disorders, such as coeliac disease.

Supplements

Vitamin and mineral supplements

Kazimierz Funk (1884–1967), a Polish biochemist, is generally credited with being among the first to formulate (in 1912) the concept of vitamins.

The word 'vitamin' is formed from the words 'vital' and 'amine' and indicates that these chemical compounds are necessary for the body's metabolism to work properly. They are usually inadequately produced by the body and therefore extra must be included in our diet or taken as a supplement. Vitamins are widely recommended in the treatment of ME/CFS, but there is no evidence that mega doses of vitamins and minerals will relieve any of the ME/CFS symptoms. However, the antioxidant action of vitamin C has been shown to improve the body's immune response. With patients taking no more than 500 mg per day there have been no reported toxic side-effects. Similarly, the vitamin B group is known to improve the health of the nervous system. Functional deficiencies of the B vitamins pyridoxine (B6), riboflavin (B2) and thiamine (B3) have been shown to occur in ME/CFS[12] and patients may therefore be advised to take one full and complete vitamin B-complex pill per day, provided that no complications are reported. As discussed in Chapter 3, some ME/CFS patients have genetic mutations affecting the methylation cycle, important for energy and all metabolic pathways. These patients with a methylation SNP need to take methylated B complex.

Some doctors specialising in ME/CFS give high doses of vitamin C and folic acid intravenously which is safe if closely monitored by the prescribing physician. I, however, err on the side of caution and advise a 500 mg daily oral supplement of vitamin C and one complete vitamin B-complex pill to increase the patient's resistance to overall infection and improve cell energy production and the functioning of the nervous system.

Supplements and the mitochondria

Since one of the main symptoms of ME/CFS is a lack of energy, it follows that many researchers have looked at the energy production in the body as a possible explanation of the disease. The powerhouses of our cells (and those of all other animals) are known as the mitochondria and it is in these organelles that a major cycle of different reactions take place, the Krebs cycle, which is an essential biochemical pathway that helps our cells produce energy. To provide the key cofactors required for optimal energy output we also need good methylation.

The building blocks of proteins are known as amino acids. Specific amino acids are needed to produce different proteins, such as neurotransmitters which send messages from one nerve to another. Different neurotransmitters are produced by slight differences to the amino acids, usually by the addition of a methyl group onto the existing amino acid; this process is known as methylation. A methyl group consists of one carbon atom attached to three hydrogen atoms and is derived from the methane molecule with one hydrogen atom missing.

Methylation is a vital metabolic process that takes place in every cell in our body, occurring more than a billion times per second throughout the body. It is not only important for energy production but vital for the body's genetics, immunity, detoxification and brain function. The reactions that occur when one molecule passes a methyl group to another produce chemicals vital for healthy energy metabolism, such as creatine, L carnitine, coenzyme Q10 and homocysteine, which ultimately leads to the production of glutathione. These chemicals produced in the methylation cycle help power the **citric acid cycle** (CAC) – also known as the **tricarboxylic acid (TCA) cycle** or the **Krebs cycle**, mentioned above, which is a series of chemical reactions to release stored energy through the oxidation of acetyl-coenzyme A, derived from carbohydrates, fats and proteins, into carbon dioxide and chemical energy by a process that ultimately converts the energy molecule adenosine triphosphate (ATP) into adenosine diphosphate (ADP) plus energy.

The biochemical details of these two cycles are quite complex so let me borrow an analogy from one of the experts in this field, Dr Sarah Myhill, who like many believes that mitochondrial dysfunction lies at the root of ME/CFS. Dr Myhill likens the methylation cycle to the starter motor in a car with the Krebs cycle being the engine. You need the starter motor to power up the engine which is required to run the car.

Likewise, the methylation cycle produces the required chemical reactions necessary to produce the chemical changes that help drive the main Krebs cycle[13].

As well as energy production, methylation is important for many other vital bodily functions, such as immune function, detoxification, balancing moods and reducing inflammation.

In my earlier days of attending international ME/CFS conferences there were a few characters at these events who stood out of the crowd. One such delegate was Rich van Konynenburg, a larger-than-life nuclear physicist, who formally proposed a biochemical model of stress-induced glutathione depletion in the disorder at a ME/CFS Conference in Wisconsin in 2004.

Rich, who sadly died in 2012, maintained that glutathione, the master antioxidant in the body and a key player in the cellular energy production system, was depleted in the cells of ME/CFS patients, and he believed this leads to many of the dysfunctions found in ME/CFS. After much research and attending numerous conferences and seminars, Rich came to believe that a methylation block was at work in both ME/CFS and autism, two disorders he became convinced had similar underlying causes.

In 2007 he re-engineered his theory, and called it the 'glutathione depletion – methylation cycle block hypothesis' to incorporate his new understanding, and he created a simplified methylation protocol specifically for ME/CFS patients, derived from a complete treatment programme developed by naturopathic doctor Amy Yasko, for disorders that are also thought to involve methylation cycle block and glutathione depletion. Dr Yasko's treatment is described in her book *The Puzzle of Autism*. Rich's theories and treatment are now used by some leading ME/CFS specialists around the world.

Rich Van Konynenburg identified methylation as essential to produce vital molecules, such as CoQ-10 and L carnitine, and many other essential chemicals. It is also important in the production of myelin which forms electrically insulated sheaths around many nerves. He found it important in DNA expression and as part of folic acid metabolism, which also switches on synthesis of new DNA and RNA. The methylation cycle is also essential for cell-mediated immune function carried out by T lymphocytes and it requires many minerals and nutrients to work correctly, the main ones being magnesium and vitamin B12, which are often advised by naturopaths and nutritionists for ME/CFS as well as creatine, L carnitine, CoQ10, and glutathione.

In the body CoQ10 (ubiquinone) is converted to the active form, ubiquinol, which is a more active compound, so I often recommend patients to take ubiquinol directly to improve their energy. In a clinical trial, CoQ10, also known as bio-quinine, has been shown to help reduce fatigue, help restore mitochondrial function and bioenergetic metabolism, and reduce oxidative stress in ME/CFS when taken together with a powerful form of vitamin B3, the coenzyme NADH[14].

As has been discussed in Chapter 3, research into genetic problems leading to ME/CFS is under way throughout the world. Some people have a problem with MTHFR (methylenetetrahydrofolate reductase) which is an important enzyme required for a chemical reaction converting forms of the vitamin folate (vitamin B9) and folic acid into an active form that the body can use during methylation. The MTHFR gene provides instructions for making methylenetetrahydrofolate reductase. This enzyme plays a part in processing amino acids, the building blocks of proteins and important for structure and functioning of the entire body.

All is not lost if one has the MTHFR gene mutation. There are certain strategies that can help, such as avoiding folic acid-blocking drugs, such as birth control pills or methotrexate. Other advice is to avoid antacids as they block absorption of vitamin B12 and other nutrients. Supplements that contain high levels of methyl B complex which includes methylated forms of B9, B12 and B6 are often used to help patients with a MTHFR gene mutation. If there seem to be a few members in the family with similar symptoms of ME/CFS or fibromyalgia it is worth having a genetic test done.

Another genetic variation that is linked with the predisposition to ME/CFS and FMS is the COMT gene[14a]. COMT provides instructions for the body to produce another very important methylation enzyme called catechol-O-methyltransferase. This enzyme is involved in the breakdown of catecholamines, which are the hormones made by our adrenal glands, such as dopamine, adrenaline (epinephrine) and noradrenaline (norepinephrine).

Noradrenaline (norepinephrine) is one of the main transmitter substances in the autonomic nervous system. Many people have the slow variation of the COMT gene known as 'COMT Slow' which leads to greater levels of noradrenaline as well as high levels of cortisol and HPA-axis dysfunction affecting the body's ability to calm itself and de-stress, which is frequently seen in ME/CFS and FMS.

A diet such as the Paleo (Stone-age) diet, with a higher level of protein, often helps ME/CFS and FMS patients. However, if a genetic test reveals a COMT Slow gene, then these patients should reduce protein-rich foods to avoid excess production of catecholamines. This is also another reason why patients with ME/CFS and FMS must reduce caffeine and abstain from alcohol as these stimulate catecholamine activity. I advise all my ME/CFS and FMS patients to take a supplement of vitamin B complex. Increasing vitamin B, especially B2, B6, B9 and B12, will help COMT methylation as will a supplementation of magnesium.

A well known physician, Dr Sharon Meglathery, in Tucson Arizona has researched the genetic link of ME/CFS and related conditions in view of her own ill health, developing ME/CFS, mast cell activation syndrome (MCAS), postural orthostatic tachycardia syndrome (POTS), raised intracranial pressure and a host of other potentially disabling syndromes in 2009. Although there are no major studies yet to back her theory, she suggests that patients who have genetic CYP21A2 mutations develop a 'wired and fired', high achieving, hyper-focused, highly stressed profile she calls CAPS (CYP21A2 mutation associated neuropsychiatric syndrome). CYP21A2 (steroid 21-hydroxylase) is part of the SNP RCCX which is a common cluster of four gene mutations. It is highly unstable and can mix and match, which leads to family histories filled with the chronic illnesses that are associated with these genes, such as ME/CFS and FMS and comorbidities such as EDS, POTS and MCAS discussed in detail in Chapter 6.

Dr Meglathery holds that individuals with CAPS are at higher risk of chronic illness, especially when an individual has inherited copies from both parents, which she claims is much more common than people would think. She theorises that 'people with CAPS are attracted preferentially to other people with CAPS'. This is likely to result in more children with two copies of the CYP21A2 mutation. This may explain why individual families seem to have multiple members with these disorders.

Magnesium supplementation

Magnesium deficiency, besides its effect on energy, is also associated with disorders of neuromuscular and psychiatric functioning and an inability to cope with viral infections[15]. In 1991 a randomised controlled trial was conducted which showed that 20 ME/CFS patients had significantly lower red blood cell magnesium levels compared with healthy controls[16]. Further studies have supported the introduction of magnesium supplementation in the treatment of ME/CFS, especially to help with energy production and with muscle pain and fatigue[17, 18, 19, 20].

The two main forms of magnesium compound taken orally are magnesium malate and magnesium citrate. In my experience it all depends on personal preference, but I usually advise magnesium maleate (or 'malate' in the US), which is a combination of the mineral magnesium and malic acid. Malic acid is a naturally occurring substance that aids energy production in the body. Some patients may find the citrate or other versions work better than maleate, and, as I keep emphasising, every patient is different and will find many different supplements that work best for them.

Fibromyalgia patients have been shown possibly to have difficulty creating malic acid. A study of 24 people with FMS suggests that magnesium maleate taken for at least two months may relieve the pain and tenderness associated with the condition[21].

Magnesium citrate is preferred by some practitioners and is the product of magnesium combined with citric acid. Magnesium citrate is often used in liquid form as a saline laxative to treat constipation, or to completely empty the intestines prior to surgery, but it can be found in capsular form. There are some superior products with a combination of different forms of magnesium to account for the way different compounds are absorbed into the blood.

The problem with most magnesium supplements is that, while a product may have a label claiming to contain magnesium citrate, it may actually use magnesium oxide as a base to boost the label claim for the elemental amount of magnesium, and blend this with a carrier such as citrate. You need to ensure that the product contains *fully reacted* magnesium, which should be clearly stated on the label.

Magnesium oxide is both *inorganic* and *insoluble*, meaning that it is extremely poorly absorbed and simply passes through the gastrointestinal tract (often resulting in unpleasant laxative side effects). Patients should look for products that are fully reacted and which are directly bound to the carrier, with no magnesium oxide. Some products may be buffered, which combines fully reacted magnesium with magnesium oxide, but at least they are better than blends. A low dose of magnesium taken several times a day is better absorbed and retained.

One should seek medical advice before taking magnesium, especially if you have any kidney disorder. Magnesium can potentially interact with certain medications, including high blood pressure medicines and some antibiotics.

Chelation (the detoxification of heavy metals)

Magnesium malate also has chelating properties in that it can bind to toxic heavy metals, such as lead and mercury or many lighter metals, such as aluminium, which are still highly neurotoxic and respond well to many chelation agents, reducing the toxic overload[22].

Chlorella

As well as magnesium maleate, an excellent chelation agent that I recommend is *Chlorella pyrenoidosa*, a blue-green algae. Chlorella contains large amounts of vitamin K, a nutrient that helps the body's clotting function (but may interfere with blood-thinning effects of certain medications, such as warfarin and others). If you are severely immune compromised, or if you take immune-suppressive drugs, or if you have a heart condition, seek medical advice before taking chlorella supplements.

Coconut oil

Together with chlorella, I recommend taking two teaspoons of coconut oil per day. It can be added in cooking, used as a spread or eaten off the spoon. The coconut oil absorbs the chlorella and heavy metal combination. However, some readers may question why taking the extra cholesterol found in coconut oil will help, given the long-running debate that too much cholesterol in the diet can lead to too much in the blood, which is associated with an increased risk of getting heart and circulatory diseases. This debate is not for this book but it is worth noting that while coconut oil is about 90% saturated fat, it also gives 'good' HDL cholesterol a boost.

Most of our cholesterol is made in the body by the liver. It is also found in many foods, including oils. It plays a vital part in how every cell works and is also needed to make vitamin D, some hormones and bile for digestion. Cholesterol is carried in the blood attached to proteins called lipoproteins. There are two main forms, LDL (low density lipoprotein), the 'bad unhealthy cholesterol' and HDL (high density lipoprotein) the 'good protective cholesterol'. Coconut oil is one of the healthy oils that is high in natural saturated fats which increase the healthy HDL cholesterol in your body.

Saturated fat is divided into various types, based on the number of carbon atoms in the molecule, and about half of the saturated fat in coconut oil is the 12-carbon variety, called lauric acid. That is a higher percentage than in most other oils and is probably responsible for the unusual HDL effects of coconut oil. But plant-based oils are more than just fats. They contain many antioxidants and other substances which help ME/CFS and FMS patients.

Psyllium husks

Psyllium or ispaghula is the common name used for several members of the plant genus Plantago. Psyllium is mainly used as a dietary fibre to relieve symptoms of both constipation and mild diarrhoea and occasionally as a food thickener and is totally gluten free, which is important. Taking a supplement of psyllium husks acts as roughage that helps with the removal and passage of the coconut oil, chlorella and heavy metal mix out through the alimentary canal. In some cases, one has to be careful about using psyllium, as it has been known sometimes to clog up the bowel. Basically, one should take the psyllium for the first month to 'get things moving' and avoid it completely if prone to constipation.

Activated charcoal

The ingestion of charcoal has also been used for centuries to help remove toxins from the body. Activated charcoal is produced at much higher temperatures than standard charcoal and is much more porous. Therefore, it is more effective in filtering impurities than standard charcoal. Takesumi, or carbonised bamboo, has been shown to be very helpful in the detoxification of many poisons, including food additives, heavy metals and other biotoxins that are found within the body. It does also have some antifungal and antibacterial properties[23].

Vitamin B12

Vitamin B12 is often prescribed for ME/CFS and FMS together with magnesium and there is evidence for its benefits combined with B9[24]. However, how the magnesium and vitamin B12 are administered depends on each individual practitioner and differs from case to case. Vitamin B12 injections, usually into the thigh or upper arm, in the form of either cyanocobalamin or hydroxocobalamin are probably the most efficient way of increasing your vitamin B12 levels.

A diet that includes meat, fish, eggs and dairy products can provide natural sources of B12 in the form of hydroxocobalamin, which is why B12 deficiency is very common in vegans. However, in numerous ME/CFS and FMS sufferers there is a problem in the absorption of the vitamin in the stomach and small intestine, so many cannot rely on diet alone.

Symptoms of vitamin B12 deficiency include depression and mood disorders, fatigue, memory failure, anaemia, low blood pressure and nerve damage in the hands and feet. Follow the advice from your doctor as each case is different and some patients may be severely deficient and others may not have a problem at all, which is again another complexity of ME/CFS and FMS in that nutritionally no patient requires the same supplementation and all dietary needs are different. Be aware, however, that B12 blood levels can be misleading as haematologists now recognise that only a proportion of B12 in the blood is 'active'.

Since the B vitamins and vitamin C are water soluble, unlike the other vitamins which are fat soluble, they are rarely found in excess in the body as too much passes out of the body. However, when the metabolism is at fault and/or fluid intake is low, one might overload on vitamin B12 which could cause flushing, diarrhoea, nausea, and vomiting.

Iodine

Due to the hormonal aspect of this disease, with the hypothalamus being affected by neurotoxins, many ME/CFS patients have been found to have thyroid problems. This is compounded by the problem of iodine deficiency, which is a global problem. In the early part of the twentieth century, iodine deficiency was reduced by adding it to flour and salt.

However, many people were found to be sensitive or allergic to iodine, with excess iodine resulting in thyroid inflammation. Therefore, in the 1980s it was removed from flour production and one rarely finds iodised salt, plus over the last few years salt intake has reduced around the world.

A study in 2011 by the British Thyroid Association UK Iodine Survey Group showed that a high number of girls in the UK were iodine deficient[25].

Iodine is an essential micronutrient with a deficiency associated with goitre and hypothyroidism and pregnancy loss plus congenital anomalies and intellectual impairment in children born from iodine-deficient mothers.

Seaweed such as kelp is one of the best natural sources of iodine and can therefore be used to help some thyroid problems. However, one does not wish to overload the iodine content for the reasons stated above, so don't have too much kelp. Advice from a nutritionist will be important.

Increased salt intake

The disturbed metabolism in ME/CFS can affect salt intake. Besides the iodine deficiency linked with reduced salt intake, sodium deficiency can produce an array of similar signs and symptoms to ME/CFS and is associated with a form of low blood pressure that occurs as one stands up after sitting or lying, called neurally-mediated hypotension (NMH). This drop in blood pressure corresponds with a drop in heart rate when tested on a tilt table[26].

However, although an increase in salt intake is advised with some patients, this may lead to severe, if not fatal, consequences if they suffer from high blood pressure. It is always best to check with the GP before increasing sodium in the diet.

ME/CFS notoriously often overlaps with other medically unexplained syndromes due to the disturbed sympathetic nervous system as detailed later in Chapter 6. One of them is known as 'orthostatic intolerance' which refers to a group of clinical conditions in which symptoms worsen with upright posture and are reduced when lying down. The severe form of orthostatic intolerance is 'postural orthostatic tachycardia syndrome' (POTS) and this is discussed in more detail in the next chapter (page 172).

Essential fatty acids

Omega-3 and omega-6 fatty acids are hugely important in the regulation of inflammation and immune function. Long-chain omega-3 fatty acid EPA (eicosapentaenoic acid), which is mainly found in fish oils, helps reduce inflammation and is necessary for many biological processes in the body so it must be constantly replenished. Due to increased demands by ME/CFS patients and also the metabolic damage from viral infections, the patient usually doesn't have enough EPA, or enough of the anti-inflammatory omega-6 fatty acid GLA (gamma linolenic acid), which is found mostly in vegetable oils, especially evening primrose oil. Many people nowadays have a diet low in EPA but high in pro-inflammatory omega-6 AA (arachidonic acid) which in excess produces what is known as a low omega-3 index (the ratio between omega 3 and 6). This has been linked with increased inflammation and the reduction of normal immune function, aggravating symptoms of ME/CFS.

In a study carried out at the ME/CFS Unit at Vall d'Hebron University Hospital, Barcelona, Spain, a leading ME/CFS expert, Dr Jesus Castro-Marrero and colleagues, showed that 92.6% of ME/CFS patients showed a low mean omega-3 index (5.75%)[27].

Central to the basis of the Perrin Technique is the fact that in ME/CFS the hypothalamus is usually overactive, leading to an overloaded autonomic system. Nerves transmit their signal via chemicals known as neurotransmitters, as has been described. Too much of one of the main neurotransmitters, acetylcholine, breaks down into acetate and choline. Thus, when originally formulating my theory in 1989 I hypothesised that one day scientists would discover too much choline in the body.

As mentioned in Chapter 2, an increase of choline has indeed been found in ME/CFS sufferers by Professor Basant Puri of Hammersmith Hospital and Imperial College, London[28], who has also discovered a deficiency in fatty acids which are important for the healthy maintenance of cell membranes, especially in the brain. This can be remedied by increasing the intake of EPA, which converts in the body to another omega 3 fatty acid, DHA (docosahexonoic acid), again as described earlier. This combines with the choline to heal the cell membranes and restore normal function of the brain. (This is fully explained in Professor Puri's book *Chronic Fatigue Syndrome – a natural way to treat ME* – see further reading.)

It is of further significance that in a study by the Federation of American Societies of Experimental Biology into the effect of omega 3 fatty acids on the neuro-lymphatic/glymphatic system, there was better drainage from the brain to the lymphatics when the intake of omega 3 polyunsaturated fatty acids was increased[29].

Guaifenesin

Guaifenesin is a pharmaceutical agent found in many cough medicines and is usually used as an expectorant, increasing the volume and reducing the viscosity of secretions in the passages of the lungs. It also has been shown to help relax muscles and has anticonvulsant properties. It is thought to do this by acting as an NMDA receptor antagonist[30]. As discussed in Chapter 2, in ME/CFS and fibromyalgia there is over-activity of the neurochemical NMDA in the thalamus of the brain due to neuro-toxicity and so guaifenesin may help some of the symptoms. By reducing the action of NMDA it may help reduce the production of neuropeptide P which will help with pain. Plus, it may help with sinus congestion, which plagues many patients. Although there are no clinical trials to support its use in ME/CFS or fibromyalgia, I have known ME/CFS patients who have had relief from headaches and general aches and pains from taking this medication.

Immunological therapies

An alternative term for ME/CFS in the USA used to be chronic fatigue and immune dysfunction syndrome (CFIDS), an acknowledgement that dysfunction of the immune system is a major feature of the disease. However, many immune modulatory treatments are expensive and not freely available, produce unpleasant side effects and yield inconclusive results (see Chapter 4).

As mentioned previously in Chapter 4, antiviral and antibiotic therapies have also been tried over the past 50 years, proposed by many in the medical profession who are sure the cause is microbial, as suggested by the older names for the disease, such as post-infectious fatigue, post-viral syndrome, Tapanui flu or chronic Epstein-Barr syndrome, the latter name given when it was assumed that it was caused by the Epstein-Barr virus that initiates glandular fever, also known as infectious mononucleosis or 'mono'.

Over the years, I have stressed that although there may be some viral or other infections that preceded the onset of the major symptoms, when you look back at the history of the patient you inevitably find many difficulties in their health, and earlier symptoms that eventually built-up over the years to a trigger, which is usually a viral infection, that leads to ME/CFS. The problem I believe is pre-viral and the virus, bacteria, fungi, parasites or many other stressors are the final triggers of the disease and never the singular cause. After all, many millions of people are infected with Epstein-Barr virus and although they may be unwell for weeks after, they do fully recover. My own wife, Julie, suffered from ME/CFS severely for seven years after contracting typhoid in Mexico, which is a bacterial infection. With the appropriate antibiotic therapy she should have fully recovered within a few weeks. So, what prevents ME/CFS patients from recovering like most other people?

The clue is in the name: post-viral or post-infectious fatigue. After the invading organism has infected the body, the immune system sends out large protein signalling cytokines to activate immune cells to destroy the virus or other infectious antigens. These cytokines then require removal via lymphatic drainage. This process we know is compromised and reversed in ME/CFS and FMS as discussed extensively throughout this book.

This is why drugs that are claimed to help ME/CFS patients or even cure them are often no help and may aggravate the condition. Antivirals such as Ampligen, may have helped some patients who are part of a particular subgroup of ME/CFS patients who have been infected by viruses. There are some doctors and scientists over the years who have presented convincing arguments for their belief that ME/CFS is caused by one specific virus, such as the retrovirus xenotropic murine retrovirus (XMRV) or a group of viruses such as enteroviruses[31].

Sometimes the theories have been proven wrong, such as the famous exposure of suspected cases of XMRV turning out to be due to contaminated samples from lab mice[32].

The reason for all these various theories is that there are many subgroups related to trigger-factors rather than to actual causation. There is more and more evidence for such subgrouping in ME/CFS[33] and it is important to know which subgroup a patient belongs to so that they can receive a more specific drug regime or a tailored management plan.

However, I believe that all the subgroups have a common physical disorder – the disturbed neuro-lymphatic system – so the physical diagnosis and treatment using the Perrin Technique is not specific to any subgroups. Subgrouping will help the practitioner know what other approach to adopt in addition to the Perrin Technique, rather than as an alternative, and an integrative combined approach will speed up the overall improvement in the patient's health.

This whole concept of an underlying common biomechanical problem affecting all ME/CFS patients also explains why the majority of people who are infected by EBV or other major viruses and bacterial infections, such as *Borrelia burgdorferi*, do not develop ME/CFS. They are lucky that their neuro-lymphatic drainage works as it should.

As we know from the SARS outbreak of 2003, as mentioned in Chapter 3, coronavirus A seemed to follow the olfactory pathway into the brain along the main route of the neuro-lymphatic drainage. This may also be the case with Covid-19, which is possibly why some people succumbing to this virus are exhibiting a known feature of ME/CFS – namely a large build-up of cytokines known as a 'cytokine storm'. Most people don't suffer too badly when infected with Covid-19, since their neuro-lymphatic drainage works correctly.

As I am writing this in April 2020 during the height of this terrible pandemic, I continue to treat some ME/CFS and FMS patients and I am advising all my patients who are self-isolating to be vigilant with their self-massage treatment, as described in Chapter 10. This will aid the neuro-lymphatic drainage which I believe could be so important to help reduce the severity of the disease and many other infections.

I suppose only time will tell if I am correct and post mortems reveal the neuro-lymphatic nature of the pathogenesis of Covid-19, but I am absolutely certain that when the pandemic is over, after a vaccine or effective treatment has been found, many new cases of post-viral ME/CFS will emerge in the survivors, and the Perrin Technique will be more needed than ever around the world.

Another drug that has been the subject of clinical trials and looked like being helpful for some ME/CFS patients is rituximab (Rituxan). This drug is used primarily for some lymphatic cancers and the relief of some autoimmune diseases, such as rheumatoid arthritis. Two Norwegian oncologists, Øystein Fluge and Olav Mella, discovered this potential by accident in three ME/CFS patients who had been treated for B-cell lymphoma. As well as helping their lymphoma symptoms, their ME/CFS significantly reduced with the treatment.

As mentioned in Chapter 4, antibodies are created by the body's immune system in response to an antigen that has entered the body. Rituximab is a monoclonal antibody which means it only targets a specific antigen, the CD20 antigen on normal and malignant B-cells, and is used in 'targeted' cancer therapy. The body's natural immune defences are then recruited to attack and kill the marked B-cells. Stem cells in the bone marrow that will develop into the various types of cells do not have the CD20 antigen. This allows healthy B-cells to regenerate after treatment. Thus, rituximab is believed to work by depleting the dysfunctional B-cells to correct the immune imbalance and improve ME/CFS symptoms.

It has been shown that neurotransmitters released by sympathetic and parasympathetic nerve endings bind to their respective receptors located on the surface of immune cells and initiate immune-modulatory responses[34]. It is this mechanism that is thought by to be targeted by rituximab.

Scientists working with Fluge and Mella in Norway demonstrated an association of autoantibodies with immune markers connected to autonomic activity which could also explain various clinical symptoms of ME/CFS[35].

So, in lay terms, what may be happening in a subset of patients with ME/CFS is that the hypothalamus in their brain becomes dysfunctional owing to a build up of neurotoxins. This then leads to a disturbance of autonomic control affecting the levels of the neurotransmitters acetylcholine and noradrenaline. This then causes disruption in some receptors of these chemicals on a group of B-lymphocytes, affecting their immune control. Therefore, in this sub-group of patients with ME/CFS, their symptoms should improve with this targeted approach. Figure 14 demonstrates the possible

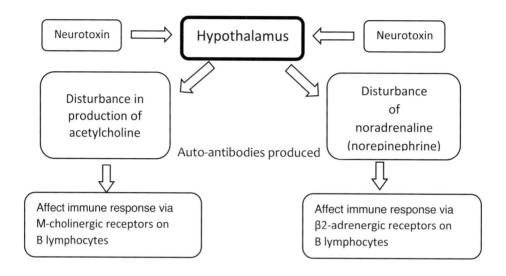

Fig. 14 The impact of neurotoxins on the hypothalamus.

immune disturbance in ME/CFS which is targeted by drugs such as rituximab.

In earlier trials, I did express my concern that it would be dangerous to treat a wider group of ME/CFS patients with a drug that depletes part of the immune system for a period until new B cells are functioning, and the drug has been known to have obvious side effects due to the increased chance of systemic infections. More worryingly was that one of the known side effects of rituximab was death! If a patient has a life-threatening disease, such as cancer or severe crippling rheumatoid arthritis, one can understand them being given a drug with such risks. However, for most ME/CFS patients, I believe taking such a drug poses an unnecessary danger to their health.

The planned larger trial went ahead, despite my protestations. However, just as I feared, it was announced in October 2017 that the larger scale research trial had failed. When an announcement comes out about failed research before it has been published, it is almost certain that there have been one or more serious adverse events.

In the published article in the *Annals of Internal Medicine*, it was revealed that rituximab was given to 77 ME/CFS patients with no significant improvement compared with a control group who received a placebo, and disturbingly but not surprisingly, 26% of them displayed serious adverse reactions[36].

Apheresis, plasmapheresis (TPE) and immunoadsorption

Apheresis is a process developed in 1972 where blood is passed through a machine that separates out one particular constituent and returns the remainder to the circulation. Plasma, the fluid part of the blood, is a light yellow liquid composed of water, salts and enzymes which helps in the removal of waste from the body as well as carrying all parts of the blood through the circulatory system.

Plasmapheresis, also known as 'therapeutic plasma exchange' (TPE), is the removal of plasma from the patient and separation by a machine into component parts, some of which are returned to the patient. This procedure may be effective in some cases of both ME/CFS and FMS when regulation of the immune response is disturbed and auto-antibodies are present, as shown in some other serious illnesses[37].

One should be cautious before beginning with this technique as during plasma exchange, blood pressure is lowered and so the technique is not suitable for patients who already have lowered blood pressure. Drinking lots of water in the days before treatment can reduce common reactions such as nausea and dizziness. Some patients have suffered from bleeds and other allergic reactions following plasmapheresis,

Immunoadsorption is another method that may help ME/CFS and FMS patients; it uses a different type of machine to remove specific antibodies from the blood without the need for TPE[38]. In ME/CFS it has helped some patients by removing autoantibodies against ß2 adrenergic receptors of the sympathetic nervous system[39], which has been suggested as a possible mechanism that leads to autonomic neuro-immune dysfunction and was the basis for testing the drug rituximab as mentioned above.

Low-dose naltrexone

Another medical approach that has been shown to help some patients with their symptoms is low-dose naltrexone (LDN) which is the 'off-label' use of the medication naltrexone at low doses for diseases such as multiple sclerosis and fibromyalgia[40, 41]. Naltrexone is typically prescribed for opioid or alcohol dependence, as it is a strong opioid antagonist. Opioid receptors modulate pain reception in the body and also increase the production of the body's natural endorphins. They have also been shown to be important in the immune system by regulating cell proliferation in certain cells, such as T and B lymphocytes and tumour cells[42].

At the 2020 online conference of the International Association of ME/CFS, Dr Jane

Mckay, reported on a pilot study on patients with ME/CFS and FMS at the Women's Hospital and Health Centre, Vancouver Canada. She and her colleagues administered very low doses of 0.25–4.5 mg of naltexone to the patient group, which resulted in increased energy, improved sleep and cognition and decreased pain in most of the patients, with little side effects[43].

The reason LDN also helps is that it may act as an anti-inflammatory agent in the central nervous system, especially on the glia[44] which contain many pro-inflammatory cytokines and other neurotoxins that build up in ME/CFS and FMS.

Adaptogens

Adaptogens are botanical medicines that have been used for centuries by eastern traditional medicine to help the body cope better with all forms of stress. Examples of adaptogens that have been shown to help ME/CFS patients include rhodiola, Siberian ginseng and liquorice[45].

Rhodiola rosea decreases cortisol levels in stress and reduces fatigue as well as increasing concentration.

Eleutherococcus senticosusm (also known as Siberian ginseng) supports the adrenal glands and increases lymphocyte activity helping the immune system. When I was heavily involved in sports medicine in the 1980s and 1990s, I used to treat many athletes who took Siberian ginseng to boost their performance, which was commonplace at that time. The World Anti-Doping Agency (WADA) classified ginseng as a permitted substance for athletes as it did not cause a positive doping test result. So, it may also help with energy in ME/CFS patients, but don't start trying to run the 4-minute mile or the 100-metres in under 10 seconds.

Liquorice root has known antiviral properties.

Ashwaganda: Another well-known adaptogen is ashwagandha, which has also been shown to have good antioxidant properties aiding the immune and nervous systems and therefore helping the body cope better with stress[46].

In a major review, Ajay Semalty and colleagues formulated a comprehensive list of herbal medicine that may help symptoms of ME/CFS and FMS[47]. Below, I have listed a selection of some other medicinal plants that they suggest may help. I have seen in clinic the improvement in some patients after taking one or more of these natural remedies. However, before you buy every adaptogen mentioned in this book, you should always consult with a qualified herbalist or doctor before taking any medicines, even plant-based ones, to ensure that you take the correct dose and to avoid any side effects or adverse reactions that may occur if you are on any other medication or have a co-existing health problem. I usually advise ME/CFS patients to start small regarding any herbal remedy as many patients are highly-sensitive to anything they put into their bodies. So, starting with the lowest dose is always a good idea to help prevent any severe adverse reactions occurring. If even the lowest dose causes a problem, stop immediately and seek your practitioner's advice.

- *Aloe vera* for gut and immune support.
- *Angelica sinensis* promotes blood circulation and modulates the immune system. It is also helpful in reducing PMS.
- *Aralia mandshurica* benefits the mind and body by helping with stress, anxiety and fatigue and to stimulate the immune system and improve stamina.
- *Echinacea purpurea* helps the immune system to fight viruses. It also helps lower blood pressure, control blood sugar and manage anxiety.
- *Gingko biloba* is a favourite of mine in helping brain fog and cognitive dysfunction. It has been used in Chinese medicine since ancient times to help brain function as it has a high flavonoid and turpenoid content that, as well as aiding signalling properties in the brain, also has antioxidant properties so is excellent in aiding the immune system.
- *Matricaria chamomilla* is used by many people to help with sleep, as a mild sedative, and to lower anxiety. It can also help reduce painful periods and other abdominal pain.
- *Pinus Maritima* (pine bark) extract helps the immune system, aids blood flow and boosts brain function as well as reducing inflammation.
- *Schisandra chinensis* (Wu Wei Zi berries/seeds) increases energy and helps reduce fatigue and has antioxidant and anti-inflammatory properties.

WARNING: It is extremely important to realise that the list of adaptogens and supplements in this book are a general guide and not set in stone. Even herbal supplements and natural botanical products can have serious side effects, especially if combined with other prescribed medicines. For example, Gingko biloba and SSRIs together may cause a potentially dangerous condition known as serotonin syndrome that is due to too much of the neurotransmitter serotonin. It is important to check with your doctor first before taking any products mentioned in this book to ensure that any drug interactions or chemical overloads are avoided.

Exercise

Exercise often helps fatigue associated with an overall lack of fitness and with depression, but excessive activity always exacerbates fatigue in patients with ME/CFS. In fact, too much physical activity can trigger a relapse in someone who is on the road to recovery. The simple question every practitioner needs to ask when initially examining a possible ME/CFS patient is, 'Does exertion ever improve the symptoms, or does it aggravate the condition?'. If the latter is true, even if at the time of exertion, the patient feels good, it is possibly ME/CFS.

Patients suffer from what is commonly known as post-exertional malaise (PEM), or post-exertional neuro-immune exhaustion (PENE). As stated in the international consensus criteria (ICC) for ME/CFS: 'Normal fatigue is proportional to the intensity and duration of activity, followed by a quick restoration of energy. PENE is characterised by a pathological low threshold of physical and mental fatigability, exhaustion, pain, and an abnormal exacerbation of symptoms in response to exertion. It is followed by a prolonged recovery period'[48]. This differs totally from the usual beneficial effects of exertion in some psychiatric disorders, such as clinical depression.

Professor Lenny Jason and colleagues at De Paul University, Chicago, found that when questioning participants in a study on ME/CFS, there was much confusion as to what PEM meant and how it differs from the term PENE used in the international criteria[49].

It is important clinically to note that if the patient feels occasionally improved following exertion, there could be an element of clinical depression. However, the patient may be suffering from both conditions at one time.

People often confuse the term 'exertion' with 'exercise'. In clinic, when I ask a patient if exertion helps or worsens their condition, sometimes the patient will say they feel better after a stroll, or a gentle cycle. There are plenty of patients with less severe symptoms who do benefit from keeping active without overloading their bodies. This is not exertion! Exertion is when a person feels that they have pushed their body more than they can cope with. With ME/CFS this will inevitably lead to the overall symptom picture worsening and, as Lily Chu and colleagues found out, during a Stanford University research study, some patients with ME/CFS don't feel the post-exertional malaise immediately but only later on and in some cases three days after exerting themselves[50].

A positive approach is important in fighting any disorder, but the horrible irony of ME/CFS is that it usually affects people who are determined, positive characters who would usually beat most illnesses with willpower alone. It is no secret that a strong willpower has been shown to help combat all types of diseases, even some potentially fatal conditions, such as cancer. The power of the mind appears to be a vital tool in overcoming pathology, by improving the immune system though neuro-immune connections. However, the neurological pathway that is involved in this phenomenon is part of the sympathetic nervous system, the very system that breaks down in ME/CFS. Thus, the more the patient tries to beat the illness by pushing themselves, the worse the symptoms become.

GET (graded exercise therapy)

Some psychologists believe that patients with ME/CFS 'perceive' greater fatigue during exercise as a result of the interaction of psychological distress, physical de-conditioning and/or sleep disturbance. They believe that the patient's fear of making their symptoms worse may lead to their reducing their activity and that the resultant physical de-conditioning can spiral into chronic disability, which leads to adverse psychological effects. Graded activity is the process of gently increasing activity to counterbalance physical de-conditioning. Patients are expected to follow the prescribed exercises, irrespective of any worsening in the symptoms and to fight against their 'perceived' fatigue.

The idea of graded exercise seems quite unsuitable for those patients who are struggling just to achieve basic activity at work or home. There is a ceiling, above which activity is counterproductive in many cases. Friedberg and Jason[51] advise that exercise should be prescribed on an individual patient-by-patient basis, while many clinicians do not recommend it at all. However, significant improvement in functional capacity was noted in a year-long study in 1997[52] involving a graded exercise regime. Unfortunately, nearly half of the patients studied were taking antidepressants throughout the trial, which, in my view, undermines the validity of the study because, as exercise has been shown to help in clinical depression, it is likely that some of the patients who improved with exercise had been suffering from the latter rather than ME/CFS.

I believe that the reason why graded exercise has been shown to help in some cases is that, when the underlying disorder (ME/CFS) has receded, a patient who has been ill, perhaps for many years, may be severely lacking in stamina and de-conditioned. Exercise will improve their stamina and help reconditioning of the body, but over-exercise will worsen their ME/CFS. It is important to understand the difference, as, if the graded activity is implemented too early in the patient's period of recovery, the illness will be exacerbated.

Pacing

One teenage patient was a keen footballer (soccer player, for American readers) before she was ill. After a few months of treatment, she had recovered enough to stand and walk around and told me she was kicking a football around her garden, which was aggravating her symptoms. She was well enough to take a few steps but definitely not healthy enough to kick a ball.

I told her, 'If you continue to kick a ball around the garden then you will only be able to kick a ball around the garden! However, if you rest and pace yourself properly, then you will eventually be able to play a whole football match'. She eventually listened and went on to make a full recovery.

The most important advice that can be given to ME/CFS sufferers is **pacing**[53]. As I explained earlier (page 9), I usually recommend doing half the activity the patient feels that s/he can cope with. Pacing is recommended not only by me, but an ME Association survey of 2010 placed it at the top of the list of the most helpful strategies recommended by patients. By the way, it does not mean, as one doctor I met at a conference thought … 'pacing up and down in a corridor'.

I swam against the tide in 1989 by advising patients with ME/CFS to pace and reduce their activity, an approach which I have championed ever since. However, significant improvement has been shown when patients are advised to avoid too much activity and carry out only 50% of their perceived capabilities. In the early 1990s, when most of the medical fraternity believed ME/CFS was just lack of general fitness or a form of depression and were therefore advocating exercise for ME/CFS, when patients who could hardly walk were advised to get fitter, I was instructing all ME/CFS sufferers to stop and pace themselves, doing just half of whatever they felt they were capable of, whether it was walking, talking or watching TV.

My 'half rule' remains a major influence on the patient's overall improvement with my treatment. If the patient overdoes things during the course of treatment they may never fully recover; indeed, their health may worsen. Some patients tell me they find it difficult to gauge what half is. Often, they have realised that they are doing too much after the particular activity and it is too late. One patient who was a keen swimmer was given the go-ahead to go back into the pool as part of her reconditioning programme and instead of keeping to the half rule she swam 50 lengths on her first dip. Her symptoms raised their ugly head and it took her weeks to recover. I asked her did she think she could have done 100 lengths? She admitted that she couldn't have managed 60, so she should have swum a maximum of 25 – that is, half of what she felt capable of doing – and even then, I would have suggested starting with just a few lengths.

The best way of following the 'half rule' is by thinking double. If you walk 0.5 km, ask yourself, 'Can I honestly walk 1 km with no problem?' If the answer is no, 0.5 km is too much. If 1 km receives an emphatic 'yes' with no worsening of the symptoms, 0.5 km is fine. If you are uncertain, even 0.5 km may be too much, and you should reduce the distance. The same applies to any activity – for example, having a conversation: if half an hour is too much, engage in only 10-minute chats at one time. If a two-hour film is too long, use the device you are watching it on to view half-hour sections at a time, provided that you feel you could watch an hour without adverse effects. This strategy prevents you from overstressing your sympathetic nervous system and, although it is difficult to implement, I have found this to be the golden rule that may make the difference between just helping a person a little to actually getting them back to good health. As the patient improves, then they can gradually increase activity safely as long as they stick by the 'half rule' … as I constantly tell my patients 'half or more is still more!'

Far infrared (FIR) saunas

A FIR sauna heats your body directly via infrared waves on the far end of the light spectrum as opposed to traditional sauna that uses heat to warm the air around your body. An infrared sauna stimulates sweating and increases heart rates at lower temperatures than does a regular sauna.

Several studies have shown some evidence that using an infrared sauna is beneficial in the treatment of chronic health problems, such as high blood pressure and Alzheimer's disease. The gentle warming process of the whole body stimulates more parasympathetic activity whilst reducing the sympathetic overloading leading to increased β-endorphins and relaxation[54]. FIR has also been shown to improve heart and lung function, helping endothelial cells.

Researchers from Kagoshima University in Japan have developed a specific treatment known as Waon therapy using FIR saunas that may be beneficial. The process is carried out for two to six weeks and involves warming the entire body for around 15 minutes once to three times a day for three to five days a week in an infrared sauna, after which the patient rests under blankets for an additional 30 minutes. This is followed by drinking an amount of water that corresponds to body weight lost through perspiration[55].

Saunas generally stimulate sweating, which can increase detoxification. However, every sweat gland has a sympathetic nerve attached to it and FIR for ME/CFS and fibromyalgia should be done gently and for only around 10 to 15 minutes maximum at a time whereby you get the benefit of FIR without sweating profusely and so reduce the possibility that you will overstimulate the sympathetic nerves and aggravate your symptoms.

Antidepressants

When one is very poorly with any protracted illness, there is a recovery mountain to climb in order to get better. When one embarks on any treatment programme and symptoms start to improve, it is akin to climbing a mountain. As patients get higher and higher, they look down and feel sad and depressed that they were so ill. When they look up, their anxiety increases as they realise how much further they have to go until they reach 'the summit'. So, patients' moods will often change as they improve. It was noticeable in the clinical trials that we carried out at Salford University in the 1990s that, as the treated patients' fatigue, pain and cognitive function improved, their anxiety and depression scores dipped in the middle of the year-long trial, but picked up again when the summit became closer and the patients showed further improvement, helping reduce the anxiety and depression in the long term. This, at least, showed that ME/CFS is not a psychological disorder in which the other symptoms would correspond to depression or anxiety scores. However, antidepressants are sometimes used in ME/CFS treatment.

Treatment of fibromyalgia often involves the use of antidepressants, together with anti-inflammatory drugs[56]. This treatment has been clinically shown to help the muscular pain in that condition. The soreness in fibromyalgia resembles the pain in some ME/CFS cases and, accordingly, similar treatment has been advocated[57, 58].

Low doses of tricyclic antidepressants have been shown to improve the sleep patterns of some patients[56]. However, some of the older generation of antidepressants are habit-forming and may result in significant physical and psychological side effects, while certain foods have to be avoided while taking some antidepressants as they can cause harmful reactions. There are fewer such problems with today's antidepressants. However, if you are prescribed medication that aggravates your symptoms, you should return to your doctor to discuss the option of an alternative antidepressant. This is the same for all pharmaceutical approaches to treatment, including herbal remedies. In other words, if a drug reduces one or more of the symptoms with no major side effect, it may prove helpful in the battle against ME/CFS. However, if the reaction to the medicine outweighs the overall benefit or if it worsens the symptoms, you should immediately consult your GP or specialist in order to review the alternatives.

One of the best natural antidepressants is tryptophan, which is contained in many foods such as nuts, seeds, tofu, cheese, red meat, poultry, fish, oats, beans, lentils, and eggs. One can also take a much stronger dose of tryptophan in the form of 5HTP which you can buy over the counter without a prescription.

Another natural antidepressant is the plant St John's wort (*Hypericum perforatum*), sometimes sold as just 'Hypericum'. It contains the ingredients hypericin and hyperforin, which are used for their antidepressant properties. Both tryptophan and hypericum stimulate the release of the neurotransmitter serotonin, reducing depressing thoughts, and should be taken with your doctor's knowledge and, hopefully, guidance.

There are plenty of antidepressant medicines known as SSRIs ('selective serotonin reuptake inhibitors') which allow serotonin to stay in the brain for longer and so can help, but if one definitely needs to be prescribed antidepressants I recommend patients ask their doctors for one in the group of SNRIs which should be taken in the morning. This group includes duloxetine, which has helped some of my patients by inhibiting the reuptake of noradrenalin (also known as norepinephrine) as well as serotonin, so it stimulates more brain activity. Since we now know that in health the hypothalamus–locus-coeruleus axis is switched off at night to help drain the brain from toxins, it makes sense to stimulate noradrenalin production in the morning, not at night when we want a more 'relaxed' switched-off brain to help improve restorative delta wave sleep.

Talking therapies

The old adage 'a problem shared is a problem halved' is so true in most cases. It is often helpful to talk over problems with those close to us. However, sometimes the problems need professional advice and that is where talking therapies come in. Talking therapies can help you work out why you have negative thoughts or feelings and may help you cope better with stress. A humorous but poignant summary of talking therapies can be seen in the box below.

Ask yourself

Do you have a problem? No … then don't worry!
Do you have a problem? Yes.
Can you do something about it? Yes … then do that something and
    don't worry!

Do you have a problem? Yes.
Can you do something about it? No.
If you can't … why worry? That won't change anything … so don't worry!

In other words, worrying doesn't change a thing except to aggravate symptoms and problems. Learn to accept the worry as a problem that you can't change but that maybe will sort itself out or somebody else will.

I know this might sound selfish but, if you can pass the buck … do so! Let somebody else who is healthier than you worry about a problem that you can't sort out. Bosses who delegate always seem happier because they give all the problems to their staff and then can close their office door behind them, put their feet up and pour themselves a whisky. Do the same without the alcohol. Find something to take your mind off any problem, find your figurative 'office door' that you can close and shut out any problem and let somebody else deal with it if possible. Learn how to change the way you cope with problems and stressful situations. One frequently-used method for helping reduce the harmful effects of stressful thought is cognitive behavioural therapy (CBT).

Cognitive behavioural therapy (CBT)

CBT is a type of psychotherapeutic treatment that helps patients understand the thoughts and feelings that influence behaviours. It is commonly used to treat a wide range of disorders, including phobias, addictions, depression and anxiety. The underlying concept behind CBT is that our thoughts and feelings play a fundamental role in our behaviour[59].

The goal of CBT is to teach patients that, while many aspects of their life and the world around them are out of their control, they can regulate how they interpret and deal with these.

The basis of CBT is demonstrated by the following conversation between a CBT therapist and a patient.

Therapist: 'I am thinking about you. Am I thinking good thoughts or bad thoughts about you?'

Patient: 'Obviously I hope you are thinking good thoughts.'

Therapist: 'Well, in fact, I am not thinking about you at all. I was actually wondering what I am having for dinner tonight.'

The therapist was using this to show it doesn't really matter what people are thinking about the patient. What matters to the patient is how they perceive others thinking about them.

If you believe others think badly about you, then you will feel sad. However, if you believe people think good things about you, then you will feel happier. In reality, it doesn't matter if everybody is thinking about their next meal or who is going to win the football match.

The effectiveness of CBT in the treatment of ME/CFS has been comprehensively reviewed [60, 61, 63, 64]. It has been shown to be more effective when delivered by properly trained practitioners in specialised clinics[60]. The use of CBT for ME/CFS is based on the belief that psychological factors are maintaining ME/CFS in all patients. Such factors may include faulty beliefs, ineffective coping behaviour and negative mood states[62]. Distorted thought patterns may lead to anxiety and depression[61].

My view, which is shared by many, including some psychiatrists, is that the depression and anxiety often seen in ME/CFS sufferers are secondary to the underlying physical symptoms of the condition. Depression and anxiety create a heightened sense of frustration and guilt in the patient, who in any case feels him/herself to be a heavy burden on those close to him/her. Some family and friends, and even certain healthcare providers, who do not acknowledge the existence of ME/CFS, may exacerbate this frustration. However, CBT may help patients to deal with secondary feelings of guilt and worthlessness and has been found to be a good coping strategy in many conditions.

In 1996 a randomised study[63] took place on ME/CFS patients diagnosed using the Oxford criteria (see Chapter 2). The group receiving CBT were functionally improved, but many reported continuing fatigue. However, in a separate study reported four years later, patients in the CBT group demonstrated significant improvements in physical functioning and substantial reductions in fatigue[64]. Some patients in the latter study had a current psychiatric diagnosis and others were receiving additional antidepressant therapy[64]. In a further study that took place in Australia using criteria that excluded psychiatric diagnosis, few differences were noted between the CBT treatment group and the controls who did not receive CBT[65].

It is probable that ME/CFS patients who have difficulty in coping with their illness will benefit from CBT. In common with other chronic illnesses, positive coping strategies and lifestyle management approaches may reduce depression and anxiety levels, but there is little evidence that CBT has a significant effect on other symptoms of the illness[65].

In 2010, the ME Association of the UK conducted a patient survey to see what treatment the patients themselves recommended. This national charity, supporting thousands of ME/CFS sufferers in the UK, listed their top 25 treatments as expressed by patient preference sorted by the percentage of people who improved:

- First was pacing, which as mentioned earlier, is an excellent coping strategy, reducing strain on the sympathetic nervous system and a necessary aid in the recovery process.
- Second favourite was relaxation and meditation, which again reduces strain on the sympathetic nervous system.
- Third most popular was the Perrin Technique which was the top actual treatment modality in the list.
- CBT was 22nd on the list.
- Graded exercise therapy (GET) was voted second bottom in 24th place with only 22.1% improved and unfortunately 33.1% reporting much worse symptoms following GET.
- (Bottom of the list for those curious was ENADA/NADH supplement, which is a coenzyme of vitamin B3 that only seemed to help 4.5% of the patients.)

When I started writing this second edition a massive trans-Atlantic battle reigned. In the UK the National Institute for Health and Care Excellence (NICE) guidelines continued to recommend GET and CBT, following the results of a controversial British study known as the PACE trial which was published in Lancet[66]. In the USA, and indeed around the world, the validity of this study has been questioned[67].

However, in 2017, following a petition from thousands of sufferers in the UK, NICE announced they would review their diagnosis and treatment guidance, including looking into the Perrin Technique. They hopefully will come to a similar conclusions as the Centers for Disease Control and Prevention (CDC) in the USA which, on 11 July 2017, updated its website information for ME/CFS, removing previously recommended treatments, CBT and graded exercise therapy.

On 16 January 2018 at a stakeholder meeting in London, which I had the privilege to attend, NICE announced they were disbanding the old criteria and starting the process of developing new guidelines for diagnosis and treatment which have been delayed owing to the COVID-19 pandemic and are due for publication in 2021.

In March 2018, an open paper published in *BMC Psychology* by an international group of academics and scientists questioned the significance of the findings in the PACE trial. The paper's authors, Carolyn Wilshire from New Zealand, Tom Kildon from Ireland, Robert Courteney and Keith Geraghty from the UK, Alem Matthees from Australia, David Tuller from Berkeley University, California and Bruce Levin from Columbia University in New York, examined all the evidence and procedures following a Freedom of Information Request to the PACE trial authors and concluded, when looking at the trial as a whole, that it did not significantly show that either CBT or GET were efficient at treating ME/CFS[68].

So, should you bother with talking therapies at all? Over the years many patients have told me about this talking therapy and that talking therapy that worked for a friend or somebody on the web or featured in a tabloid newspaper. The truth is, all talking therapies share one basic truth. There is no 'one size fits all' and they will work only if the patient engages with the counsellor and therapist. In my Manchester clinic we have a group of counsellors and talking therapists who are there to help patients cope. I use the word 'cope' intentionally, because no talking therapy will cure ME/CFS, but by reducing the emotional stress one can decrease a major source of inflammatory changes in the brain which is emotional or mental stress. Talking therapies reduce the strain on the brain's emotional centres, also known as the limbic system (see page 17), and so help dampen the dysfunctional effects of upregulated neurochemistry that we see in ME/CFS. This heightened emotional system is sometimes referred to as 'limbic kindling' and is thought to be a major feature of ME/CFS[69].

The following section describes some of these talking therapies in more detail.

Neuro-linguistic programming (NLP)

NLP is a method of communication, personal development and psychotherapy developed through the initial work of Richard Bandler and John Grinder in California in the 1970s. They claimed that neurological processes (*neuro*), language (*linguistic*) and behavioural patterns learned through experience (*programming*) are all connected, and these can be changed using certain techniques to achieve better mental health and to attain life goals. It was a system influenced by the work of therapist Virginia Satir, widely regarded as the 'mother of family therapy', and psychiatrist Fritz Peris, founder of Gestalt therapy, which is aimed at increasing sensation, perception, bodily feelings, emotion, and behaviour, in the present moment. It also draws on some of the concepts of psychiatrist and hypnotherapy expert Milton Erickson to change bad patterns of thought into hopefully good ones[70].

To demonstrate how effective NLP techniques are, let us try a little experiment that I often perform in my workshops. To make this work, read the instructions aloud to somebody else in the room.

Look around the room you are in and find three green things (could be ornaments or items of clothes or furniture etc). Focus on these three green things and remember what three green things you have chosen.

Now, once you have definitely remembered the three green things, close your eyes and do not open them until you are instructed to at the end … this is very important!

Still keep in your mind the image of these three green things and say to yourself what these three green objects are. Do you remember what these three green things are?

Now, whilst keeping your eyes closed and not opening them until after the experiment is over, say aloud the three green things that you have remembered.

Now keeping your eyes closed tell me three blue things that you saw in the room. (Most people will not remember, or will struggle to remember, any blue objects. Even if there are plenty, such as a blue top you or they might be wearing etc.)

Now open your eyes and look at what blue things there are in the room…

So, why did the person find it difficult to remember any blue objects? In just a minute or so they were blinded to every colour other than green due to the NLP-based VAK technique, which stands for:

- visual: they were asked to look at three *green* things
- auditory: they heard your instructions
- kinesthetic: they turned their heads whilst they looked around the room.

Using the VAK principal one can tap into different parts of the brain and encourage better neurotransmission and improve function in the higher centres. This can help the higher centres work in a more balanced way and can reduce the effects of certain unhelpful thought patterns. It can also be used to help you believe you can get better if you are stuck in the 'I'm never going to recover' mode that does affect many chronically ill people, including some ME/CFS patients.

Another well-known NLP technique is to become your own life coach and say STOP when you want to change a certain thought. This can help train your brain to think in a much more positive way and improve your emotional wellbeing.

The Lightning process (LP)

Some believe that the power of the mind, using a similar approach to NLP, can help their physical wellbeing and therefore improve physical health as well as emotional. This is the basis of the Lightning process (LP).

LP is one of the most controversial of the talking therapies for ME/CFS and, although the claims are that it combines neurolinguistic programming (NLP) with an osteopathic component as part of its philosophical foundations, I am unsure where osteopathy comes into it.

As this book shows, ME/CFS is a very real physical disease; however, some people as they improve physically are rightfully worried about overdoing things. This can sometimes create a fear of moving on into good health. It isn't a phobia but a real fear, based on the fact that if you overexert yourself with ME/CFS you end up with post-exertional malaise. If you have been ill for a long time, and many ME/CFS patients have been, then it is natural to be scared of doing too much as you start to recover. As mentioned above, NLP techniques help because, through visual, auditory and kinesthetic processes (VAK) – that is, seeing, hearing and movement methods – one can retrain the brain's patterns and reduce pathways of stress.

LP employs similar methods to stop patients thinking they are ill anymore and helps them start to think of moving along the pathway of health. Any thoughts of being unable to move on are quickly stopped by the process and replaced with positive thoughts. The claims are that patients in just three days should be able to do things they thought impossible before they started the process.

I have always been open to many different views and theories concerning the treatment of ME/CFS, but one thing I am absolutely certain of is that it is a chronic long-term disorder of the nervous system, usually involving many other systems, such as the immune, cardiovascular, hormonal and/or gastrointestinal systems, and you cannot change years of dysfunction in a few days. The toxins will still be there from many other sources and one has to improve the overall neuro-lymphatic drainage to bring about a more permanent solution; otherwise, if patients exert themselves, the toxins will build up and eventually there will be a relapse in the disease.

The Gupta programme

There are many other treatments out there based on NLP. These include the Gupta Programme, also known as the 'Gupta amygdala retraining programme', which can be a useful tool to some as a home-based coping strategy which comes with a DVD that teaches the patient the techniques that may help reduce symptoms. It was developed by Ashok Gupta, who suffered from ME/CFS himself before curing himself of it, and then conducting research into the brain neurology of these illnesses. His research led him to conclude that these conditions are caused by abnormalities in the brain, especially structures called the insula and the amygdala, which are both part of the limbic system involved in controlling emotions. The amygdala is one of groups of cell bodies in the brain known as the basal ganglia which, as discussed in Chapter 2, has been shown to be affected when toxins do not drain out of the brain as they should[71]. The latest findings in brain neurology, and specifically what is known as neuroplasticity, show that the brain is inherently capable of being re-wired, and the Gupta Programme claims to help to re-wire the brain's responses to restore health.

There are many other mind-body techniques which all have helped some of my patients over the years, such as such as the 'Mickel therapy' and 'Reverse therapy' which are techniques that address feelings and emotions which are built up in the body. The principle behind these techniques is that they help change the brain's errant core emotional patterns and restore some stability in the hypothalamic and autonomic control mechanisms, thus helping ME/CFS and FMS.

As far as I am concerned, anything that can reduce stress and balance the nervous system will help patients with ME/CFS, but – I repeat – talking therapies in general are not cures for this disorder, although they should never be dismissed and should be considered as part of the integrative approach that may be necessary to achieve the best results for some patients.

Dr Sarno's approach

John Ernest Sarno Jr (1923–2017) was Professor of Rehabilitation Medicine at New York University School of Medicine. Sarno is most famous for his controversial approach to many conditions, including ME/CFS and fibromyalgia, which he regarded as forms of 'psychosomatic disorder', in other words the mind affecting the physical. He coined the term 'tension myositis syndrome' (TMS), which he explained was also the cause of many other disorders.

According to Sarno, TMS is an illness that is a product of emotional issues hidden deep in the subconscious which would be too painful if they surfaced. The neuroendocrine system, controlled by the brain, leads to actual physical symptoms as a way of protecting patients from this inner 'rage'. The repressed unconscious emotions lead to abnormal autonomic activity which results in reduction of local circulation of blood, known as 'ischaemia'. The ischaemic changes lead to mild oxygen deprivation that can cause muscle and tendon pain, nerve pain and numbness, tingling and weakness, which are familiar symptoms to patients with ME/CFS and FMS. Sarno's strategy was to make the patient aware of what the body was trying to do via a daily study programme and, if necessary, psychotherapy. Sarno's belief was that when the symptoms are seen for what they are, they then serve no purpose and will go away.

In 2007 a published study of TMS treatment showed a 54% reduction in the average pain intensity scores for a group of 51 *chronic* back pain patients, whose average pain duration before the study was nine years[72].

His approach obviously does work for some forms of back pain, but it isn't a cure for patients of major disease processes, such as ME/CFS and fibromyalgia. This is because the autonomic dysfunction seen in these disorders is due to many different predisposing factors, not just an underlying subconscious 'rage'. This is despite, as I have said in Chapter 4, my name for ME/CFS being TPOS (thoroughly p****d off syndrome) which is a name that, although it usually brings a smile to my patients' faces, resonates with them as they often feel helpless and frustrated beyond belief; they want to but cannot get on with their lives, as any attempt to try and beat the disease is often hit by a brick wall … a very large and impassable brick wall.

Granted, previous emotional trauma or issues that are hidden away in our subconscious mind do affect our general health and may lead to a build-up of neurotoxicity. As I constantly tell my patients, emotional stress is a major cause of neuro-inflammation.

Recent research has confirmed that neural inflammation due to increased levels of pro-inflammatory cytokines plays an important role in stress-induced depression. ME/CFS and fibromyalgia are not forms of depression; however, one of the symptoms of these conditions is secondary depression. Partly it is due to the illness being such a disabling and cruel disorder which stops very active people, often in their prime, from getting on with their lives. But the build-up of many pro-inflammatory cytokines in the brain of ME/CFS and fibromyalgia patients can disturb messages to and from the limbic system in the brain, which is the centre of emotions.

The link between inflammation and depression has been known of for some time. As mentioned in Chapter 4, cytokines, which are signalling protein molecules, are an important part of the immune system, signalling the body's defences to attack invading organisms such as viruses and bacteria. Increased levels of pro-inflammatory cytokines have also been found in the blood of patients suffering from depression, leading to activation of the glial cells in the brain of depressive patients.

Psychological stress caused by social and environmental factors can trigger a variety of changes in both mind and body. Extreme stress can lower our cognitive functions, cause depression and elevated anxiety, and is a risk factor for many illnesses, including ME/CFS and fibromyalgia.

A research team at Kobe University in Japan, led by Professor Furuyashiki, found that repeated stress induced the gene-expression of inflammation-related cytokines, such as interleukins and interferons. This led to the atrophy and impaired response of neurons in the area at the front of the brain known as the medial prefrontal cortex, causing depressive behaviour[73]. These findings, according to Professor Furuyashiki, demonstrate the role of neural inflammation caused by the innate immune system in the build-up of stress-induced depression.

This can lead to the mood swings commonly seen in ME/CFS. It is also of interest that at the annual meeting of the Radiological Society of North America in December 2019. Kenneth T Wengler and fellow scientists at Columbia and Stony Brook Universities in New York State, showed a disturbance of the blood–brain barrier in patients with clinical depression. Also, at the same meeting it was announced that neuroradiologists at the University of North Carolina had discovered dysfunctions in two regions of the brain that are significant in the symptoms of ME/CFS and fibromyalgia. One was the dorsal lateral prefrontal cortex, which is important for cognitive functions and directly linked to the amygdala. The other region of the brain that the team from North Carolina had found plays a major part in depression was the thalamus. We know from the research into the 'glymphatic' system (see page 94) that when the drainage of neurotoxins is impaired, the build-up of fluid takes place around the region of these two structures.

The amygdala and the thalamus are directly linked to the hypothalamus and all form the central core of the brain's limbic system which is important in the regulation of the subconscious and moods.

Hypnosis

Years ago, when I saw many stressed individuals attending my clinic with pain and other symptoms that were not being helped by manual therapy, I decided to attend a therapy course which included hypnosis. I found it an excellent tool that continues to help many patients relax and, besides pain relief, can help improve the quality of patients' sleep. Hypnosis may be often viewed as a showman's trick for the stage. However, it can be a useful tool in reducing stress and helping people cope with all manner of traumas. It has been tested in a pilot study on ME/CFS patients who reported that hypnosis helped in muscle pain management, both at rest and after exertion, with a slight improvement in quality of life, but unfortunately there was no increase in cognitive ability[74].

Wellbeing therapy

Wellbeing therapy (WBT) is another method of improving patients' levels of psychological wellbeing, using cognitive-behavioural techniques. In CBT (page 136), the therapist attempts to change distorted thought; however, with WBT the patient is initially guided to concentrate on occasions that make them feel good, showing them that all is not lost and any interrupting bad thoughts are consequently analysed and addressed so they don't reduce the feeling of wellbeing. The initial focus on thoughts of wellbeing is the reason that this form of therapy may be more beneficial than CBT, although it is much less practised around the world[75].

Tapping/emotional freedom technique (EFT)

Using a structured approach, by tapping your fingers on certain meridians around the body, has been shown to reduce anxiety and depression in some people. It was based on 'thought field therapy' developed in the 1980s by psychologist Roger Callaghan, primarily for the treatment of phobias using his knowledge of the mind combined with Chinese medicine. In the 1990s he tutored an engineer, Gary Craig, who developed the basic technique that we have today.

In EFT, the patient taps with their fingertips five to seven times on each of nine specific meridian points of the body that are used in acupuncture, while focusing on negative emotions or physical sensations. This helps to calm the nervous system, rewire the brain to respond in healthier ways, and restore the body's balance of energy. As with the other therapies to help the limbic system, which is the centre for emotions in the brain, this simple technique can help reduce the results of stress[76, 77].

EMDR therapy (EMT)

Eye movement desensitisation and reprocessing (EMDR), also known as 'eye movement technique' (EMT), is an interactive psychotherapy technique developed by psychologist Francine Shapiro in 1987 after observing that moving her eyes from side to side appeared to reduce the disturbance of negative thoughts and memories. It has been shown to be an effective treatment for trauma and post-traumatic stress disorder (PTSD)[78]. The complete EMDR therapy is in eight separate stages that involves visual and talk therapy to help reduce stress. However, I have adapted one part of it for my patients, which in three minutes helps them relax and can be simply carried out to reduce anxiety and aid sleep in patients with ME/CFS and fibromyalgia.

Most patients of mine do not like the sensation caused by moving their gaze from side to side. It usually makes them feel dizzy or nauseous. To avoid unpleasant sensations but utilise the principle of alternating brain activity, instead of eye movement patients can use alternate tapping of the left and right index fingers on a surface such as their thigh, in a slow rhythmic pattern for three minutes. This is known as resource tapping and is derived from EMDR, combining imagery with bilateral stimulation.

EMDR has been successfully shown as a do-it-yourself technique to reduce pain, fatigue, anxiety and depression in fibromyalgia patients by leading psychologist Dr Fred Friedberg, who has served for many years as president of the International Association of ME/CFS (IAME/CFS)[79, 80].

I find this technique works better with both ME/CFS and FMS patients if they, with their hands placed lightly on their thighs, close their eyes whilst focusing only on their alternately tapping index fingers. Although it is a tapping technique, it is much simpler than tapping on the meridians as in EFT and it is the alternating fingers that produce a therapeutic rhythm as the neurological impulses to and from the brain switch from side to side.

The technique can be done sitting or lying, and after only a three-minute session the patient should notice that any stressful events should elicit less anxiety and will not bother them as much.

Changing patterns of brain activity is a fundamental rationale behind how hypnosis and NLP work, and the effect of resource tapping and eye movement in EMDR could produce similar results very quickly. EMDR could also have an overall benefit in improving brain function by re-integrating the brain with the rest of the   nervous system and reorganising mind–body connections, much as we see marching and cross-crawl help improve coordination in patients (see Chapter 10).

Mindfulness

Mindfulness is a therapeutic meditation technique that improves mental wellbeing by focusing on the present moment as well as calmly acknowledging and accepting one's feelings, thoughts, and bodily sensations plus awareness of the world around one. It has been shown by psychologists at two top universities that it can help some of the symptoms of ME/CFS and fibromyalgia. It is done in a relaxed sitting position and takes about half an hour once a day for at least eight weeks.

Researchers at Oxford University examined whether mindfulness helped ME/CFS symptoms and showed that there were improvements in levels of fatigue, anxiety, depression, quality of life and physical functioning following the training programme[81].

Meanwhile, a study at Harvard University has linked mindfulness to grey-matter volume increase in the areas of the brain related to learning and memory, emotion regulation and sense of self[82].

Acceptance and commitment therapy (ACT)

Acceptance and commitment therapy (ACT) is based on concepts and values of mindfulness and was developed by American psychologist Steven D Hayes, who explained in a 2005 interview: 'ACT… grew out of my own experience with panic disorder and treating other clients with anxiety problems. I'd been trained as a cognitive behavioral therapist. But when I realized that cognitive behavioral therapy (CBT) wasn't helping me deal with my own problems with anxiety, I returned to some of the more Eastern ideas. If I don't focus on my symptoms, what do I want to be doing with my life? That's where the role of commitment came into ACT.'

Using ACT, the patient accepts and makes room for any challenges life may throw at them rather than fight them, while practising mindfulness, distress tolerance and emotion regulation. In CBT, patients are trained to challenge distressing thoughts. In ACT, the thought is accepted as a thought and then defused using a variety of techniques.

As already explained, if the main cause of neuro-inflammation is emotional stress, ACT helps the person be present in the moment and learn to accept painful or stressful thoughts and emotions. It is a useful tool for many people struggling with mood, thought, anxiety or personality disorders, but it has also been shown to help reduce chronic pain[83].

In chronic pain, the main activity to promote the pain has been shown to shift from the standard neural pathway seen in acute pain to the areas in the brain more involved with the emotions. In other words, in acute pain, receptors around the body known as nociceptors send messages up the spine to the pain centres in the brain, including the thalamus. The nociceptors seem to have much less influence on chronic pain, which is experienced due to areas in the brain such as the amygdala being very active

ACT trains the person to notice an uncomfortable emotion or thought and acknowledge it, but to let it flow by, without holding on to it or letting it drive actions in that moment. So, when one has chronic pain the best thing to do is not to try and fight it head on or to simply ignore it. To reduce the pain, accept it and focus on any other goals you have now and let the pain flow by. It is difficult for severely ill bed-ridden patients to have any goals to focus on other than their illness, but the meditation and mindfulness aspect of ACT has helped many people escape from a life of misery with unending pain.

I have been asked by some patients over the years how I have managed to keep cheerful and positive when facing many stressful and challenging periods in my life. I use a similar approach to ACT. I call it the 'Perrin Woosh'. I let stressful events pass me by going 'Woosh!' right over my head, not stopping to make their mark but not ignoring them either. It might look as though I don't care, but it isn't that at all. I just focus on the things that are going in the right direction and accept the things I cannot change at the time and let them 'Woosh' by, away from any immediate harm to yours truly.

Another strategy I employ is what I term 'optimistic pessimism'. If things are not going right in my life, I imagine the very worst-case scenario. It might seem a crazy way of coping, but when the very worst doesn't happen – and invariably it doesn't – … I am happy.

It reminds me of a famous quote from the legendary American actor and comedian George Burns who lived to be 100. When he reached his 90th birthday he was asked by a journalist, 'Mr Burns, how does it feel to be 90?' He dutifully replied 'Well, I'll tell you. I get up every morning and read the obituary column. If my name's not there I eat breakfast'.

Warning: As you can see, there are many forms of talking therapy available but, as I emphasise again and again in this book, patients also require a physical approach for a physical illness. Words alone via the psychological approach may reduce stress and help patients cope better but will not rid them of ME/CFS or FMS. Patients should be aware that some talking therapists may encourage them to do far too much too soon, or worse, lay the blame on them, the patient, if the approach doesn't work. Patients should never blame themselves or force themselves to increase activity because they have been told that this is the best way forward.

Acupuncture

Some fibromyalgia patients of mine have benefited from this ancient Chinese form of medicine, which can be done as an adjunct to the Perrin Technique. By inserting fine needles under the skin, western medical acupuncture stimulates the body's natural endorphins that reduce pain and promote healing.

A course of acupuncture can lead to longer lasting pain relief, often after a single treatment. Traditional acupuncture is based on the belief that a 'life force' or Qi (pronounced 'chee') flows along pathways of the body known as meridians. The ancient Chinese belief is that stagnation of Qi leads to disease and that acupuncture can re-establish the flow of this energy, and restore health. Perhaps the Qi in some way is related to lymphatic drainage which, when stagnated, or flowing the wrong way leads to diseases such as ME/CFS and fibromyalgia … food for thought,

Myofascial trigger-point dry-needling

Fascia is the connective tissue, primarily formed of collagen, found beneath the skin that attaches, encloses and separates muscles plus other internal organs. The myofascial tissue is the fascia that is attached to the muscles and contains a rich network of lymphatic vessels. In ME/CFS and especially fibromyalgia, the myofascial layers are tight and cause much of the superficial pain.

Myofascial trigger-point dry-needling, simply known by many as dry-needling or intramuscular stimulation (IMS), is similar to acupuncture as it uses needles on certain myofascial trigger points which are specific tender points that can become tight and often painful when there is mechanical disturbance in the area. Dry-needling can treat a dysfunction of skeletal muscle and connective tissue, minimise pain and improve or regulate structural or functional damage.

Ozone therapy

We often hear on the news that the ozone layer in the atmosphere, which protects us from the sun's harmful rays, is being affected by planetary pollution. Ozone is formed naturally following lightning in thunderstorms and is actually a molecule of the oxygen we breathe (O_2) with an extra oxygen atom attached (O_3). Ozone is a formidable steriliser and a powerful antimicrobial agent. The extra atom of oxygen creates a reactive form of the gas and via the process known as oxidation (see page 98) destroys the walls of bacteria and viruses and afterwards reverts back to the harmless oxygen that we breathe.

Ozone therapy can be a useful in treating inflamed and painful tissue by targeting and destroying the cells responsible for the damage.

Some patients who have connective tissue and hypermobility disorders, such as Ehlers-Danlos syndrome, discussed in detail in the next chapter (see page 174), have been helped using a treatment known as prolozone therapy. Prolozone therapy uses injections of nutrients to increase the amount of collagen and cartilage in a weak or damaged region of the body, thereby regenerating new tissue together with ozone to destroy the damaged ligaments. The action of prolozone therapy helps strengthen hypermobile painful joints. By repairing the damaged tissue, it can reduce the chronic pain that causes misery to so many patients with ME/CFS and especially FMS[84].

Alexander technique

The Alexander technique is a teaching programme based on postural balancing that helps you change long-standing habits that cause unnecessary tension in the body. It was discovered in the 1890s by an Australian actor, Frederick Matthias Alexander, who initially developed what he called 'the work' to help his vocal problems.

An Alexander teacher will help you learn how to improve your health via the natural balance of your head, neck and back, what Alexander called 'the primary control'. The technique works through re-establishing this natural balance to promote easy upright posture and improved functioning of the body and mind.

It may not be that much of a coincidence that it developed just after osteopathy officially came into being in 1885 as many concepts of Alexander's are very osteopathic in nature. As a way of continuing any postural improvement gained from the Perrin Technique, on top of the exercises given by the practitioner, ME/CFS and FMS patients are encouraged to seek a local Alexander teacher if they have any ongoing postural problems or just to maintain the balance.

Neural therapy

Developed in Germany in 1925, neural therapy is used by some doctors to treat pain and disease by injecting local anaesthetics into nerves, scars, glands, trigger points, and other tissues. It is based on the theory that areas of disturbed electromagnetic fields cause illness and that these fields can be disrupted by a pain-killing injection, allowing the body to heal. However, there could be unpleasant side effects from the drugs used. Also, many local anaesthetics contain adrenaline/epinephrine which acts as a vasoconstrictor and slows systemic absorption, thereby prolonging the anaesthetic effect. Since adrenaline has similar effects to the main sympathetic neurotransmitter, noradrenaline/ norepinephrine, any local anaesthetics used on ME/CFS and fibromyalgia patients must be non-adrenaline based to avoid overloading the sympathetic nervous system and thus worsening the symptoms, as described earlier (page 93)[85].

Electrotherapy

Electromagnetic waves are emitted from every substance in the known universe, including our cells. Unhealthy cells or organs emit altered electromagnetic waves. The basis of any form of electrotherapy is that, by changing these waves back to normal, the damaging effects of disease will be reduced, thus promoting a healthier internal environment.

The Rife machine

The Rife machine developed by scientist Dr Royal Raymond Rife (1888–1971) is a form of electrotherapy using sound and light to control and destroy microbes. Rife machines use a certain frequency that matches a resonance of the pathogen, known as the 'mortal oscillatory rate' that kills off bacteria or viruses. A Rife machine can therefore be a useful tool in the arsenal when treating ME/CFS and fibromyalgia if there are known to co-infections, such as borrelia bacteria or herpes viruses.

Earthing

Earthing is based on the fact that the Earth's surface contains an endless number of electrons and its negative potential can help the neutralisation of free radicals in the body, similar to the action of antioxidants, helping restore balanced health. It has been scientifically shown that by walking barefoot on the outside ground and using specially produced conductive products, such as earthing mats, a more harmonious balance is achieved in the electromagnetic fields within the organs that can improve health. Fluctuation of the strength of the Earth's potential may also help regulate a person's biological clock. Coming into contact with the Earth also energises the body plus aids the regulation of the autonomic nervous system, reducing the sympathetic overload seen in disease processes. This could aid neuro-lymphatic drainage and reduce many of the symptoms in ME/CFS and FMS[86].

Colonic irrigation (colonic hydrotherapy)

Colonic irrigation is a form of hydrotherapy that involves flushing waste material out of the bowel using water sometimes containing herbal preparations and is often more effective than using an enema. It should always be carried out by a trained practitioner and under the guidance of your doctor, as there are some known side effects such as anaemia and it is not recommended for inflammatory bowel disorders and some other serious diseases. Of course one has to replace the healthy gut bacteria removed in the process and so probiotics are required after the colon has been irrigated. By cleansing out toxins stuck in the bowel this method could prove useful for some ME/CFS and FMS patients and has been shown to help symptoms of irritable bowel syndrome, such as pain, constipation and diarrhoea[87].

The magic bullet?

Will there ever be a pill to cure ME/CFS and FMS? This question is raised again and again by patients, doctors and scientists. In my opinion, based on over 30 years of clinical research into this field, unfortunately but unequivocally, NO! This is because every ME/CFS patient and every FMS patient is different, with different toxins affecting different neurochemical pathways affecting different sections of the central nervous system causing different metabolic disturbances leading to a different array of symptoms. This view, as you can imagine, makes me hugely popular at scientific meetings and ME/CFS and FMS conferences ... Not!

Of course, nobody wants to hear this, or read this for that matter, and for the patient it looks as if all is lost.

It isn't!

It just means that we have to approach the treatment of ME/CFS and FMS in a different way to most diseases. As I mentioned in Chapter 2, leading Canadian ME/CFS physician, the late Dr Bruce Carruthers, once said, 'Treat the dis-ease and not the disease!'

'Big Pharma', a colloquial term for leading pharmaceutical firms that produce most of our medicines today, don't like to hear this. If there is not a huge return on the amount of investment by the drug companies, they may not be motivated in helping research into disease treatment in the first place. If there is not a magic bullet at the end to kill the bug or sort out the biochemical problem, then they won't see the point of funding studies that go on for years and years before any successful pill or potion may be developed.

There are, however, blood and other lab tests and drugs that have and are being developed that will identify and help some sub-groups of patients, such as targeting an aspect of the immune system or reducing the upregulated stress response. These may help some patients, but unfortunately worsen other individuals with ME/CFS or FMS who have a different symptom picture with other metabolic disturbances.

There are two major and complex problems that continue to beset the diagnosis and treatment of ME/CFS. The first is that two or more conditions can exist at any one time in one patient. It is sometimes difficult for doctors, for example, to distinguish between depression and ME/CFS, particularly in those cases of ME/CFS in which depression is an additional feature. The second problem is that because there is no universally accepted means of diagnosis, by tests such as blood or urine analysis, most doctors diagnose ME/CFS by exclusion. In other words, the patient will be diagnosed as suffering from ME/CFS only when all other possible diagnoses have been excluded. In my view, this is a hazardous method of diagnosing any disease. Can you imagine if a doctor were to tell a patient, 'Well, after all the tests, we cannot find anything else wrong with you, so it must be cancer'. Yet thousands of people around the world are being told that they have ME/CFS, using the exclusion method of diagnosis.

Some medical experts on ME/CFS have touched upon the neurological effects of the disease, and how the immune system and the body's hormones are affected. However, the treatment recommended by these specialists is to improve the immune system by pharmacological methods or hormonal and chemical balance by dietary means, supplements or hormone replacements and, if necessary, by psychiatric drugs or psychotherapy. These treatments do help symptom relief in many cases and often I will recommend supplementation and agree with many pharmaceutical approaches to help certain symptoms, but if this is all that is done to treat the patient, then these practitioners are missing a crucial point: they are treating just the symptoms rather than aiming at the root cause of the disease. The neurological system that controls the hormonal and chemical balance of the body is the autonomic nervous system and the system that is the main factor in drainage of major toxins from the body as well as a major part of our immune system is the lymphatic system. If these two systems were working correctly, the body would cope with extra stresses and strains due to chemical, physical, mental, immunological and emotional exertion. Only then might pharmacological approaches, psychotherapy and healthy hypoallergenic diets bring about a permanent improvement in patients with ME/CFS.

Sadly, in many people with ME/CFS, there is little or no recovery, despite many and varied dietary and chemical approaches to treatment. The key to finding a complete and lasting remedy is to find a treatment that helps the body cope. This concept is in keeping with modern medicine's approach to the management of other types of disease. For example, the use of vaccinations to increase the body's immunity, and thus resist the effects of certain types of infection.

If one regards any stress factor as an infection, the obvious course of action is to increase the body's defence in staving it off. The fortification of the body is controlled by the autonomic nervous system. The centre of this elaborate web of nerve tissue primarily is found in the hypothalamus and the limbic system of the brain, down to the brain stem, and from the spinal cord spreading throughout the body. As already described in Chapter 3, American neurophysiologist, Dr Irvin M Korr, anatomist Professor Frank Willard, plus German neurophysiologist Professor Wilfred Janig, have all made major contributions to the study of the autonomic nerves[88, 89, 90, 91, 92, 93, 94] and how mechanical stimulation of this system has a major effect on the body as a whole. My treatment programme and my theory as to the cause of ME/CFS is influenced greatly by the work of these scientists who are all luminaries in the field of osteopathic principles and philosophy.

Many sportsmen and women – such as the cyclist Mr E, described at the beginning of Chapter 1 – exert more strain upon their dorsal (thoracic) spine in the pursuit of their sport than the average individual. Golf, yachting, cycling and weightlifting are just a few other different disciplines that put extra stress on the upper back. In some individuals this could further lead to irritation of the sympathetic nervous system, resulting in the development of ME/CFS.

Since the early 1990s many people suffering from this debilitating disorder have arrived at my practices in the north-west and south-east of England, desperate for help and a sympathetic ear. At first I thought it unlikely that I would be able to help, but, as more patients came, I began to notice a familiar pattern. There were common postural and mechanical factors shared by the patients. These similarities, consequently, led to the establishment of my manual system of diagnosis and treatment for this disease.

Case: Mr J

Originally, I knew Mr J socially. We saw each other at a party where he told me that he had been forced to take time off from his law studies at college due to ill health. He explained that he had initially suffered from a viral infection six months earlier. Since then, he had felt very lethargic, complaining of aches in all his limbs and palpitations. His symptoms were aggravated by exertion. His doctor had diagnosed ME, and he enquired whether I had heard of it.

I told him of my research and the fact that I was writing a book about the subject. A few days later, this 19-year-old man was lying on my treatment table, hoping I would perform miracles. He had been convinced nobody could help him and that he just had to rest at home until he felt well enough to return to his studies. I knew that my methods had worked on others and was genuinely convinced that I could treat him successfully.

His dorsal spine was restricted, and his posture was typical of a student who bent over his books at home and slouched in a lecture hall during the day.

After nine treatment sessions over four months, Mr J returned to college, almost back to normal, and his symptoms of ME/CFS had abated. Through a chance meeting at a party he was able to return to healthy, active life. Now he is a successful city lawyer with a large family, and he has been symptom-free for well over 20 years.

Chapter 6

Defining fatigue

The first virtue in a soldier is endurance of fatigue;
courage is only the second virtue.

Napoleon Bonaparte (1769–1821)

Case: Keith's story

I was a very active 57-year-old. I went to the gym four evenings a week after work, twice for heavy sessions aiming to build stamina and twice for more power-related work. A good day out was a big mountain walk. Then in the spring of 2013, after a stamina work-out and too soon after suffering a virus, I simply failed to recover as I normally did from my exhausted state. After two months of gradual further decline I was forced to stop work and become an invalid at home, able to do very little. At that stage my GP had diagnosed post-viral fatigue, which changed to chronic fatigue syndrome in the autumn when I was seen by the local NHS consultant specialist. I was offered the usual mix of antidepressants, cognitive behavioural therapy and graduated exercise therapy. Given that I was assured that CFS was not a mental issue, that mix seemed strange.

Fortunately for me, although not for her, my sister-in-law was suffering her second bout of CFS and had discovered the Perrin Technique, which was proving helpful. Fortunately also, I discovered that there was a Perrin practitioner, Marika Harding, within reasonable travelling distance of home. I was struck that the Perrin Technique was the only treatment on offer for CFS that was based on a theory of what CFS actually was, and that this theory had been, and was being, critically academically studied. What struck me most, however, was how some of my historic health issues linked into this theory of CFS: I have an unusually straight thoracic spine and had an old rugby injury exacerbating things at T2; I used to bounce quickly back to health after viruses, but no longer did; my upper back below my shoulder blades was puffy and tended to be itchy.

The most important aspect of the Perrin Technique was having a therapist who understood my predicament and who offered support that, although physically based, was actually psychological as well.

Marika warned me that treatment would initially make me feel worse, and it did, but after six weeks I did start to feel less bad. After a couple of months, I could get out and do a little gardening: I allowed myself eight minutes a day. After six months I felt fine providing I was not doing anything. So, I started up what I considered to be a gentle exercise regime; unfortunately, it was not a gentle exercise regime and so I returned to Step 1. About this time, I learnt that I had lost the job I loved. I had suicidal thoughts but felt that through Perrin there was still hope. With Marika's help I started again.

Over the next two-and-a-half years we made progress with lymphatics, CRI and the chronic state of my spine to achieve a state where I was physically fine. I found the technique's self-help aspects incredibly important. So also, the 'half rule', although this struck me as illogical because if you never push yourself to the limit, how do you know what half is? I interpreted this as NEVER pushing myself and NEVER tiring myself through activity. I found this very difficult as it meant being unable to visit family and friends, and I lost some of the latter as a consequence. But I felt, as an active man, that life in a CFS state was not worth living and the consequence of that was a single-minded determination to get better against all the odds. Being told that only a small minority of people of my age fully recovered from CFS simply meant that I had to ensure that I was in the small minority rather than my chance of a full recovery being low.

Once physically better, I very gradually increased my level of activity, which I kept very uniform, as my sympathetic nervous system learnt again to respond correctly to stimuli, always under the guidance and restraint of Marika. Patience really was a virtue.

By Christmas 2018, I had fully recovered from CFS. Now I can again go on holiday with my wife. I can again visit friends and family. I have again climbed 3000-foot mountains in batches. I have become a dedicated cyclist, going out over the last year two or three times a week for typically 40-mile rides, sometimes with as much as 1000 metres of vertical ascent. I again enjoy my active life. I know that my back is not 100%, and I look after it; I know that my lymphatic system is not 100%, and I look after it. But it is not an exaggeration to say that I owe my life to Marika Harding and the Perrin Technique, and I shall always be grateful to them both.

Mr W Keith Hamflett of Bromsgrove, Worcestershire
Patient of Marika Harding, Registered Osteopath and licensed Perrin Technique practitioner, Worcestershire, UK

What do we mean by the term 'fatigue'? According to a dictionary definition[1], fatigue is:

FATIGUE sb [a. Fr fatigue fem, f. fatiguer]
Lassitude or weariness resulting from either bodily or mental exertion.
Physiologically as: A condition of muscles, organs or cells characterised by a temporary reduction in power or sensitivity following a period of prolonged activity or stimulation.

English author Samuel Butler (1835–1902) once said that 'Life is one long process of getting tired'. Chronic fatigue syndrome is so much more than just being tired. ME/CFS and fibromyalgia patients tend to express their feelings of fatigue as aches in muscles, severe pain in joints, weakness in one or more limbs, and/or an overall lack of energy and vitality. Patients may feel that they have just run a marathon when they have only walked round the block, or that picking up their suitcase is as hard a task as trying to lift a ton weight. In other words, the effort and the resultant aches and pains are apparently unjustified in relation to the physical stress on the body.

What happens in fatigue?

A muscle fibre contracts due to stimulation from the nerves known as motor nerves. These form part of the somatic nervous system, which is involved in the conscious control of voluntary movements within the body. When over-exercising individual muscles, the contractile power within the muscle fibres is eventually depleted until a state of fatigue exists. This loss of power may be caused by a breakdown at different stages of the muscle-reflex pathway. In other words, there could be a failure in the transmission of somatic nerve impulses to the muscle, or it could be a collapse in the actual contractile mechanism inside the muscle.

Fatigue in ME/CFS

Fatigue is often regarded by practitioners as being psychogenic in origin. It may result from severe physical and/or mental activity, or lack of sleep. The degree of the fatigue will vary according to the personality and stamina of the individual. Experiments have shown that if a movement of the hand is continued for long enough to initiate a state of fatigue, and at this stage the blood flow into the hand is stopped by inflating a cuff around the upper arm, although the somatic motor nerves are still functioning, there is no recovery of power until the cuff is released and normal circulation is restored[2].

The blood flow to muscles is under the influence of the sympathetic nervous system. Thus, if the sympathetic nerves are not functioning correctly, it could lead to a reduced blood flow to certain muscles. One would then reasonably assume that these muscles would be likely to suffer from some form of fatigue.

In ME/CFS the normal activity within the sympathetic nervous system breaks down, as we have seen. The effect may be systemic, causing widespread aches and pains throughout the entire body, or it may limit the fatigue to one or two muscle groups.

As we have already discussed earlier in the book, the sympathetic nervous system also controls the lymphatic system and in ME/CFS the dysfunction of the sympathetic nervous system leads to a backflow of toxins.

As anybody taking part in sports, especially endurance athletes such as marathon runners or road cyclists, knows, when muscles have been over-working for too long, they may get cramps, possibly severe spasms and pain. This is due to a build-up of lactic acid. When we exert ourselves, we begin to breathe faster to supply more oxygen to the body. There are two forms of exercise: aerobic (using oxygen) and anaerobic. As long as we breathe and we exercise gently, we use oxygen, which combined with glucose produces the energy needed by our working muscles. During exertion, the body may not deliver enough oxygen to supply the extra demand, which leads to anaerobic respiration.

This process yields energy from glucose being broken down into a substance called pyruvate which, in the absence of oxygen, converts into a substance called lactate. Lactate allows glucose breakdown and thus energy production to continue. The working muscle cells can continue this type of anaerobic energy production at high rates for only a couple of minutes, before high levels of lactate amass.

High lactate levels lead to an increase in the acidic state of the substance – that is, lactic acid. The high acidity within the muscle cells leads to disruptions of other metabolites. The same metabolic pathways that permit the breakdown of glucose to energy perform poorly in this acidic environment. This prevents permanent damage during extreme exertion by slowing the key systems needed to maintain muscle contraction. Once the body slows down, oxygen becomes available and lactate reverts back to pyruvate, allowing continued aerobic metabolism and energy for the body's recovery from the strenuous event.

Contrary to popular opinion, lactate or lactic acid build-up is not responsible for the muscle soreness felt in the days following strenuous exercise. Rather, the production of lactate and other metabolites during extreme exertion results in the burning sensation often felt in active muscles (a 'stitch'), though which exact metabolites are involved remains unclear. This often-painful sensation also gets us to stop overworking the body, thus forcing a recovery period in which the body clears the lactate and other metabolites.

An earlier clinical trial that I carried out with colleagues at the University of Central Lancashire concluded that a possible major cause of the muscle fatigue in ME/CFS is lack of lymphatic drainage of the muscle due to sympathetic dysfunction. This would lead to an excess of lactic acid among other metabolites in the muscles of ME/CFS patients[3].

In 2013, researchers in Newcastle, UK, showed, using advanced brain scanning technology, that disturbance in cerebral vascular control associated with sympathetic dysfunction in the brain is directly related to excess lactic acid in skeletal muscle leading to fatigue in ME/CFS. The cells from ME/CFS patients produced on average 20 times as much lactic acid when exercised, suggesting an underlying cause for the aching muscles that patients often experience as soon as they begin to exercise. 'We have found very real abnormalities', said Professor Julia Newton, the head of the research[4].

Muscles like other tissues of the body need a healthy lymphatic system. Otherwise there will be no way of dealing with the excess lactic acid that Newton and her colleagues discovered. If the drainage was going in the wrong direction it would lead to further increase of lactic acid and metabolites in the muscles and further pain and discomfort. Elevated lactate levels have also been found in patients with fibromyalgia[5, 6].

It is also important to realise that this build-up of lactic acid in the muscles of ME/CFS and FMS patients follows exertion with the effects often delayed until the patient tries to utilise the muscles later on. As was mentioned in Chapter 2, a pivotal study by scientists in California demonstrated the post-exertional malaise only by testing and then re-testing the muscle the following day.

Neuro-inflammation

Throughout the book you will encounter many references to inflammation. Whilst inflammation in the spine remains a contentious issue among some ME/CFS experts who insist on calling ME 'myalgic encephalo-myelopathy' and not '-myelitis', there is always some neuro-inflammation occurring in ME/CFS and fibromyalgia. It may not always affect the spine and, in some cases, can only be found in some parts of the brain, but there is now much evidence to support my original theory that pro-inflammatory cytokines and other neurotoxins pass through the blood–brain barrier and into the glial cells of the brain, leading to neuro-inflammation[7].

Neuro-inflammation is a symptom of many diseases, including Alzheimer's disease, Parkinson's disease, and multiple sclerosis[8]. Neuro-inflammation has also been shown to be caused by disturbance in the neurotransmitters produced by the brain[9]. Other scientists are now finally talking my language, arguing that ME/CFS is due to inflammatory molecules entering the brain through opened sections of the blood–brain barrier[10]. This process can continue for long periods and predispose a hypersensitive and over-active central nervous system, leading to further inflammatory and immune changes in the brain.

Neuro-inflammation may also be related to excess oxygen and nitrogen molecules in tissues. This can cause oxidative stress, leading to tissue damage which is discussed in Chapters 4 and 5. Adverse effects can occur when nitric oxide (NO) is also affected by oxidative stress. NO is a signalling molecule in many physiological and pathological processes. The free radicals that can lead to oxidative stress can also affect the levels of nitrogen availability, leading to many bodily disorders. This process is known as nitrosative stress and has been shown to be a major factor with oxidative stress in the build-up of many of the symptoms of ME/CFS and fibromyalgia.

Dr Martin Pall, Professor emeritus of biochemistry and basic medical sciences at Washington State University, maintains that ME/CFS is due to the build-up of nitric oxide (NO) acting through its oxidant form peroxynitrate (ONOO). This NO/ONOO cycle occurs during oxidative stress and creates havoc in all the metabolic pathways in the body, affecting mitochondrial function, increasing inflammation and producing excessive NMDA activity in the brain among many consequences[11].

The immune system in the body contains different types of cell, as described earlier. Natural killer (NK) cells are important in the body's immune system, recognising and responding to infected cells. NK cells possess receptors allowing them to sense and respond to molecular patterns of bacteria, viruses, parasites and fungi, including 10 different types of protein; these NK receptors are known as 'toll-like receptors' (TLRs). They also react to certain environmental toxins.

It has been shown that high amounts of stress or a previous injury can predispose the TLRs to be more sensitive and release inflammatory molecules more readily in response to an immune stressor[12]. The activation of TLRs to the oxidative and nitrosative stress pathway leads to the production of more inflammatory molecules, which creates a vicious cycle[13, 14].

The renin–angiotensin system (RAS)

Renin is an enzyme that is released into the circulation by the kidneys. Its release is stimulated by:
1. sympathetic nerve activation

2. reduction in blood pressure into the kidney
3. decreased salt (sodium chloride – NaCl) transport within the kidney.

Renin release has also been shown to be stimulated by an increase in prostaglandins in response to the reduced NaCl transport.

When renin is released into the blood, it acts upon angiotensinogen to form angiotensin type 1. Angiotensin converting enzyme (ACE) is found in the walls of the blood vessels, especially in the lungs and heart, and transforms angiotensin 1 to angiotensin 2. The main function of angiotensin 2 is to cause the constriction of blood vessel walls, leading to increase in blood pressure. It also stimulates sodium reabsorption in the kidneys, increasing salt and water retention by the body. It acts on the adrenal glands to release the hormone aldosterone, which also leads to increased sodium and fluid retention in the kidneys.

Angiotensin 2 stimulates the release of vasopressin (also known as antidiuretic hormone, ADH) from the neurohypophysis – the posterior lobe of the pituitary gland – which increases fluid retention by the kidneys. It also stimulates thirst centres within the brain and, most importantly in the pathogenesis of ME/CFS, it facilitates noradrenaline (norepinephrine) release from sympathetic nerve endings and inhibits the noradrenaline re-uptake by nerve endings, thereby increasing the adrenaline-mediated function of the sympathetic nervous system. As we know, in ME/CFS we want to dampen sympathetic activity to help reduce symptoms and also improve neuro-lymphatic drainage.

Doctors prescribe 'ACE inhibitors', such as enalapril, fosinopril, lisinopril and ramipril, to help with blood pressure and cardiac problems, such as coronary artery disease. They are also often advised for diabetes, certain chronic kidney diseases and migraines. The ACE inhibitors help relax the veins and arteries to lower blood pressure.

Side effects may include a dry cough, fatigue, dizziness from blood pressure going too low, headaches and loss of taste. ACE inhibitors can cause fluid retention in tissues, so basically one needs to maintain the correct balance of angiotensin 2 in the body to maintain overall health of the cardiovascular and respiratory systems and much more.

Sometimes angiotensin receptor blockers (ARBs), such as losartan and telmisartan, are prescribed for cardiovascular disease, and sometimes aldosterone receptor blockers, such as spironolactone or eplerenone, have been helpful in heart and circulatory disorders.

Interestingly, it was shown that the coronavirus that caused SARS in 2003 attached to ACE 2 receptors, especially in the lungs; plus there is evidence that Covid-19 does the same. Patients treated with ACE inhibitors and ARBS have increased numbers of ACE 2 receptors free in their lungs for coronavirus spike proteins to bind to. These are the very large crown-shaped viral membrane proteins that give the virus its name and enable the virus to invade the host cell[15].

As mentioned above, angiotensin acts on the posterior lobe of the pituitary gland, which is one of the areas of the brain known as the circumventricular organs detailed in Chapter 4. Angiotensin also works on three more of these natural gaps in the blood–brain barrier that make them vulnerable to infiltration by large toxins. These are the area postrema, the subfornical organ, and the organum vasculosum[16], which have a critical role in maintaining blood pressure regulation and volume homeostasis via various nuclei located between the third ventricle and the brainstem. The brain renin–angiotensin system (RAS) works independently to the hormonal renin–angiotensin–aldosterone system (RAAS) and is involved in the regulation of water intake, salt appetite, blood pressure and autonomic functions. Up-regulation of angiotensin receptors in these nuclei has been shown to reduce baro-reflex sensitivity (that is, the speed with which signals from receptors in the aorta and carotid arteries control the brain's response to changes in blood pressure) and increase sympathetic tone, thus contributing to the development and maintenance of hypertension and heart failure. This disturbed baro-reflex sensitivity explains why some patients with ME/CFS and FMS can also suffer from neurally mediated hypotension and orthostatic intolerance, as discussed in Chapter 2. It can also lead to a more severe condition known as POTS which is discussed further on in this chapter (page 172).

The increase of sympathetic activity in heart failure is accompanied by a reduced parasympathetic tone. The renin-angiotensin system has not only multiple interactions with the sympathetic nervous system but may also influence blood vessel tone directly by angiotensin 2[17].

The renin-angiotensin system also has an effect on the parasympathetic nervous system via angiotensin 2 receptors on the cholinergic nerve terminals in the smooth muscle of the airways in the lung[18].

It is now accepted that the brain has a significant influence over angiotensin-induced hypertension and that an overactive brain renin-angiotensin system plays a vital part in the development and maintenance of neurogenic hypertension (nerve-induced high blood pressure).

The renin–angiotensin system is also a factor in the production of neuro-inflammation. Angiotensin 2 has been shown to induce inflammation with hypertension via the activation of T cells and promoting the vascular infiltration of leukocytes.

These immune cells then interact with the circumventricular brain regions mentioned above, especially the subfornical organ, to promote inflammation and oxidative stress by free radicals such as superoxide dismutase (SOD)[19]. A healthy drainage of the circumventricular organs via the CSF (cerebrospinal fluid) is paramount in reducing the neuro-inflammatory damage to these regions of the brain and beyond. This explains why in ME/CFS and FMS, a reversal of the neuro-lymphatic drainage leads to a breakdown in the renin-angiotensin system and an increase in the neuro-inflammatory process.

Other neurochemical changes in ME/CFS

Neuro-inflammation or neuro-degeneration also affects the regulation of several other chemicals, such as choline within the brain which has also been seen in ME/CFS, as discussed in Chapter 5 (page 122).

Years ago I had the pleasure of hearing a lecture at one of the international conferences for ME/CFS by neuroscientist Professor Jarred Younger, formerly of Stanford University, who now runs the Neuroinflammation, Pain and Fatigue Lab at the University of Alabama. He discussed how his team had discovered the presence of pro-inflammatory cytokines in the glial cells of the brain and how he believed that neuro-inflammation played a major part in ME/CFS and FMS.

After the lecture I approached him and invited him to dinner at the conference hotel where we exchanged ideas and thoughts over a long and enjoyable meal, and I realised that I had finally met a kindred spirit. Like myself, Younger believed that ME/CFS and fibromyalgia are both triggered by oversensitive microglia in the brain. He was focusing on immune activation that led to this state of inflammatory hyperarousal, to such an extent that the glial cells start pumping out inflammatory factors at the first sign of a stressor. Younger and colleagues used a newly developed method that produced a heat map and a chemical signature of the entire brain.

It turned out there was not one specific region, but many different areas or groups of areas, in the brain that were abnormal in ME/CFS. He found that the basal ganglia and thalamus were two regions with high levels of lactate and inflammation. There was a high heat signature in another area of the brain, the interior cingulate cortex. Disturbance in this region leads to malaise, fatigue and pain and it had been found to be dysfunctional in both ME/CFS and fibromyalgia studies in the past.

Younger holds that immune cells are breaching the blood–brain barrier in multiple areas; like a flood overwhelming a dyke, they are essentially pouring through gaps across the brain. However, I maintain that the toxic overload in the brain is not only due to a build-up of cytokines but also due to possible environmental toxicity and emotional and physical stressors.

Meanwhile, at the time of writing this edition there are claims of a newly developed, highly accurate blood test for fibromyalgia. It examines the RNA profile of patients to determine the levels of cytokines in the blood. The test results show that most FMS patients have a lower level of cytokines than in the blood of healthy people. This is probably also the case in many patients with ME/CFS, as the cytokines are pumped by the lymphatics away from the blood in the reverse direction and into the central nervous system via the neuro-lymphatics. However, with some fibromyalgia patients, as with ME/CFS, there are other co-infections that lead to overstimulation of the immune cells and a heightened level of cytokines in the blood.

This seems to be very confusisng! Are FMS or ME/CFS diseases of immune overload similar to autoimmune diseases such as lupus or rheumatoid arthritis, or due to an underactive immune system, as is the case in viral infections or cancer?

The answer is, both!

ME/CFS and FMS are both diseases of immune imbalance due to the dysfunction of the autonomic nervous system's control of the immune system and lymphatics, leading to immune over-reaction and under-reaction. This is why a meta-analysis of serum cytokine levels in FMS patients has revealed conflicting results[20].

The test for cytokine profiles will produce different results for different patient subgroups. Also, there are plenty of other diseases that will lead to similar results with this blood test, so it is not specific enough, although the test does highlight the importance of immune dysfunction in FMS and demonstrates that FMS is not just tight painful muscles.

Patients with FMS may suffer from fatigue, but it is widespread pain all over the body that is the principal symptom, just as post-exertion malaise is the main symptom with ME/CFS. As I stated in Chapter 3, I have very rarely found patients with fibromyalgia who do not also fulfil the criteria for ME/CFS and I feel they are both neuro-lymphatic disorders. The difference in the pathophysiology between the two diseases is determined by the area of the brain affected and by the type of toxins. In ME/CFS, many neural pathways that are involved in the processing of information, sleep, cognition, and especially the regions of the thalamus and basal ganglia that relay messages to and from the frontal area of the brain (the thinking part) to the back of the brain (the doing part), become disturbed by the toxins. In fibromyalgia it is probably nuclei in the posterolateral area of the thalamus that are mainly affected as these regions of the thalamus and the basal ganglia play a major part in the central regulation of pain, as already discussed in Chapter 2.

With around one hundred billion (100,000,000,000,000) neurons in the brain, and trillions of synapses between these nerve cells that each produce chemicals that transmit different messages, it is easy to see how toxic exposure from thousands of different pollutants and other chemicals, microbes such as bacteria, viruses, mycotoxins produced by moulds, and inflammatory activity in the brain and spinal cord, produces such an array of symptoms. It also explains how every ME/CFS and FMS patient in the world is different, with a unique set of causes, triggers and symptoms. At the time of writing this new edition, in the 30 years plus I have so far worked in this field, having seen thousands of ME/CFS and FMS patients, I have yet to see the same exact presentation in two patients. This is why these disorders are so confusing to most of the medical world as doctors can't place them into a box where they know exactly what diagnostic tests need to be done and what pills and potions need to be prescribed. Usually, all that the laboratory can achieve is to show that there are specific gene expressions or that some part of the patient's metabolism isn't working well and to exclude other diseases. The heterogeneity of the condition means that pharmacological treatment of ME/CFS and FMS is given for symptomatic relief but does not address the root biochemical cause, since every patient has their own unique biochemical pathway disruption.

By addressing the neuro-lymphatic pathway and improving the drainage of the central nervous system one can achieve better long-term health in most sufferers of ME/CFS and FMS.

As with ME/CFS, the sympathetic nervous system lies at the root of FMS. Evidence from biopsy has revealed a major source of pain in fibromyalgia is due to an increase in sympathetico-sensory innervation – that is, more communication between the sympathetic and sensory nerves[21]. As already explained in Chapter 3, in disease states pain is often produced due to signals from sympathetic nerve fibres crossing over to adjacent sensory nerves in what are known as ephapses. This explains why in fibromyalgia there seem to be quite random symptoms, not seemingly following a sensory nerve pathway. For instance, if one has a prolapsed intervertebral disc, commonly known as a 'slipped disc', in the lower lumbar spine at the base of ones back, this would usually irritate and maybe even trap a nerve, or nerves, leading to pain radiating down the side and back of the thigh and down the lower leg to the feet.

This is due to an irritation of the sciatic nerve roots leading to what many refer to as 'sciatica'.

With FMS and ME/CFS, it is sympathetic nerves that often are being irritated, in the thoracic spine and upper lumbar region. However, sensory nerves may also be irritated, spreading pain all over the back and down the extremities. This is why I sometimes see patients with 'crawling' sensations, numbness, tingling, pins and needles or stabbing pains in any part of their anatomy that cannot be simply explained when viewing the normal anatomical pathway of sensory nerves. One needs to examine the thoracic and upper lumbar regions of the spine, which is where the sympathetic nerves spread out from the spine to control the body, but much more importantly, receive messages from the body into the central nervous system.

This brings us to another long-held view in the medical world that has been turned virtually upside down by science. The autonomic nervous system, for centuries has been looked on as mostly an efferent system – that is, one sending messages from the brain and the spine to the different parts of the body. For instance, sympathetic nerves generally control the circulation via efferent nerves sending messages to smooth muscle walls of the blood vessels. Very little importance has been placed on the afferent or sensory component of autonomic nerves, until the last few decades. As mentioned in Chapter 3, Professors Willard and Janig showed around 80% of the influence of sympathetic nerves is afferent, being much more important in the messages coming into the central nervous system.

This is why the thoracic-spinal component of the Perrin Technique is so important in both the examination and diagnosis. It is also why treatment to this region is a seminal part of the Perrin Technique, especially the region where the sensory nerves enter the spinal cord, known as the dorsal root ganglia. The treatment of this region will be discussed in more detail in Chapter 10. However, three tragic cases of ME/CFS patients in the UK offer physical proof that the dorsal root ganglia are affected.

- **Lynn Gilderdale** was bedbound with ME for 17 years and took her own life in 2008. Whilst still a minor, Lynn was held in a secure unit at Guy's Hospital London until the medics requested permission to use force on her. Her parents refused and discharged her. This case was brought to the world stage by the terrible events following Lynn's assisted suicide, when her mother Kay was accused of her murder. Thankfully, Kay was acquitted and went on to write a moving book about this awful tragedy (*The Last Goodbye*). When Lynn's body was examined post mortem, inflammation of the dorsal root ganglia was discovered.

- **Sophia Mirza**: Similar findings were also discovered in 75% of the spinal cord during a post mortem examination organised by Criona Wilson, the courageous mother of Sophia Mirza, who tragically died in 2005 at the age of 32 from acute renal failure after suffering severely from ME/CFS for six years (see www.sophiaandme.org.uk). Sophia's death was the first ever case to have ME/CFS officially recorded as a contributing factor in the cause of death.
- **Merryn Crofts**: More recently, at an inquest in May 2018, 21-year-old Merryn Crofts, who had tragically died the year before, became the second person in the UK to have ME/CFS officially recorded as a causative factor in her death. Merryn's family donated her brain and spinal column for research and dorsal root ganglionitis was yet again discovered in her spine.

Many other disorders can cause fatigue symptoms. Most sufferers of ME/CFS reading this will hopefully have had extensive tests to eliminate the possibility of a wrong diagnosis. ME/CFS is often judged to be the cause of the fatigue only when these other diseases have been ruled out, and all other possible explanations have been explored. Although ME/CFS is a possibility in all cases of fatigue, one should always ensure that no other serious condition is at the root of the problem.

The effect on the body from neurological and hormonal changes following long-term wear and tear is known as allostatic load. How the body achieves balance via the endocrine and neuro-immune mechanisms and copes with these changes is known as allostasis. The control of the natural balance of metabolic pathways in the body, i.e. homeostasis, is orchestrated by the autonomic nervous system, with the hypothalamus at the helm. Therefore, any aspect of metabolism can be disturbed when the hypothalamic function is directly affected by allostatic load, which may take the form of any type of stress or disease process, and this is precisely what is going wrong in ME/CFS and FMS. Most research teams around the world are looking for more biomolecular evidence rather than looking at the body as a whole. So, it is inevitable that as the tests become more sophisticated they will eventually find metabolic disturbances with every chemical pathway in the body. The study of a set of metabolites within the organism tissue or cell is known as metabolomics. Projects involving metabolomics in ME/CFS are taking place in laboratories run by scientists such as Robert Naviaux in San Diego[22] and other researchers from across the USA[23].

I am in awe of these amazing scientific breakthroughs. These tests are looking for microscopic signatures that will help diagnose ME/CFS, which I applaud. However, I feel that the more scientists examine the metabolomic profiles or the genetic signatures, the more likely it is they will eventually reveal many different subsets of ME/CFS patients all with slight differences, so it will become increasingly difficult to use the tests to help diagnose this one disorder.

At present there are many tests that doctors around the world carry out to confirm or exclude the most common disturbances in the body that can lead to a state of fatigue. Without going into the detail of every test that can be performed to see if the body as a whole is functioning, I have included in the Appendices an explanation of the most common tests that can be carried out to check the general health of the patient (page 395). Most blood and other pathological tests that I have seen with ME/CFS patients tend to record slightly higher or lower results than the norm, but within the parameters of what is considered normal.

If they have levels that are very high or very low, it usually means that something else is going wrong as well as the ME/CFS. However, the changes of one or more element within the blood may reflect long-term health problems that are directly due to the ME/CFS. For instance, as discussed in greater detail later in this chapter, a blood test could show that your thyroid T4 (the hormone thyroxine) levels were low. This could be due to a separate condition that the patient has due to many different possible factors, but in many cases of ME/CFS it is dysfunction of the hypothalamus, which then sends the wrong messages to the pituitary gland, which in turn fails to regulate the amount of thyroxine that is produced by the thyroid gland in your neck, leading to a disturbance of many metabolic functions, such as heart rate, and can be a further cause of fatigue.

Metabolic dysfunction can lead to many other conditions that occur together with ME/CFS and I have rarely met patients who have been ill for many years with ME/CFS or fibromyalgia who don't have what are known as comorbidities – that is. other diagnosable conditions. This makes a total mockery of the old diagnostic criteria which state that one should only diagnose ME/CFS when all other conditions have been excluded.

An example of how wrong it is to diagnose by exclusion can be seen in the hypothetical case of an unfortunate individual who suffers from a brain tumour. If that person was ever attacked by an axe and they were stretchered into a hospital with an axe stuck in their head, I doubt very much that the doctors would send him home saying that the headache was already known to be due to the brain tumour and not related to the extra appendage sticking out of their cranium!

To be fair, the earlier diagnostic criteria which diagnosed by exclusion, such as the 1998 CDC revised criteria[24], were developed for research purposes only and not really intended for clinical use. In research studies, it is imperative that you do not include comorbidities, otherwise you do not know if a treatment procedure tested is affecting the specific illness. However, in clinical situations, as I have explained, comorbidities should never lead to excluding the diagnosis of ME/CFS.

It is equally wrong to assume that all symptoms are a result of ME/CFS or FMS once they have been diagnosed. A patient may have two, three or even more conditions affecting their body at the same time causing similar symptoms; this makes treatment more difficult and usually worsens the prognosis of the illness. The multiple illness case scenario in ME/CFS is much more common than people think and increasingly I am called upon to treat patients with what I call ME/CFS PLUS.

Fatigue due to comorbidity

So, what are the common comorbidities with ME/CFS? All the conditions below that can also cause fatigue and other similar symptoms are found occasionally together with ME/CFS, which can, as I have said, be very confusing for the practitioner, since it isn't always clear which condition is responsible for the individual symptoms.

Postural orthostatic tachycardia syndrome (POTS)

In Chapter 5 I have already mentioned that POTS is related to the autonomic nervous system disturbance present in all ME/CFS. POTS occurs when the autonomic nervous system fails to compensate for upright body posture and causes fainting and dizziness due to low blood pressure on standing. The condition has been recognised since at least 1940, affecting millions worldwide aged 15–50 years, with a female to male ratio of around 5:1[25, 26].

Professor Peter Rowe, a world-famous paediatrician, who is head of paediatrics at Johns Hopkins University Hospital in Baltimore has found that many young patients with ME/CFS also have POTS.

Researchers at the University of Newcastle, UK, studied haemodynamic responses of ME/CFS patients when standing for over two minutes. Professor Julia Newton, who led the research team, concluded that POTS was relatively common in ME/CFS patients, and patients' clinical evaluation should include autonomic function tests, such as the response to standing – POTS is indeed an under-recognised condition in ME/CFS[27].

Diagnosis

POTS is confirmed by lying on a head-up tilt table (HUT) in a specialised clinic which is then tilted upright to a 60–80-degree vertical angle for approximately 45 minutes and blood pressure and heart rate are measured.

The standing test is another test for POTS which can be done in any clinic, with the patient being asked to stand upright without any assistance, so s/he must supports his/her own weight and maintain balance.

In ME/CFS and FMS, as I have said earlier, many patients suffer from orthostatic hypotension, also known as postural hypotension, which causes dizziness if one gets up too quickly from lying or sitting. This is due to disturbed sympathetic control leading to a blood pressure which is not high enough to pump sufficient blood into the head when standing up. This form of postural (standing up) hypotension (low blood pressure) is also known as neurally-mediated hypotension. POTS is a more serious version of this problem and is diagnosed if the heart rate increases to 120 beats per minute or by 30 bpm (40 bpm in patients aged from 12 to 19) in five to 30 minutes after standing up, and the disorder has lasted at least six months with no other obvious cause of the symptoms, such as bleeding, other heart conditions or a side effect of medications.

Since the sympathetic nervous system mainly uses the neurotransmitter nor-adrenaline (norepinephrine) to transmit impulses, a high plasma level of noradrenaline seen in sympathetic disturbances is also considered useful to identify some POTS patients[28].

Treatment

There is no universally accepted treatment for POTS, with some doctors prescribing beta blockers or steroids such as fludrocortisone or some other medication to increase blood pressure, but there are many other non-pharma measures that may help.

People with POTS should eat small regular meals and drink 2 litres of fluids and increase salt intake to about 2–3 teaspoons a day[29]. However, you should avoid the increase in salt if you suffer from high blood pressure or kidney problems. If in any doubt about health risks, it is best to check with your doctor before increasing your salt intake.

Orthostatic intolerance is common to many ME/CFS and FMS patient without full blown POTS and is due to the effect on the autonomic control of blood pressure and volume due to the shift of large amounts of blood volume from upper to lower body and is traditionally treated with intravenous saline but has complications if used long term.

Oral rehydration salts (ORS), which usually contain glucose plus sodium and potassium salts are available online or from pharmacies as convenient sachets of pre-formulated low-concentration granules. These are effective, inexpensive, safe and convenient; when mixed with a litre of water they will rehydrate the body fast, regardless of the cause. One should buy only those that follow the WHO formula – a tried-and-tested sodium and glucose mixture that has been used by the WHO in cholera outbreaks. Researchers in New York have shown that ORS improved short-term orthostatic tolerance exhibited by patients with POTS[30].

However, some patients with either ME/CFS or FMS have problems with their insulin levels or issues with excess yeast, such as candida, and risk aggravating the condition by the addition of glucose in any form, so I would tread very carefully and again seek advice from your GP.

Keeping as active as possible is beneficial, but is not always possible if one also has ME/CFS, but total inactivity will make both conditions worse so it is important to try and maintain some muscle strength, especially in the legs, so regular gentle exercise even if it is just clenching the buttocks for a few minutes a day, will be of use. When lying down one should always elevate the head end of the patient's bed. Never get up from bed quickly, which is also a golden rule for ME/CFS patients. Sit on the side of the bed for at least a minute before standing and always avoid long periods of standing still.

Dizziness or feeling faint can be helped by lying down and raising your legs. If you are unable to lie down, you can cross your legs in front of each other while standing and squeeze your legs together, or rock up and down on your toes. Clenching other parts of the body, such as buttocks and tummy muscles and/or even your fists, may help, and in some cases compression tights may also help.

Joint hypermobility/Ehlers-Danlos syndrome (EDS)

Many patients seen in clinic with ME/CFS have extraordinary mobility in their joints. The hypermobility is sometimes found to be due to Ehlers-Danlos syndrome which is now known to be a group of connective tissue disorders that are mostly inherited and are varied both in how they affect the body and in their genetic causes. EDS patients also may have skin that can be stretched much more than normal.

At the time of writing, EDS is classified into 13 subtypes. Each EDS subtype is classified by slightly different clinical symptoms and identifiable variants in genetic testing. However, some patients are diagnosed as having EDS on signs and symptoms alone without a confirmed genetic abnormality.

Patients with EDS have loose/unstable joints which are prone to frequent dislocations and joint pain, hyper-extensible joints and often an early onset of osteoarthritis. The fragile skin may lead to severe bruising and scarring with slow and poor wound healing. They may also have fragile arteries, intestines and uterus, and often have a poor spinal posture, with a thoracic spine which is bent forward with some side-bending (kyphoscoliosis), poor muscle tone, heart valve problems and gum disease.

Connective tissue is what the body uses to provide strength and elasticity and is found all over the body. Normal connective tissue contains strong proteins that allow tissue to be stretched but not beyond its limit, and then safely returns that tissue to normal. The connective tissue in EDS is badly constructed or processed, with some or all of the body affected, and can be pulled beyond normal limits, which causes damage to the tissue. Being a genetic disorder, the same symptoms run in families. (NB: There are some rare cases where the EDS has been a caused by genetic mutation and is not familial.)

There is an assessment tool used by many practitioners to confirm a hypermobility state. It is known as the Beighton scale[31], which is included below and gives scores related to the severity and extent of the hypermobility. However, the scale was developed as a research tool to indicate general hypermobility. Often a score over six is used as a diagnosis of generalised hypermobility but does not mean a person has EDS or any other disease process. Joints not evaluated on the Beighton scale can be hypermobile so sometimes a low score does not indicate the severity of the condition.

The Beighton score is calculated as follows:

- One point if, while standing, when bending forward you can place the palms of your hands on the ground with legs straight and no bending of the knees.
- One point for each elbow that bends backwards (extends) 10 degrees or more.
- One point for each knee that bends backwards (extends) 10 degrees or more.
- One point for each thumb that touches the forearm when bent backwards.
- One point for each little finger that bends backwards beyond 90 degrees.

I am not the only person to have carried out a clinical study into mechanical problems in ME/CFS. In a leading university in Baltimore, USA, in the 1990s, a study led by Professor of Pediatrics, Peter Rowe, at the Johns Hopkins Children's Center, was carried out. Their findings suggested either that hypermobility itself is an important factor in the development of ME/CFS, or it is associated with another factor that predisposes a person to ME/CFS.

The primary feature of EDS is abnormal connective tissue, which can also affect the walls of blood vessels, leading to veins distending excessively in response to ordinary pressures from the blood flow. This in turn leads to increased pooling of the blood in swollen veins and many associated symptoms. These include frequently fainting or feeling very dizzy all the time, especially when standing still and even worse in a hot shower. Connective tissue disorders can also affect the integrity of lymphatic vessels and may also contribute to the backflow of lymph and varicose megalymphatics (grossly enlarged lymph vessels – see page 249) seen in ME/CFS and FMS.

Research by Rowe and his team suggests that hypermobility and connective tissue abnormalities should always be examined in patients with ME/CFS together with screening for orthostatic intolerance syndromes, such as POTS, as mentioned earlier in this chapter.

The research team examined 116 children aged 10 and older, for joint hypermobility. Sixty per cent of those with ME/CFS showed joint hypermobility, compared with 24% of the healthy children. Rowe and colleagues had previously reported that many patients with orthostatic intolerance also had EDS[32].

Cranio-cervical instability (CCI)

In some severe cases of EDS there is also the possibility of cranio-cervical instability (CCI), also known as occipito-atlanto-axial (OAA) hypermobility syndrome or atlanto-axial instability (AAI). This condition is the due to weakness and hyperlaxity of ligaments that join the occipital bone at the bottom of the skull with bones at top of the neck. The first cervical vertebra is also known as the atlas and the second, the axis. Instability in this region may lead to damage and dysfunction of the upper part of the spinal cord or, worse, the brain itself. One of the structural effects seen in AAI can be a Chiari malformation, which is where there is a downward displacement of part of the cerebellum at the base of the brain.

The diagnosis of CCI/AAI is usually made following an upright MRI and rotational three-dimensional CT scans and then confirmed by a reduction of symptoms when the head is gently pulled up from the neck and worsened by pushing the head gently down. Other physicians and neurosurgeons, such as Dr Dan Heffez of Wisconsin, USA, have seen the connection between FMS and Chiari malformation and upper cervical problems[33].

Treatment for CCI sometimes involves surgery, although this should only be considered in the most extreme cases. My professor of orthopaedics at the British School of Osteopathy, Professor Tony Andreason, used to famously say: 'Surgery is terminal'. In other words, the effects of surgical procedure good and bad, last for life. In most cases of CCI the treatment of choice is support with a cervical collar. I recommend a soft cervical collar to be used for an hour at a time where the patient can rest their chin comfortably on the top of the front part of the collar taking the strain off the upper neck. This should be used in combination with frequent applications of cold and warm compresses, as mentioned in Chapter 10 (page 273). Very gentle specific isometric exercises are also given in Chapter 10, which will gradually strengthen the suboccipital region. The exercises need to be done in very short gentle bursts but have to be carried out frequently, at around every three hours throughout the day, and like all exercises for ME/CFS and especially FMS, they must be painless. If even the slightest tightening of the muscles elicits pain, then the patient should stop. As I say to all my students in my workshops: 'PAIN = NO GAIN'. Pain is the enemy of ME/CFS and FMS as the neural pain pathways will aggravate already heightened pain control centres in the brain.

There are practitioners who have successfully treated more severe CCI for years without surgery. They use a type of injection technique for joint hypermobility known as prolotherapy. It utilises a sclerosing injection which is designed to irritate the joint and sounds like it shouldn't help because, as it says on the bottle, it irritates the joint! How can this oxymoron be explained? With a skilled practitioner the injection, which usually has an analgesic and possibly an anti-inflammatory component, will also contain a saline or sucrose solution which, by irritating the ligaments, causes them to tighten, resulting in an improvement in joint strength and less hypermobility.

Some practitioners use prolozone injections, mentioned in the previous chapter (page 150), which contain ozone to achieve the same results as prolotherapy, but which practitioners claim is a quicker method with fewer side effects.

Case: Miss L

This case illustrates the diagnostic confusion that surrounds ME/CFS.

Miss L, a 12-year-old child, had been severely disabled with an unknown disorder for the previous eighteen months. She had been wheelchair-bound for some of the time and unable to attend her regular school for more than a few hours a week. She had mostly spent the days at home, cared for by her devoted single mother, who had two other young children to look after. She had been taken to a local health authority school for a few hours each week; even that had often been too taxing for her ailing body.

The postural disturbance of the thoracic spine in most cases of ME/CFS is usually not too severe, often with evidence of old osteochondrosis with a flattened upper thoracic region. However, Miss L was born with a syrinx (cyst within the spinal canal), as seen in this MRI image (Fig. 15(a)). This is rare but demonstrates the extent of possible spinal dysfunction.

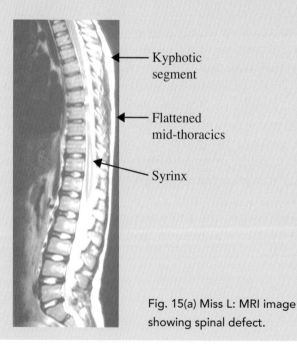

Kyphotic
segment

Flattened
mid-thoracics

Syrinx

Fig. 15(a) Miss L: MRI image
showing spinal defect.

A syrinx within the spinal cord usually leads to a condition known as syringiomyelia. This neurological condition leads to a loss of pain sensation and reduction in normal sensory function on one side of the body. In other words, a different set of symptoms to ME/CFS. Miss L also had a defect at the top of her neck. A small section of her brain was slightly protruding down into the spinal canal (see Fig. 15(b)).

As mentioned earlier, when there is a noticeable protrusion down the spine it is known as a Chiari malformation and is responsible for many symptoms common to ME/CFS as it affects normal spinal cord function.

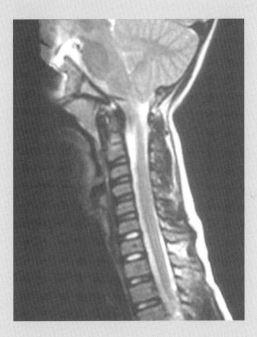

Fig. 15(b) Miss L: Upper cervical defect.

Chiari malformation often presents in patients who have a syrinx.

A defect at the uppermost region of the cervical spine and other cases of Chiari malformation and cervical stenosis, in which the spinal canal has narrowed, have been observed by others in ME/CFS patients[34]. This leads to the health and function of the spinal cord and even the brain being compromised.

The MRI scan in Fig. 15(b) shows a partial herniation of the cerebellar tonsil into the spinal canal.

So, Miss L had two conditions that could have caused major neurological problems, but her symptoms, which included severe fatigue, headache, lack of concentration, sleep disturbance, irritable bowel and irritable bladder, sore throat and pains in her neck, back, chest and extremities, were diagnosed at her local hospital as mostly psychological. The syrinx, in their opinion, had nothing to do with the symptoms and the upper spine problem was not severe enough to be classified as a full Chiari malformation and was considered to be unrelated to her condition.

ME/CFS was never mentioned and when her mother brought her in to see me. I found it difficult to believe that the only treatment Miss L was receiving was regular sessions with the hospital psychologist. Miss L's paediatric neurologist dismissed the idea that she had ME/CFS. However, as her treatment with me slowly progressed and her symptoms started to improve, Miss L's doctors began to take notice. I explained to them how the girl's spine was extremely flattened in the upper part of her back. Her breastbone was slightly malformed, showing a slight concavity, which would have affected her respiratory mechanics. She had lymphatic swelling in her chest and neck as well as the tender areas familiar to all the ME/CFS patients that I had seen (see Chapter 8). Although Miss L's doctors continued to be sceptical, they could see the encouraging results of my treatment and they then included me in Miss L's case-management meetings at the hospital.

I have been in touch with Miss L's family recently and they have informed me that she made further recovery over time and managed to complete a bioscience degree, and years on now works in the lab of a major UK hospital. She has settled down with her partner and they recently had their first child. She has finally got her life back – without surgery.

This case demonstrates that even when there is a clear visible hindrance to normal cerebrospinal flow, the idea that physical problems can have any possible link to the symptoms of ME/CFS is often just simply ignored.

As well as Chiari, the upper cervical bones may compress the spinal cord, leading to the head feeling too heavy for the neck to support it and head pain aggravated by any movements in the upper neck and affected by any activity changing the cerebrospinal fluid flow in the head such as coughing, sneezing, yawning and crying. All the symptoms of autonomic disturbance seen in ME/CFS patients will be exacerbated due to the brain stem irritation seen in most cases of CCI/AAI.

Ankylosing spondylitis (AS)

Another comorbidity that I have occasionally seen in clinic affecting the spine is ankylosing spondylitis (AS), which is a chronic inflammatory arthritis of unknown origin but is thought to be a type of autoimmune disease linked to a particular gene known as human leukocyte antigen B27 (HLA-B27).

AS causes inflammation in the spine, often in the thoracic spine and the sacroiliac joints in the pelvis. It therefore leads to further inflammatory toxins building up in the spinal cord, aggravating the symptoms of ME/CFS and FMS. Over time this can damage the spine and lead to the growth of new bone which in severe cases can cause parts of the spine to fuse (ankylosis).

The gene HLA-B27 has been linked to the development of *Klebsiella pneumoniae* bacterial infection as a predisposition to AS. So, in cases where an inflamed thoracic spine becomes gradually stiffer and stiffer, especially if there are also problems affecting the pelvis, it is worthwhile having a blood test for this gene and also testing for *Klebsiella pneumoniae*[35].

If ankylosing spondylitis is diagnosed it means that it is more difficult to keep the spine inflammation-free and as mobile as it needs to be. This will affect the prognosis in ME/CFS and FMS but I have helped many patients with AS by regular treatments and gentle exercise aimed at maintaining as much movement in the spine as possible and reducing the inflammation, following the same protocol as described in Chapter 10.

Idiopathic intracranial hypertension (IIH)

IIH, previously known as 'benign intracranial hypertension' or 'pseudotumor cerebri', is a condition of unknown cause leading to an increase in pressure within the brain.

Like ME/CFS and fibromyalgia, it most commonly affects women and leads to daily diffuse, non-pulsating head pain which is aggravated by coughing. The most common finding is papilloedema, which is an eye condition that happens when pressure in the brain makes the optic nerve swell, affecting vision. However, recent research has looked into the possibility of a lesser, more common form of IIH, causing headaches and other symptoms but not papilloedema. A group of doctors who carried out research at Cambridge University have highlighted that this could explain many of the symptoms of ME/CFS[36].

The rationale behind this idea makes so much sense. Higgins and colleagues argued that the most common presentation of most known diseases is always the mild case of the disorder. For instance, take asthma. It is a very common condition and affects many people who need the occasional puff on an inhaler but can manage their life without too many problems. However, there are some very severe cases that can hospitalise patients and even be a cause of death; thankfully these are much fewer than the minor cases. However, with the present accepted criteria for IIH, the more severe cases when there is headache and papilloedema and severe nausea, are the cases usually diagnosed, with less severe cases without papilloedema rarely diagnosed. This is very unlikely to be so, and therefore there must be many people with minor cases of IIH never correctly diagnosed.

The Cambridge team had already shown in 2013 that some ME/CFS patients had symptom relief following a drainage of cerebrospinal fluid (CSF) using a lumbar puncture[37]. Although the lumbar puncture demonstrated the elevated intracranial pressure in the ME/CFS patients, in most cases I would not recommend sticking a needle into the spinal cord to remove fluid as it could worsen the condition. It has actually caused a major relapse in the symptoms of many of my ME/CFS patients over the years who have had a lumbar puncture for investigative purposes only. However, in some severe cases when nothing else is working and the patient presents with unremitting headache with nausea, a lumbar puncture may be worth considering as a final option.

IIH has been clearly demonstrated in some patients with ME/CFS but this could equally be the case with many fibromyalgia cases where severe headaches are a major symptom, which has been discussed in a recent paper by a group of Belgian researchers[38].

Lyme disease

Lyme disease is named after Lyme, Connecticut in the USA, where the disease was first identified. It is an illness that is becoming much more commonly diagnosed. It is a bacterial infection that usually originates from a tick bite, most commonly from a deer tick. The disease has a variety of symptoms, including changes affecting the skin, heart, joints and nervous system. It is also known as borrelia (the infective bacterium is *Borrelis burgdorferi*) or borreliosis. A diagnosis of Lyme disease is more likely if the patient can remember a tick bite and has the characteristic erythema migrans (bull's eye) rash (see Figure 16).

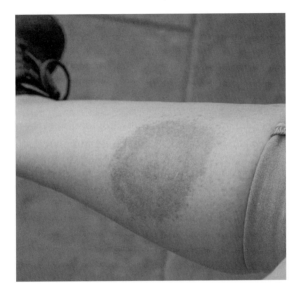

Fig. 16 A bull's eye rash (see also colour plate 1).

To make a diagnosis, the doctor may take a blood sample to determine whether or not the patient has developed an antibody towards Lyme disease. The usual blood test done in the UK is known as the ELISA test which, unfortunately, is not very accurate so many patients are wrongly cleared for borrelia. A plate-based assay technique, ELISA (enzyme-linked immunosorbent assay) is designed for detecting and quantifying substances such as peptides, proteins, antibodies and hormones.

Many specialised clinics in the USA and many European countries use a second screening tool to confirm the diagnosis if the ELISA test is positive. This is known as the Western Blot test. This two-tier-test is used to more accurately detect several antibodies to proteins of *Borrelia burgdorferi*.

The Western Blot is a method commonly used to detect and analyse proteins. Originally known as the immunological pathogen detection test (Immunoblot), it was used for the first time in 1807 by Moscow State University professors Peter Ivanovich Strakhov and Ferdinand Frederic Reuss to demonstrate a spread of molecules due to the presence of a charged interface between the particle surface and the surrounding fluid. This process is known as electrophoresis.

Unfortunately the ELISA and Western Blot tests have been shown to miss up to 60% of cases of Borrelia[39]. However, there are laboratories across the world that offer more precise testing, including in Germany, which favour a different test known as an Elispot test which is much more sensitive than either the Elisa or Western Blot tests. The Elispot assays use a form of ELISA that is specially treated with chemical reagents that basically clean up the sample to make it a much more accurate diagnostic test.

As mentioned in Chapter 4, the antibody immunoglobulin G level is raised in long-lasting infections. Therefore, if there is a long-term co-infection such as Lyme disease, then the IgG will usually be high. So, if one has possibly been infected years before it is important that tests are carried out to determine the level of Borrelia IgG when investigating Lyme disease.

Also, according to the Centers for Disease Control and Prevention (CDC) in the USA, often tests in the first few weeks of the illness show up as negative, since antibody numbers haven't built up enough in the blood to be detected. This is why the guidelines of the International Lyme and Associated Disease Society (ILADS) advise experienced practitioners to use their clinical judgement even when tests are negative[40].

My own theory of severe, chronic Lyme disease is that it is a subset of ME/CFS, but triggered by a Borrelia infection, which has led to high levels of cytokines and the bacterium itself travelling into the brain, leading to what is known clinically as neuro-borreliosis. In other words, millions of people around the world may have been bitten at some time by a tick. Many get infected by *Borrelia burgdorferi* but don't get the major effects because their immune system kills off the bacteria and the lymphatics drain the infection and the inflammatory toxins away and break them down. However, if a person has a problem with their neuro-lymphatic system and the Borrelia and cytokines flow backwards into the central nervous system, then the severe chronic disease with major neurological problems ensues.

With Lyme disease, the best defence is prevention. As mentioned, the highest risk comes from deer ticks which usually occur in wooded areas. When in these areas, cover up your exposed skin and make sure your trousers are tucked into your socks.

If you find a tick attached to your body do not pinch or swat it. Use tweezers to remove it, grasping the tick as close to your skin as possible and slowly pull the tick straight out, then wash the bitten area well with a mild soap and use an antibiotic ointment on the wound.

If infected, early treatment with antibiotics, such as doxycycline, amoxicillin or daptomycin, will usually be enough. The antibiotic course often needs to be repeated and quite lengthy to be effective and there is a reluctance in various countries to pay for this long-term approach. However, if not promptly diagnosed and correctly treated, those infected with Lyme disease can develop severe chronic neuro-borreliosis.

There are many different treatment strategies that have helped chronic Lyme patients; however, I have yet to find the one that helps all. It is, as with all cases of ME/CFS, a matter of trying different protocols and finding which gives the best relief. Besides the Borrelia affecting different parts of the brain and the body there can be many co-infections from a tick bite, such as Babesia, Rickettsia and Ehrlichia, plus many human herpes viruses that can accompany Borrelia with chronic Lyme disease.

However, what I am trying to make the medical world understand is that it is not the species or the infection that is the issue, but the body, and particularly the brain's way of dealing with infections that is the core problem. If the body's lymphatic system, and especially the neuro-lymphatics, were working properly there would not be a build-up of these pathogens and the body would simply kill the infection and drain away the post-infectious toxins naturally. However, if there is a backflow then these nasties end up in the central nervous system, which results in the symptoms of ME/CFS.

If the symptoms become chronic, you might consider seeking consultation with a naturopath or herbalist. There are some clinics around the world that specialise in the treatment of Lyme and other chronic infectious diseases using antimicrobial and immune-supportive herbs (with and without antibiotics) and with acupuncture to regulate immunity and manage pain. In a 2017 study, researchers found that essential oils, including oregano, cinnamon bark, clove buds and wintergreen, killed Lyme bacteria even more potently than any pharmaceutical antibiotic.

One of the active ingredients of garlic, allicin, has been shown to exhibit antibacterial activity against a wide range of gram-negative and gram-positive bacteria; antifungal activity, particularly against *Candida albicans*; antiparasitic activity, including against some major human intestinal protozoan parasites; and antiviral activity[41].

This has led to allicin becoming a very important component of natural anti-Lyme treatments. I have personally seen the benefit of a long-term dose of allicin as part of the treatment protocol for Lyme disease, but one should always follow advice from a trained naturopath or herbalist. As wonderful as garlic is, it is also important to know that it can increase risk of bleeding as, like fish oils, it has anti-clotting properties. Therefore, as a precaution, garlic and fish oil supplements should be stopped at least two weeks before any planned surgical procedure[42].

In a new study, Professor of Molecular Microbiology and Immunology Dr Zhang and his team, at Johns Hopkins University, Bloomberg School of Public Health, found that five essential oils, including garlic, helped destroy the Borrelia bacteria in their lab. The herbal combinations worked better than the individual natural remedies and have been shown to be more effective in combination. More work needs to be done before a herbal treatment containing the essential oils they tested can be prescribed to the public so it is still early days, but it is promising that leading universities are looking beyond standard pharma for the answer to major infectious diseases such as Lyme disease[43].

To support the immune system, I often advise patients with Lyme disease to use the herb cilantro, which is the name given to the leaves and stems of the coriander plant. Interestingly, there is evidence that coriander leaves also help rid the body of the yeast infection *Candida albicans*[44], which, as stated in Chapter 5, is prevalent in ME/CFS.

To find the appropriate dose of these herbal remedies and supplements it is best to start with the minimum dose and consult your local herbalist or pharmacist to see what the optimum and maximum dose you should take is. It is also always important to discuss any possible drug interactions with the doctor before taking any new remedies even though they are only supplements and herbs.

The Cowden protocol

The Cowden protocol is one of the most tried and tested self-administered herbal protocols for treating Lyme disease and recommended by naturopaths and herbalists around the world. Dr Lee Cowden MD from Dallas Texas, co-founded the Academy of Comprehensive Integrative Medicine in 2008 is a USA board-certified cardiologist and internist who is internationally known for his knowledge and skill in practising and teaching integrative medicine.

He developed several liquid herbal formulas that contain special local herbs from South America. Known as the Cowden protocol, this treatment takes five to nine months. During that time, patients take combinations of 13 different herbal formulas, including pinella, which is a herb extract from the Peruvian plant *Pimpinella anisum* that helps cleanse the brain and reduces brain fog.

Other herbs and natural products advised by Lee Cowden include burber, serrapeptase and samento:

- Burber aids lymph drainage and detoxification and comes from the Peruvian manayupa plant.
- Serrapeptase, also called Serratio peptidase, is an enzyme from the silkworm that helps the body break down non-living tissue and has been shown to have strong health benefits for arthritic back pain, headaches, sinusitis and breast engorgement.
- Samento or 'cat's claw' is a herb that I have known to help many patients fight infection and reduce inflammation. It is a very useful antimicrobial that helps beat many coinfections.

Parasitic infections

Besides viral, bacterial and fungal infections, one must not ignore parasitic infections that can also cause symptoms of fatigue, confusion, lethargy and muscle weakness. Specialised private labs around the world can run tests to exclude these.

There are parasites that may lead to ME/CFS, and some parasitic infections may be due to a deficiency of an enzyme – chitinase – which should break down chitin. Chitin is a major portion of the cell walls of fungi and the exoskeleton of insects and some parasites, such as the minute roundworm *Varestrongylus klapowi* (Vk) discovered by Dr Larry Klapow, an American biologist, after suffering from ME/CFS.

These roundworms secrete a hormone, vasoactive intestinal polypeptide (VIP), which is involved in regulating blood pressure and blood flow, and hippocampal cholinergic neuro-stimulatory peptide (HCNP), believed to be involved in memory and immune function. Vk larvae have been discovered by Dr Klapow in the nasal mucosa of ME/CFS patients and there is a possibility that the larva migrates into the brain via the perivascular spaces which run along blood vessels supplying the olfactory nerve.

Dr Klapow suggests a treatment that is based on supplementing a chitinase enzyme deficiency which occurs in around 6% of the population due to a mutation in the Chit1 gene which controls macrophage secreted chitinase. There are several diseases associated with the mutation, according to Dr Klapow, and Vk-related CFS is one of them. It is interesting that Dr Klapow understands that killing off the worm is only part of the answer, and that drainage of the parasite out into the lymphatics is a crucial part of overall treatment, which is what the Perrin Technique is designed to do.

Toxoplasmosis

Toxoplasmosis is caused by Toxoplasma, one of the world's most common parasites. It can be picked up by eating contaminated meat or by exposure to infected cat faeces. Testing looks for antibodies to toxoplasma.

Giardiasis

The most frequent parasites in humans are protozoa (single cell organisms) such as *Giardia lamblia*, which causes giardiasis, also known as 'beaver fever', and typically leads to abdominal symptoms such as diarrhoea, flatulence, stomach cramps and nausea.

Babesiosis

Babesiosis is a malaria-like illness caused by the parasite *Babesia*. It is also known as nuttallia. It is usually transmitted by a tick bite and often occurs at the same time as Lyme disease.

Mast cell activation syndrome (MCAS)

A mast cell is a type of white blood cell with many granules containing chemical mediators such as histamine and tryptase, the most common enzyme found in mast cells. Histamine is a nitrogen-containing chemical that has properties influencing the body in many different ways, including affecting smooth muscle in the body, for instance in the walls of blood vessels and lymphatics. When mast cells are activated by an allergen, they also release our old friends the pro-inflammatory cytokines.

Although best known for their role in allergies, mast cells are important in protecting the body by supporting the immune response. They are the only blood cells found throughout the brain, communicating with neurons and glial cells, and they also help the blood–brain barrier function correctly[45, 46].

The National Institute of Health in the USA has discovered a genetic abnormality that leads to high levels of tryptase. It is during mast cell activation syndrome (MCAS) that these and other mediators are over-produced, creating an over-active allergic response. This leads to an array of symptoms such as rashes like urticaria, more commonly known as hives, swelling, flushing, itching, abdominal pain, nausea/vomiting, loose bowels and difficulty breathing, which are all strangely familiar to many ME/CFS patients.

A diagnosis of MCAS is aided by blood or urine tests which show a higher level of mediators during symptomatic episodes. Treatment for MCAS is usually just to relieve the symptoms. Sometimes antihistamines and other drugs to reduce the release of the mediators from the mast cells are prescribed. In very severe cases, the patient may go into anaphylactic shock which requires an immediate injection of adrenaline.

PANS/PANDAS

I have seen some younger patients, usually in their teens or early twenties, with some major psychological symptoms, such as severe anxieties or phobias, obsessive compulsive disorder (OCD) and/or some tic disorders, as well as the usual neurological symptoms of ME/CFS. Their condition begins suddenly, usually before the onset of puberty, following an infection such as flu, chicken pox, Lyme disease or mycoplasma.

This is now known as 'paediatric acute-onset neuropsychiatric syndrome' or PANS. Some patients have begun their symptoms, or worsened, following a streptococcal infection such as a strep throat or scarlet fever, and this condition is known as PANDAS ('paediatric autoimmune neuropsychiatric disorders associated with streptococcal infections').

Streptococcal and other infections attack organs such as the brain with molecules that mimic the brain's own cells, which prevent detection by the immune system's antibodies. This molecular mimicry leads to antibodies reacting with the strep molecules, but also with the host molecules, causing a pseudo-autoimmune illness. With PANDAS, the infection and eventual mimicry have been found in the heart and the brain, taking place primarily in the basal ganglia.

As explained throughout this book, we now know that this region of the brain (the basal ganglia), which is a major part of the limbic system, controlling emotions, is affected when neuro-lymphatic drainage does not work properly[47], and is a major area of neurotoxicity in ME/CFS and FMS.

Therapy usually involves antibiotics and symptomatic relief of neuropsychiatric symptoms in specialist centres. However, there are very few clinics worldwide that specialise in the treatment of PANS or PANDAS. Due to the overlap with ME/CFS symptoms, I would advise that all the treatments given should be in conjunction with the drainage techniques for the neuro-lymphatics outlined in this book which should help speed up any recovery[48, 49, 50, 51, 52].

Electromagnetic hypersensitivity (EHS)

In recent years, with the expansion of WIFI networks across the world, I have started seeing a growing number of ME/CFS and FMS patients with electromagnetic hypersensitivity. These patients' symptoms worsen when exposed to any low-dose electromagnetic radiation, which can lead to the patient having to avoid exposure to mobile phones, WIFI and sometimes all electrical devices, making their lives intolerable.

The cause of EHS is unknown but I feel in ME/CFS and FMS it is due to the increased sensitisation of the nervous system due to neurotoxic overload. Researchers have shown that it may be due to impaired detoxification[53].

Patients have found that they can reduce the electromagnetic radiation effect on the body by taking natural detox products containing the mineral zeolite. At the nuclear disaster of Chernobyl in 1986, over half a million tons of zeolite was dropped into the reactor to absorb radioactive metals, and food containing zeolite was given to animals and humans to reduce their radiation levels.

Some patients have found painting the rooms in their house with special paint containing zeolite also helps reduce the levels of electromagnetic radiation and improves symptoms. There are more than 45 different naturally occurring zeolites, of which the clinoptilolite zeolite is safe to ingest and has been found to naturally remove radiation as well as heavy metals from the body[53a].

There are devices available online that have been shown to block harmful EMF radiation and WiFi, but one must be careful which ones to try as some of the claims are not backed by science. One should only choose radiation shields or blockers that have been properly tested to be safe and effective.

Chronic inflammatory response syndrome (CIRS)

Excess mould, following exposure to water-damaged buildings, often with visible mould growth and musty smells, can lead to the body's inflammatory response to toxins such as moulds going out of control, with a resultant cascade of inflammatory and hormonal changes – a condition called 'chronic inflammatory response syndrome' (CIRS). This often leads to fatigue, pain, gastrointestinal and neurologic symptoms, sleep disturbances, and other damaging effects to the body.

This condition was first described by a leading physician in Maryland, USA, Dr Ritchie Shoemaker. Other causes are exposure to harmful types of blue-green algae and spider bites. In CIRS, the antibodies needed by the patient's immune system are not able to recognise and break down certain toxins, such as mycotoxins produced by mould, which most frequently happens in the 24% of the population who have the genetic susceptibility known as HLA DR/DQ genotype.

Prevention is better than cure, so to reduce the chance of exposure there is a test one can have carried out on dust in your house. This test, known as an ERMI (environmental relative mouldiness index), evaluates the amount of mould spores that have settled in the dust in your house.

Hyperventilation syndrome

Hyperventilation, or shallow rapid breathing, leads to low levels of CO_2 in the blood, which can, as shown in Chapter 4, cause fatigue, pain and other symptoms of ME/CFS and FMS. However, a research study concluded that there was little association between hyperventilation and ME/CFS[54].

Hyperventilation syndrome (HVS) is due to problems that occur when a person hyperventilates for a long period, usually due to stress. The resultant physical changes, such as increases in pH in the blood (respiratory alkalosis), and constriction of cerebral arteries, lead to many symptoms such as dizziness, blurred vision, faintness, headaches, palpitations, tachycardia and cold extremities, which are all common symptoms of ME/CFS and FMS.

The muscles of the upper body become tight in patients suffering from HVS, in response to stress which places more strain on the thoracic spine and also prevents the diaphragm functioning correctly. HVS can be helped by practising gentle exercise techniques to breathe slowly and deeply and also utilise the diaphragm better by abdominal breathing exercises.

Dry eye syndrome (DES)

Dryness of the eye, known medically as 'keratoconjunctivitis sicca' is a common feature in ME/CFS and FMS as the autonomic control of the lacrimal glands that produce our tears is disturbed, leading to a problem producing tears and lubricating the eyes. Also, this condition may be exacerbated by medication taken by patients. Some types of antihistamine and antidepressant and contraceptive can affect the cholinergic control of the lacrimal ducts, leading to dry eyes. Dry eyes can also be a symptom of other eye diseases and medical conditions that affect the production of tears by the lacrimal glands, such as the autoimmune disease Sjogren's syndrome, which also causes a dry mouth and affects the salivary glands.

There is a separate condition known as dry eye syndrome (DES), with symptoms of burning sensation; itchy eye; aching sensations; heavy, fatigue; sore red eyes with photophobia; and blurred vision. Scientists in Taiwan showed in a large population-controlled study that patients with DES were five times more likely to develop ME/CFS, compared with a non-DES group[55].

The reason why DES is a risk factor for developing ME/CFS is that some of the neurotoxic drainage occurs via perivascular spaces down the optic nerve pathways. Increased inflammation in the region of the eye could overload the neurotoxic backflow in vulnerable patients, leading to ME/CFS. Increased computer use, contact lenses, ageing, menopause, smoking and frequent flying have all been shown to be aggravating or causal factors in DES. So, this is one of many reasons why I advise patients to reduce their computer use. Also, contact lenses should be replaced with glasses and smoking should be reduced if doing so doesn't cause too much stress.

Other common causes of fatigue

Anaemia

As discussed in the previous chapter, the mitochondria in cells produce energy by a series of chemical reactions utilising many enzymes which are produced when the biochemistry in the body is balanced and when one's diet contains the correct nutritional support. However, without two essential raw materials, all the other supplements, vitamins and minerals would be useless, and no energy would be produced at all. These two raw materials are oxygen and glucose.

Lack of oxygen to the tissues of the body leads to fatigue, and thus if there is a reduction in the oxygen-carrying red blood cells, or the function of these cells becomes impaired, as in some cases of anaemia, a major symptom is lethargy and weakness. A common cause of anaemia is iron deficiency, since iron is the main constituent of the oxygen-transporting element (haemoglobin) within the red blood cell. A simple blood test to determine the level of iron, or a red blood cell count, will eliminate anaemia from the doctor's investigation.

One can increase the level of iron in the blood by eating foods with very high iron content, such as broccoli, asparagus and dark leafy greens including spinach and kale. Some legumes, such as kidney beans, are also rich in iron.

The blood sugar glucose is a monosaccharide containing one sugar molecule. Glucose together with fat forms the body's main fuel and is usually derived from bread, fruit, vegetables and dairy products. The liver produces, stores and releases glucose depending on the body's need, regulated by the pancreatic hormone insulin, which helps cells to absorb glucose from the blood, and glucagon, which facilitates the release of stored glucose from the liver.

Glucose, besides being so important for energy production in the body as a whole, is also known as 'brain food'. The brain, with around one hundred billion nerve cells, is the most energy-demanding organ in the body, requiring half of all the energy produced in the body. So, a disturbance in glucose levels will aggravate any other problems with the brain's function, as in ME/CFS and FMS. It can also lead to a variety of conditions, such as diabetes and hypoglycaemia and other neurological and cardiovascular diseases.

Patients with ME/CFS and FMS often present in clinic with the condition known as 'reactive hypoglycaemia'. This, I believe, is due to neurotoxins, leading to a disturbed hypothalamic–pancreatic axis which in turn leads to overproduction of insulin after meals, causing the amount of glucose in the bloodstream to fall to a lower than normal level. Also called postprandial hypoglycaemia, the glucose levels drop within four hours after eating, leading to the person becoming ravenously hungry. As well as this extreme hunger, patients often complain of dizziness, clammy skin and increased sweating, general weakness and shakiness, often accompanied by palpitations and light-headedness.

The best advice to patients with reactive hypoglycaemia is to avoid simple carbohydrates, such as white bread, and also alcohol and to eat regular small meals throughout the day. I usually recommend to patients who suffer from reactive hypoglycaemia to divide their three meals a day into six smaller meals, having half of breakfast at the beginning of the day and a couple of hours later eat the other half, repeating this process with lunch and dinner.

As with other metabolic processes, in ME/CFS and FMS the neurotoxicity doesn't always cause an increase in hormone levels. The dysfunction can cause the exact opposite in some patients, so I have on occasion seen patients develop diabetes due to a lowering of insulin.

Heart conditions

Heart problems may lead to impaired blood flow to the rest of the body, which, subsequently, will lead to a reduced supply of nutrients and oxygen. This in turn will cause feelings of fatigue. Since pains in the chest and arms, as well as an increase in heart rate, are common signs and symptoms of cardiac disorders, the sufferer will often interpret these signs as an impending heart attack. However, these symptoms are very common in ME/CFS and FMS. After listening to the patient's heart and running other tests, such as an electrocardiogram (ECG), the doctor should be in a position to discount heart disease as the cause of the problem. I have seen some ME/CFS patients in a serious state of anxiety over their chest pains and palpitations. Practitioners should be aware of the distress these symptoms cause and ensure the patient is satisfied that a cardiac arrest is not imminent.

Lung disorders

Oxygen depletion occurs if the lungs are not functioning correctly, as in the case of COVID-19. This will result in fatigue within the muscles and since ME/CFS can leave a person feeling breathless, lung function, as well as heart rhythms, should be thoroughly investigated.

Bowel and kidney disorders

These should be eliminated from the investigation, as the resultant metabolic changes that can occur will often lead to fatigue. Many patients suffer from irritable bowel syndrome (IBS) and gut dysbiosis, as mentioned in Chapter 5.

Glandular fever

One specific disease that is frequently mistaken for ME/CFS, and vice versa, is infectious mononucleosis (better known in the UK as glandular fever), which results from infection by the Epstein-Barr virus (EBV). An analysis of the blood will reveal a large increase in mononuclear, agranular white cells. This is why another common name for the disease, especially in the USA, is 'infectious mononucleosis' or simply 'mono'. An antibody test on the blood, such as the Paul Bunnell test, or the mono spot test, will confirm if the signs and symptoms are caused by glandular fever. The test is readily available at your doctor's clinic.

EBV infection is one of the most common triggers of ME/CFS and so antibody blood tests on patients often reveal EBV IgG, which, as explained previously, shows that the patient has had the disease in the past.

Addison's disease

Addison's disease is a hormonal disorder, which can cause fatigue, and plagued American president John F Kennedy (1917–1963), for much of his life. It is due to a disturbance in the normal functioning of the adrenal glands, situated next to the kidneys. The dysfunction leads to a deficiency of the hormones produced by the adrenals, such as adrenaline (known as epinephrine in the USA, as I've said). The condition is improved by hormone replacement therapy and, often, steroids.

Patients with Addison's disease usually present with muscle wasting and a darkened pigmentation of the skin. Their blood pressure is often lowered, and sufferers may lose their appetite and experience nausea and vomiting. Although there are some similarities between this disease and ME/CFS, the skin discolouration, a drop in the serum levels of the adreno-cortical hormones and a fall in blood pressure are all signs of Addison's that are easily detectable by clinical tests.

Other hormonal disorders

In ME/CFS it is very common for hormone levels to be slightly higher or lower than normal and this is due, primarily, to the hypothalamus not functioning correctly. Many other primary hormone disorders, such as hypothyroidism, thyrotoxicosis, diabetes mellitus and hyperparathyroidism, may cause symptoms common to ME/CFS. These disorders can be verified by means of blood tests.

Thyroid function tests should be carried out to monitor the production of thyroxine (T4) and triiodothyronine (T3) in the thyroid gland. Thyroid-releasing hormone (TRH) is secreted by the hypothalamus and stimulates the production of thyroid-stimulating hormone (TSH) from the anterior pituitary gland. TSH in turn stimulates the production and release of T4 and T3 from the thyroid. Blood tests for TSH, T3 and T4 should be done in order to verify that the thyroid is functioning correctly.

When dealing with hormone problems affected by stressors, the first pathway that comes to mind in medicine is not the hypothalamus–pituitary–thyroid (HPT) axis but rather the hypothalamus–pituitary–adrenal axis (HPA). The adrenal glands are involved in the production of hormones such as cortisol, which is often referred to as the 'stress' hormone, as it is the main hormone released in stressful situations. It affects blood sugar levels, regulates metabolic processes and helps immunity plus also has been shown to support:

- memory function in the brain
- aldosterone production, important in blood pressure regulation
- DHEA, important in the production of testosterone and oestrogen
- adrenaline (epinephrine) and noradrenaline (norepinephrine), both of which are also important in the fight-or-flight response to stress and crucial in the functioning of the autonomic nervous system.

As many people know, serotonin (5-HT) is an important neurotransmitter in the central nervous system, where it modulates circuits involved in mood, cognition, movement, arousal and autonomic function. The adrenal medulla (the inner part of the adrenal glands) is now known to store amounts of serotonin and so is part of the neuroendocrine control of the body under stress. So, basically, if the hypothalamus is affected by toxic overload it can directly lead to a dysfunction of both the thyroid and adrenal glands leading to a possible fatigue state.

Endometriosis

Endometriosis is a painful condition affecting many women in which the lining of the uterus/womb (the endometrium) grows outside of the womb. A study by scientists in Stanford concluded that more than a third of women with ME/CFS suffer from endometriosis[56]. This is not surprising since the lymphatic system transports endometrial cells to various parts of the body and so, if there is a problem in normal lymphatic drainage, it could affect endometrial cell transport.

Hormone disturbances due to dysfunction of the hypothalamus in ME/CFS and FMS may cause an increase in oestrogen, which is known to be another common cause of endometriosis.

Polycystic ovary syndrome (PCOS)

Another very common comorbidity affecting many women with ME/CFS and FMS is polycystic ovary syndrome (PCOS), which again is caused by hormone imbalances, such as high levels of androgens and insulin, which can occur if there is a toxic overload affecting the hypothalamus. Androgens such as testosterone are known as 'male hormones', although all women make small amounts of androgens which are the precursors to oestrogens. However, too much testosterone, which can be due to excess insulin, can prevent ovulation, and can cause extra hair growth and acne which are common signs of PCOS.

A study at Harvard university showed that a history of polycystic ovarian syndrome, and ovarian cysts were reported more often in ME/CFS cases compared with controls[57].

Myasthenia gravis

Nerves transmit their impulses by means of chemicals known as neurotransmitters, as I have explained in relation to serotonin, noradrenaline and others. When a motor nerve, which controls muscles, enters the muscle fibre, it releases the transmitter substance acetylcholine, which stimulates the fibre to contract. In the autoimmune disorder myasthenia gravis, which affects mostly young women, antibodies impede, modify or destroy the receptors for acetylcholine at the neuromuscular junction, which prevents the muscle from contracting and results in a marked weakness. The patient feels this frailty, especially at the end of the day. The muscles in the head are often affected first, causing difficulty in swallowing and chewing. The eyelids become very heavy and even holding up the head can become arduous.

The muscular weakness in myasthenia gravis can be quickly relieved by certain medications, such as edrophonium chloride. The rapid improvement is the key to establishing the diagnosis. As discussed in Chapter 5 (page 125), during the early stages of ME/CFS there is often an overproduction of acetylcholine in the brain, leading to too much choline[58].

Gilbert's syndrome

The healthy liver directly filters the blood and breaks down around 99% of toxins. The rest are carried away in the bile which is produced by the liver from the break-down of red blood cells. The toxic substances then travel into the intestines where they are absorbed by fibre and excreted.

In Gilbert's syndrome, a benign hereditary disorder, another cause of fatigue is due to the liver's inability to process the yellow bile pigment produced by the breakdown of red blood cells, bilirubin. This leads to varying amounts of bilirubin in the blood. The intermittently high levels of bilirubin cause people with Gilbert's syndrome to complain of mild, intermittent jaundice, occasional bowel disturbances and often some weakness and fatigue, usually in the morning. A blood test, liver function test or genetic test will confirm whether or not the patient's fatigue is caused by this disorder.

Detoxification in the liver involves two phases. In phase I, enzymes directly neutralise some chemicals by oxidation, but most need further processing in phase II by action of pathways involving a process known as conjugation – that is, binding toxins with chemicals that neutralise them or make them water-soluble and thus able to pass into the urine or bile stimulated by the activity of different enzymes. One of the phase II detoxification pathways is glucuronidation, which utilises glucuronic acid as a conjugation agent. Some studies have shown that Gilbert's syndrome may be due to an inability to detox through glucuronidation. This basically leads sufferers to be less able to clear toxic loads[59]. The treatment suggested by some is to help stimulate the glutathione pathway, another phase II detox pathway. Spinach, asparagus and avocados all contain high levels of glutathione so should benefit people with Gilberts syndrome.

Unfortunately in ME/CFS and FMS, if the control of the lymphatics is disturbed as well as the autonomic control of the liver, the entire detoxification process may be affected, disrupting all the phase I and phase II detoxification pathways.

Chronic infections

Besides Lyme disease (see page 182), other chronic infections, such as toxoplasmosis, should be eliminated in the diagnostic process. This infectious disease is caused by a microscopic parasite that can live inside the cells of humans and animals, especially cats and farm animals. Diagnosis of toxoplasmosis is usually conducted through blood tests.

Early stages of HIV infection may resemble symptoms of ME/CFS and can be ruled out by a blood test. There are also plenty of human herpes viruses, most commonly HHV3, 6 and 9, that have been found in many ME/CFS patients; they can trigger the disease but also be coinfections, muddying the waters and affecting improvement in patients. As with chronic bacterial infections that need long-term antibiotics, whether natural or pharmaceutical, treatment of chronic viruses requires long-term antivirals alongside the manual drainage techniques shown in this book. The long term use of antibiotics will affect the natural gut flora, so it is important to take pre- and probiotics to maintain a healthy microbiota which, as we now know, has a major influence on the brain's function (see Chapter 4).

Many ME/CFS and FMS patients have chronic fungal infections which could come from environmental mould and, like many cases I have seen over the years, mould is sometimes hard to find in old damp houses. As well as testing the patient, their home needs to be tested as thoroughly as possible to rule out any continuing fungal exposure.

Sleep disorders

There are many different types of disorder that can stop a good night's sleep and sleep is essential for health especially, as we now know, for the drainage of toxins from the central nervous system.

If a patient has a co-morbid sleep disturbance, then it can severely affect the other symptoms of ME/CFS and FMS. The prescription of sleeping pills, muscle relaxants or low-dose antidepressants all may help but they do not treat the cause of the problem and, indeed, in the long-term may cause further damage to the patient and worsen their overall symptoms.

Patients with poor sleep should have their sleep problems properly analysed at specialist sleep clinics using a process known as polysomnography. This procedure is used to collect many physiological parameters during sleep. A polysomnogram (PSG) examines the patient's sleep overnight. The sleep clinic will attach many different monitors to the patient. The procedure is painless and uses the following technologies:

- electroencephalogram (EEG) that measures the brain's wave patterns
- electrooculogram (EOG) measuring eye movement
- electromyogram (EMG) measuring muscle activity in the rest of the body
- electrocardiogram (ECG) measuring the heart's activity
- pulse oximetry used to measure the oxygen level (oxygen saturation) of the blood
- measurements of airflow and respiratory effort.

A PSG is considered to be the gold standard for diagnosing sleep disorders such as sleep apnoea, and sleep-related hypoventilation/hypoxia, nocturnal seizures, narcolepsy, periodic limb movement disorder (restless leg syndrome) and rapid eye movement sleep behaviour disorder[60].

Neuromuscular disorders

Neuromuscular disorders include multiple sclerosis (MS), which, although it sounds like and is often confused with ME, is a completely different disorder affecting the central nervous system. MS, also known as 'disseminated sclerosis', is a chronic inflammatory disease that can cause many similar symptoms to ME/CFS. Actually, since there is also no universally accepted theory why people develop MS, one could argue the possibility that MS is another neuro-lymphatic disorder and closer to ME/CFS than we think. Scientists in the USA in 2017 who proved the existence by MRI of lymphatic drainage in the human brain have even suggested that MS may be a possible disorder of this 'newly discovered' drainage system[61].

In MS, however, the fatty layer surrounding many nerves, known as the myelin sheath, is gradually destroyed. This sheath helps signals to move along the nerve and so patches of demyelination in the brain and spinal cord in MS lead to various symptoms, depending upon which signals are interrupted. It can mostly be detected by MRI scan and analysis of cerebrospinal fluid via a lumbar puncture.

Tumours

Malignant disease, such as undiagnosed lymphomas and other tumours, should be ruled out by investigations such as blood tests and, when necessary, scans such as MRI, and obviously biopsy when necessary. I always err on the side of caution and feel that it is at all times better to rule out serious pathology as soon as possible so the worry of impending doom is abated if the tests prove negative. If, however, the tests show a malignancy, nowadays the prognosis in most cancers improves with early detection, so, if there is any query as to whether there is a tumour, then I would always immediately refer the patient on to their doctor for further investigation.

There have been links made between ME/CFS and cancer and there is some evidence that there is a higher chance of developing non-Hodgkin's lymphoma (NHL) if you have ME/CFS. This isn't surprising as, the more stagnation in the lymphatics, the nastier the illness becomes, which could have devastating ramifications and eventually lead to cancer developing within the lymphatic system itself. Cindy Chang and colleagues have suggested that NHL may occur due to an infection or chronic immune activation[62].

Post-chemotherapy syndrome

As mentioned previously, cytokines can produce nasty side effects, such as sickness and lethargy and cognitive problems, as discussed in Chapter 4. Chemotherapy often involves the injection of large amounts of interleukins and/or interferons which target the cancer cells. However, being large protein molecules, excess cytokine activity requires the lymphatic system to function well; therefore, if the flow is in reverse, cytokines will build up in the central nervous system leading to what is often described as an overall mental fogginess leading to 'chemo-brain'. Breast cancer patients may find that it lasts for six months after chemotherapy[63].

Breast cancer and ME/CFS and FMS

Over the years I have seen more than a few patients who have had breast cancer prior to ME/CFS and some who we find to have the condition during the course of treatment. Thankfully, when we examine and treat the breast lymphatics in clinic, it is a perfect situation to be able to feel for any abnormality in addition to the varicose lymphatics discussed in Chapter 8 (see physical signs, page 241). As we are able to feel possible pathological changes very early on, thankfully, over the years, many lives have been saved. However, clinically we see many women who have had mastectomies and chemotherapy following breast cancer who later developed ME/CFS or FMS. This is not just a case of bad luck. There is a definite link between the treatment for breast cancer and the trigger for ME/CFS and FMS and there are two major reasons. Post-chemotherapy syndrome, as described above, and breast-implant illness (BII).

Breast-implant illness (BII) can develop after undergoing reconstruction or cosmetic augmentation with any type of breast implant. It is also known as autoimmune/ inflammatory syndrome induced by adjuvants (ASIA)[64, 65]. Some claim that the immune system is reacting to the silicone polymers that have been dispersed from the implant into the body. However, BII can occur with any type of breast implant regardless of the shape or content. One could argue that even the saline implants have a silicon shell that could still be toxic, but this is a very controversial subject due to regular legal challenges against the implant manufacturers that are very rarely successful.

The problem probably lies with the surgery itself and that is why it doesn't make any difference what the implant is made up of. My own opinion on post-surgical problems leading to ME/CFS were clarified when I watched a breast implant operation take place and saw the surgeon cut straight through many lymphatic vessels with a sharp surgical instrument known a spatula which is used to cut and retract the breast tissue.

If the patient has had cancer, their immune system has taken a major knock. Even if the problems started after a cosmetic operation to enhance or reduce the size or shape of the breasts, if the patient had predisposing factors overloading the sympathetic nervous system together with problems in the past that have already overstrained the neurolymphatic system, then the body becomes a 'ticking timebomb'. Just one trauma, such as surgical incision across the breast lymphatics, could be the final straw and the trigger for ME/CFS or FMS.

Even when viewing BII as a psychological illness, researchers have claimed that new treatments to help women who have had implants 'warrant serious consideration'[66].

Functional neurological disorder (FND)

The illness FND is diagnosed when there is a problem with the functioning of the nervous system with no physical abnormalities detected on any investigative tests, such as scans or EEGs.

FND patients can experience a wide range and combination of symptoms that are physical, sensory and/or cognitive. All the symptoms of FND can be seen in patients with ME/CFS and FMS, including in some severe cases, muscle paresis, tremors, spasms, whispering speech (dysphonia), loss of vision or double vision, non-epileptic seizures, blackouts and faints (syncope). As with ME/CFS, FND is uncommon in very young children and is more likely to affect women than men[67].

So, when does a patient with all the symptoms of ME/CFS or FMS receive a diagnosis of FND?

As we know there are no physical tests to support a diagnosis of ME/CFS or FMS that can be carried out during the clinician's initial examination (with the exception of the physical signs I discovered, which were validated in an NHS study detailed in Chapter 8)[68]. Nor do standard clinical neurological tests help a physician diagnose ME/CFS. FND, however, is diagnosed when clinical neurological tests are positive, but no obvious causation is detected.

Psychotherapy, speech therapy and occupational therapy are approaches that may help FND patients with the retraining of abnormal brain patterns. Specialised physiotherapy techniques have also been found to be helpful in encouraging automatic rather than focused movements[69].

Future research into FND may yet reveal that a problem with the neuro-lymphatic system also lies at the root of this rare but increasingly commonly diagnosed condition.

Multiple chemical sensitivity, sick building syndrome and aerotoxic syndrome

Most ME/CFS and FMS patients suffer from sensitivity to smells and substances, including scented products (e.g. perfumes), pesticides, plastics, synthetic fabrics, smoke, petrochemicals and paint fumes. There is a condition known as multiple chemical sensitivity (MCS), also known as 'idiopathic environmental intolerances' (IEI), that can cause many similar symptoms to ME/CFS and FMS, including fatigue, nausea and headaches[70]. A similar condition to MCS is sick building syndrome (SBS)[71], which can cause fatigue, cold, flu-like symptoms and headache, dizziness, nausea, eye, nose or throat irritation, difficulty in concentration, palpitations and oedema.

As with MCS, the cause of SBS is not fully understood; however, most accept it is due to effects from environmental neurotoxins. If these conditions are actually subgroups of ME/CFS then one can comprehend all these illnesses as being due to dysfunctional neuro-lymphatic disorders. Most sufferers of SBS experience relief soon after leaving the building, although long-term problems from the neurotoxins can occur leading to full blown ME/CFS. For many years some scientists have viewed these conditions all as primary environmental illnesses[72].

A new kid on the block, as far as environmental disorders are concerned, is aerotoxic syndrome, which name was first coined by Drs Chris Winder and Jean-Christophe Balouet at the International Congress of Occupational Health 2000. They claimed that short- and long-term ill-health effects were caused by breathing airline cabin air which was full of atomised engine oils and other chemicals used in aircraft. This condition affects air crew following long-term exposure at altitude to such atmospheric contaminants. This syndrome can become chronic following moderate to substantial exposures[73].

I myself have seen ME/CFS in aircrew over the years, and in people who due to their job or lifestyle travel extensively on aircraft. One female patient of mine who was a commercial pilot, suffered such severe symptoms she had to retire from flying early on in her career, with the condition causing her to be severely ill for many years. She was confirmed as having severe ME/CFS after being hospitalised 11 years earlier with viral meningitis. Although the meningitis was the trigger for her ME/CFS, a major factor was aerotoxicity, although she had many other predisposing factors. These included postural problems leading to recurrent back pain in her teenage years and glandular fever when 19 years old, with other immune problems when growing up. As her nervous system was so overwhelmed by the aerotoxins it took a long programme of treatment, with severe symptoms in the early stages of detox. However, she slowly recovered and three years after her initial treatment is now able to live a much healthier active life … away from planes.

Many pilots fly until their retirement without any major health issues and many people live in the same house or work in the same building as sufferers of environmental disease without succumbing to the aforementioned illnesses. So how are they immune to these illnesses?… What makes them different? The case above answers this question. The people who develop MCS, SBS or aerotoxic syndrome all possess a compromised neuro-lymphatic system from prior or coexisting problems. Once the drainage system has been disturbed and autonomic control has been damaged, then the body will find it increasingly difficult to cope with the build-up of neurotoxins via perfumes, chemicals in buildings or petrochemicals from jet engines, leading to the many symptoms I see every day in clinic. So, basically these environmental illnesses are all different forms of ME/CFS, just given new modern names to reflect the nature of the source of toxicity.

Auto-immune diseases

Diseases of the immune system, such as rheumatoid arthritis, systemic lupus erythematosus (SLE) and Sjögren's syndrome, are important to consider when diagnosing ME/CFS.

SLE is a chronic, autoimmune disease of the joints, skin, kidneys, brain, heart, lungs and gastrointestinal tract. It occurs mostly in women of childbearing age. A characteristic redness on the cheeks and nose of patients, the so-called 'butterfly rash', hair loss and a history of multiple miscarriages are all symptoms of SLE; however, some ME/CFS patients have similar symptoms.

Sjögren's syndrome, which often occurs together with other autoimmune disorders, affects the mucous membranes plus the salivary and lacrimal glands, causing dry mouth and eyes. Patients with Sjögren's can suffer from prolonged fatigue, rashes and dry skin.

While many symptoms of these autoimmune conditions are the same as those of

ME/CFS and FMS, the RA, SLE and Sjögren's patients usually have joint swelling as well as stiffness and pain; ME/CFS and FMS doesn't cause generalised swelling of the joints so this is an important differentiating factor. If the patient has swollen arthritic joints, it doesn't mean that they don't have ME/CFS or FMS, as patients could, and frequently do, suffer from more than one condition, as we have seen. However, if one notices swollen joints then one has to investigate the probability that they also have a comorbid rheumatological condition. Blood tests should then be carried out to identify the antibodies produced in most autoimmune diseases.

There is an opinion held by many researchers of ME/CFS and FMS that patients display characteristics of autoimmunity and these conditions may also be classified as auto-immune disorders[74]. In FMS there has been objective evidence that disease of the small nerve fibres such as C fibres is involved[75].

A PhD student, Ryan Whelan, discussed his research in Nevada at the 2020 online conference of The International Association of ME/CFS, examining a subset of ME/CFS patients who have a comorbid autoimmunity to small fibre nerves that form the autonomic nervous system[76]. This study is supported by other recent research which examines autoimmunity, neuroinflammation and small fibre neuropathy in the pathogensis of FMS and ME/CFS and suggests ME/CFS could possibly be an autoimmune disease of the hypothalamus[77].

I do believe these scientists conclusions are correct and there are some ME/CFS and FMS patients with autoimmune problems affecting their autonomic and hypothalamic control. This would lead to dysfunction of the neurolymphatic system. However, I do not think this is the case with most and although there will be a subgroup of patients who respond well to immunoglobulin therapy or other treatments of autoimmunity, most will need other treatments not related to auto-antibodies.

More than one disease

To summarise, this chapter has drawn attention to the complexities facing clinicians when trying to diagnose and treat patients with fatigue as a major symptom. It has also highlighted that there are many other origins of fatigue, and that only by comprehensive tests can other possibilities be eliminated from the investigation. However, it is also important to realise that even if tests show other reasons for the symptoms, it does not necessarily exclude the diagnosis of ME/CFS or FMS.

As I have said earlier in the chapter, it continues to amaze and worry me how many

ME/CFS patients are diagnosed primarily by the exclusion of other, better understood diseases. It is perfectly possible, and common, for people to suffer from more than one disease or disorder at one time. This is why my discovery of physical signs that are common to ME/CFS and FMS patients (page 241) is so important, and as shown in NHS research published in *BMJ Open*[68], they provide a much-needed aid in the diagnostic procedure and will be discussed in detail later in the book.

Chapter 7

The significance of toxins in ME/CFS

Slowly the poison the whole blood stream fills.
It is not the effort nor the failure tires.
The waste remains, the waste remains and kills.

William Empson (1906–1984) English poet

Case: Cathy's story

I was an independent type 'A' personality. I was excitable and outgoing and a highly active entertainer working on stage throughout the UK as a stand-up comic, musical theatre performer and the UK's top Jessie J Tribute Act. By day I was the managing director of my own children's theatre school called the Sparkle Theatre School in Preston, Lancashire.

I trained regularly with a personal trainer in the gym and in my 'rest' time I would go to a Zumba class. It was normal for me to go to bed at 2 am after being on stage and to get up at 5 am to write my next show.

I had just completed a theatre workshop and a photographic shoot for a new TV agent. I was also painting 30 garden fences and all my indoor furniture with the windows closed and the heating on.

In February 2014, aged 39, I suddenly collapsed onto my lounge floor and couldn't move being in chronic pain. The pain was so unbearable, it felt as though I had been hit by a truck, broken every single bone in my body and then been set on fire. My head was so inflamed, it felt as though it had been inflated like a balloon inside my skull causing intense pressure and severe cognitive malfunction. I didn't know who I was or where I was. I lost all sense of reality.

My symptoms matched dementia and my memory and thought processes were barely functioning. I couldn't move, speak, see or hear properly. I was extremely sick and dizzy and had tinnitus. My heart was pounding in chronic pain and it was racing so fast that I thought I was having a heart attack. My lungs burned in pain as I struggled to breathe, and my skin was flushed red and burning hot all over.

I was totally sober, but I felt as though I was incredibly drunk, as everything was a blur. It was like being in a living nightmare. I was absolutely terrified and I believed that I was going to die.

My body, barely 7 stone in weight, felt as heavy as lead. I couldn't lift my head or my dominant right arm, which had constant tremors. I was shivering and freezing cold, whilst sweating profusely at the same time. The pain level was so intense that my skin and bones couldn't stand to touch anything. I was bed-bound with severe vertigo, acute hyperacusis (sound aversion) and extreme light sensitivity. I wore ear plugs and had blackout curtains in my bedroom, but the slightest sound seemed so loud that it was excruciatingly painful. I couldn't watch television, use the computer or even read a book, as my vision was so impaired, with vertigo.

I couldn't understand even the most basic of tasks. I just lay there in chronic pain, drifting in and out of sleep.

I started having repetitive night terrors. I would wake up drenched in a hot sweat, with rigid spasms where my joints contorted (like in a febrile fit), coupled with complete numbness in both arms and feet, which felt as though a tight band had been tied around my elbows and knees, stopping the blood flow to my lower limbs. I experienced loud bangs in my head which felt like an electric shock, and my head would momentarily spasm, with flashes of light behind my eyes and temporary blindness. I also had electromagnetic sensitivity, and holding a mobile phone caused my fingers to burn.

I had chronic IBS and gallbladder, kidney and bladder pain. I also had gastric reflux and vomiting, plus multiple food and chemical sensitivities.

I had severe back, neck, head and shoulder pain. I also had blocked sinuses and my throat and glands were so swollen that I could barely breathe. This caused frequent and very frightening choking episodes in my sleep (sleep apnoea). The level of pain and fatigue was so intense that it hurt too much to cry. I lay in bed and couldn't move.

I was misdiagnosed by my doctor with 'anxiety' and prescribed citalopram antidepressants which made my symptoms worse, so they were stopped.

It took nine months before I was eventually referred to a neurologist who told me that I had 'anxiety, likely ME/CFS'. He said 'ME/CFS is anxiety; it is all in your mind and the pain you are experiencing is not real pain'.

I had numerous ambulance visits to hospital and many hospital tests including blood tests which showed extremely low blood markers, especially vitamin D. I had a brain scan which came back as normal.

I was finally 'officially' diagnosed by a second neurologist, a ME/CFS specialist, as having 'severe 'ME/CFS and fibromyalgia' in September

2014. I was told that I was one of the most severe ME/CFS patients that he had ever seen.

Desperate to recover, I tried numerous 'alternative' treatments without success. During one of these treatments, I was told that the symptoms I was experiencing were entirely psychological and that I could now 'get out of my wheelchair and walk again as I was cured'. That night I collapsed in extreme pain and was rushed into hospital in an ambulance. I was kept in A & E overnight and given morphine.

I was eventually referred to pain management and put on a large amount of pain medication. This included morphine patches, morphine drink, codeine, opioids, diazepam, round-the-clock paracetamol, ibuprophen and antibiotics each time an infection flared.

I was additionally referred to the local CFS services to start the NHS NICE guidelines' Graded Exercise Therapy (GET). At the CFS service, with severe vertigo and chronic sound and light aversion, flopped over the side of a wheelchair, I was advised to get up and walk five minutes one day and six minutes the next. I followed the NHS NICE guidelines of CBT, GET, PACING and pain medications to the letter. I found these exacerbated my symptoms.

Two years later, in 2016, I was diagnosed in hospital with 'bilateral vestibular hypo function' (inner ear vestibular damage) which had been severely affecting my balance, hearing and vision and causing vertigo. I was told by an ENT specialist that my career on stage was over.

Two months later, a plumber discovered a broken flue pipe from a gas boiler in my kitchen which had been emitting carbon monoxide and poisoning me, probably since it had been fitted 10 years earlier. A month later, I was recommended by a patient in recovery from ME/CFS to try Dr Perrin's treatment as it had really helped her.

Dr Perrin examined me and said that I had 'very severe ME/CFS and fibromyalgia' and that my symptoms and inflammation markers were so severe, and that my head was so inflamed, that he was surprised that I was smiling. He explained that it would very likely take a number of years of treatment to recover, and that full recovery was not guaranteed. He said that I had ME 'plus' carbon monoxide poisoning, 'plus' vestibular damage 'plus' possible underlying chronic coinfections, and that would make recovery even more difficult but not necessarily impossible.

At this, I started to cry. Dr Perrin believed me. He didn't laugh at me or recommend more psychological therapy. He understood every single symptom I presented with, and not only that, for the first time in my life he could explain the reasons why I had been so sick for so long.

Prior to being diagnosed, I was asked by Dr Perrin to complete a medical and personal history form, and this included the following:
- I was a fast breach birth and had an excessive level of infections, viruses and allergies from birth, including parvo virus (aged 10 years) and glandular fever (Epstein Barr virus) (aged 17 years) plus recurrent tonsillitis for 25 years and had taken a large amount of prescribed pharmaceutical medications from birth.
- Ten years before I collapsed I had told my doctor that I had intense headaches and pressure on the top of my head which also felt like it was burning hot.
- Two years before I collapsed, I had a flu-like virus and vertigo. I pushed through and went on stage on New Year's Eve with vomiting and vertigo and collapsed after the show. I was wiped out for a number of weeks following this.
- I had been under a very high level of mental and physical stress over many years, in running two entertainment businesses, driving long distances and carrying heavy public-address speakers to and from work.
- I had been the victim of a number of assaults which were under police investigation.

- I had carbon monoxide poisoning and a high level of paint fumes exposure in my home from painting furniture inside with the windows closed and the heating on, as it was winter.

Dr Perrin explained that I am one of the most 'toxic' patients he had ever treated in 30 years. He said that he believed I had most likely had this condition for a very long time in order for it to be so severe.

In March 2020, when the Covid-19 pandemic lockdown began, my personal situation didn't change in any way, but to protect myself at this uncertain time, I stopped my treatments with Dr Perrin for almost three months. I kept up the daily self-massage [see Chapter 10] at home as well as the hot and cold treatments on the spine, under Dr Perrin's guidance, but found that my health rapidly deteriorated over this time and that the severity of my ME symptoms increased. I was in a great deal of pain, particularly in my stomach and gallbladder area, which consequently required hospital investigations.

When I was able to restart treatments with Dr Perrin, I felt safe in knowing that he had full PPE equipment and was following the strict protocols and guidelines. I felt an immediate relief in the level of pain and ME symptoms that I was experiencing, when restarting my regular treatments with Dr Perrin. It has taken several months to correct the physical decline in my health that occurred from missing my regular treatments.

Today in September 2020: Dr Perrin said that today, after four and a half years of treatments, that he is still draining toxins out of my system. He has succeeded in getting my lymphatic drainage and cranial flow moving more efficiently. The adrenaline-fuelled 'fight or flight' state which I have lived in all my life has switched off and I feel calm and at peace for the first time ever. Dr Perrin is additionally using a specialised osteopathic manual treatment to realign my spine, neck and jaw, and to unblock my inner ears. My ears have been so painful and congested with infections and fluid build-up over many years and now after these treatments the level of sinus congestion has reduced significantly. I can now breathe well through my nose.

Since starting treatments with Dr Perrin I have had numerous ENT infections, including tonsillitis, high fever viruses, gum infections with teeth extractions, ear infections and a mouth full of ulcers. I have also had weekly gastric flu-like symptoms with sneezing and coughing as everything clears, with outbreaks of hives, red spots and bruises all over my body.

My IBS symptoms and chronic gallbladder pain have reduced significantly and I no longer have gastric reflux. Dr Perrin no longer has to manually manipulate the drainage of my stomach every week in treatment.

The level of pain and inflammation in my spine, neck and head is reducing through treatments. The intense skull pressure and burning head pain, which I have experienced from childhood, have reduced significantly. I no longer take any medications at all.

I believe that had I been diagnosed with ME/CFS 40 years ago when I first started presenting with symptoms, I would not have become this severe.

My improvement with the Perrin Technique has been gradual and consistent and I am optimistic that my recovery will continue. I am very grateful for finding the Perrin Technique as this is the only treatment that has helped to improve my health.

Although Dr Perrin has explained to me that full recovery from 'long term very severe ME/ CFS' is not guaranteed, I am extremely positive and absolutely determined to return to the job I love on stage. Thanks to Dr Perrin's treatment, alongside his support and encouragement throughout, I believe that this will one day be possible.

Cathy Vandome, Preston, Lancashire UK

The word 'toxin' was coined in the late nineteenth century and is defined as 'an antigenic poison or venom of plant or animal origin, especially one produced or derived from micro-organisms and causing disease when present at low concentrations in the body'[1]. For simplicity 'toxin' is used in this book in the broader sense of any substance that is harmful to the body. Accordingly, mercury, which is a heavy-metal toxin, is from neither plant nor animal source but it is nevertheless a major toxin to the body. Nowadays there are many man-made toxins, including chemical weapons such as novichok, which is Russian for 'newcomer' but has been around since the 1970s. We definitely have a lot more to contend with today than in the 1800s!

Pollutants

Environmental pollutants have long been seen as major causative factors in neurodegenerative disorders, such as Parkinson's disease, although there may also be genetic factors that make a person more susceptible to that illness[2]. Studies have revealed major variations in an individual's ability to detoxify noxious agents and have shown that neurological disease may derive from an exceptional vulnerability to certain neurotoxins[3]. This susceptibility is to toxins from both external sources in the environment and from free radicals (see Chapter 4) and toxic chemicals normally found within the central nervous system.

A few examples of the different types of toxins are listed in this chapter. However, with over 144,000 chemicals in the environment, less than two dozen have actually been banned[4]. The US Government Office of Technology has estimated that up to 25% of all chemicals might be neurotoxic[5]. The US Department of Health has estimated that each year approximately 2000 new chemicals are produced and, no matter what safety procedures are taken, they are all – inadvertently or deliberately – introduced into the environment via the air, water or foodstuffs[6].

According to Julian Cribb, author of *Surviving the 21st Century* more than 250 billion tonnes of chemical substances a year are harming people and life everywhere on the planet. Worse still, according to the World Health Organization, around 12 million people die every year from diseases caused by the direct and indirect result of man-made pollutants.

The figures per year are frightening:
* 30 million tonnes of manufactured chemicals produced a year
* 400 million tonnes hazardous waste is generated per year

- Over 11 billion tonnes of coal, oil and gas is burned per year.

Not to mention the hundreds of billions of tonnes of waste products that are found in water and the food chain worldwide. Environmental pollutants have been discovered at the top of Mount Everest and at the bottom of the deepest oceans. Mercury is seen in the tissue of polar bears in the Arctic, and honeybees are dying globally from agricultural pesticides[7].

The sources of toxic exposure which have been implicated as potential causative factors of ME/CFS are listed below[8, 9, 10, 11, 12], with common examples. However, as one can see from the above figures, these are just the tip of the toxic iceberg that globally pervades our environment.

Air pollutants (indoor and outdoor)

- **Benzene** is a widely used chemical and is one of the top 20 chemicals produced in the USA. Outdoor air contains low levels of benzene from tobacco smoke, automobile service stations, exhaust from motor vehicles and industrial emissions. People may breathe in vapours from products that contain benzene, such as glues, paints, furniture wax and detergents. Breathing benzene can cause drowsiness, dizziness and unconsciousness; long-term benzene exposure affects the bone marrow and can cause anaemia and leukaemia[13].
- **Chloroform** is a colourless liquid with a pleasant, non-irritating odour and a slightly sweet taste. In the past, chloroform was used as an inhaled pre-surgery anaesthetic, but it is not used in that way today. Chloroform is used to make other chemicals and is formed in small amounts when chlorine is added to water. Other names for chloroform include trichloromethane and methyl trichloride. People are exposed to chloroform when breathing contaminated air and when drinking or touching the substance or water that contains it. Breathing chloroform can cause dizziness, fatigue and headaches and long-term exposure may damage the liver and kidneys. It can cause sores if large amounts come into contact with the skin[14].
- **Chlorofluorocarbons (CFCs)** are chemical compounds, consisting of gases, such as methane or ethane combined with both chlorine and fluorine. They were formerly widely used in industry, for example as refrigerants, propellants and cleaning solvents. Their use has been prohibited as they have

been held responsible for part of the depletion of the ozone layer and are now substituted by hydrochlorofluorocarbons (HCFCs) – which are now believed to cause liver disease[15].

- **Polychlorinated biphenyls (PCBs)** are a class of organic compound with one to 10 chlorine atoms attached to biphenyl, which contains benzene (see above). PCB mixtures have been used for a variety of applications, including hydraulic fluids, lubricating and cutting oil, and as additives in pesticides, paints, adhesives and plastics. People exposed to large amounts of PCBs suffer skin conditions such as rashes. Studies in exposed workers have shown possible liver damage[16].

- **Toluene**, also known as methylbenzene or phenylmethane, is used as an industrial feedstock and as a solvent. It is a clear, colourless liquid, which is found mainly in crude oil. It is also produced when making coke from coal. It causes disturbance of the nervous system. People are often affected by breathing in air in a toluene-contaminated workplace, mostly from automobile exhaust fumes, some paints, paint thinners, nail varnish, lacquers and adhesives[17, 18].

- **Tobacco smoke** contains nicotine, which is a stimulant of the nervous system leading to addiction. Medical research has determined that tobacco smoke together with its tar is a major cause of cardiovascular disease as well as respiratory diseases.[19].

- **Carbon monoxide**. A study by Knobeloch and Jackson in 1999 showed that chronic exposure to low levels of carbon monoxide (CO) can cause vague symptoms that are easily mistaken for other common illnesses. The authors argued that carbon monoxide exposure should be considered in the differential diagnosis of patients who present with chronic symptoms of headache, fatigue, dizziness, nausea and mental confusion – especially when the onset of these symptoms is during the winter heating season[20]. Furthermore, a later retrospective study was published in 2012 by Clarke and colleagues, who found that 4.3% of 1758 patients in emergency departments examined for non-specific symptoms, such as chest pain, breathing difficulties, headache and flu-like symptoms showed signs of carbon monoxide exposure that was unknown to the patient or treating physician[21].

Over the past 30 years I have seen many individual cases of patients who in their past were exposed to carbon monoxide fumes. This emphasises how important it is to have properly fitted and tested CO detectors and alarms in your home as well as smoke detectors. Those lucky enough to survive carbon monoxide poisoning may end up with a life full of physical and mental fatigue, with constant pain and a dysfunctional immune system and many more disturbing symptoms triggered by excess of carbon monoxide in their body, as seen in Cathy's story at the beginning of this chapter.

Food contaminants and additives

- **Cadmium** is a naturally occurring metallic element and present everywhere in our environment. It was first used in industrial batteries and as coatings for the protection of steel from corrosion. Under normal conditions, adverse human health effects have not been seen in the general population. However, long-term occupational exposure can cause severe harm to the internal organs[22]. It is also important to realise that cacao trees absorb cadmium through their roots and store it in their seeds which are the cocoa beans used to make chocolate. Environmental pollution and excessive use of fertilisers containing cadmium affect the levels in the soil and high amounts are also found naturally in volcanic soils. This means eating even pure dark chocolate, which is healthier than the milk and flavoured varieties, could potentially lead to a build-up of cadmium to dangerously high levels and affect your health.
- **Aspartame** is an artificial, non-carbohydrate sweetener (aspartyl-phenylalanine-1-methyl ester). It is commonly used in diet soft drinks and is often provided as a table condiment. In the European Union, it is also known under the E number (additive code) E951. Aspartame is one of the sugar-substitutes used by diabetics. Yet, along with other food additives and colourants, such as Brilliant Blue and Quinoline Yellow, aspartame has been shown to have neurotoxic properties[23].
- **Dioxins** are the common name of polychlorinated dibenzodioxins (PCDDs), which are major pollutants commonly occurring in the environment as by-products in the manufacture of some organochlorides and from natural sources such as volcanoes and forest fires. However, they are highly fat absorbable and so are found in many fatty foods and are easily accumulated in humans from diets high in fish and meat[24].
- **Bisphenols** are a group of over 40 chemicals, such as bisphenol-A (BPA), used to manufacture many forms of plastic products. They are commonly

found in food and beverage can liners, food packaging, toys and water bottles. BPA is one of the most-used chemicals in industry today and research published in 2007 has linked them to a wide range of health conditions affecting reproduction, brain and metabolic processes. So, eating fresh food is a much better option than canned or packaged food[25].

Soil contaminants

Fertilisers and pesticides used in agriculture inevitably find their way into the food chain and many, such as the weed killer glyphosate, have been linked with the predisposition to many serious diseases, for example non-Hodgkin's lymphoma[26].

As early as 1961, chronic fatigue was seen as a major symptom following long-term exposure to organophosphates[27], the main ingredient of many artificial fertilisers, so it is no surprise that organochlorides also found in many types of fertiliser have been found to be higher in ME/CFS patients compared with normal subjects[28].

Chlordane is a man-made pesticide, used from 1948, that leads to toxic exposure in farm workers, gardeners and pest control workers. Even though it has been banned in the USA since 1988, chlordane is still found, many years later, in the air of homes treated for termites. Most health effects in humans that may be linked to chlordane exposure are in the nervous system, the digestive system, the liver and the immune system[29].

Medical/healthcare contaminants

It is an unfortunate fact that pollutants can be picked up even in medical and healthcare settings, which ought to be safer than the home, workplace or external environment.

Heavy metals in dentistry and vaccines

Mercury has been implicated as a major heavy metal neurotoxin, leading to neurological dysfunction and oxidative stress. A primary source of mercury poisoning is the amalgam in dental fillings[30]. ME/CFS sufferers should be tested for mercury content in the blood. If it is high, seek out a dentist expert in replacing amalgam fillings. The most likely time during which mercury can enter the blood is during the process of inserting or extracting the filling. The procedure must therefore be carried out with the necessary safety precautions firmly in place. As already stated earlier in Chapter 4 (page 93), it is equally important that when any local anaesthetic is injected in the mouth it should be non-adrenaline-based. The usual anaesthetics administered by dentists contain adrenaline (epinephrine) which will over-stimulate the sympathetic nervous system and could have a disastrous effect on ME/CFS and FMS sufferers.

Long before the issues concerning the MMR vaccine were raised, mercury poisoning had been implicated in problems with vaccinations in general. Mercury is present in the preservative thimerosal (also known as thiomersal) that used to be the most common preservative in stockpiled vaccines. Vaccinations against cholera, tetanus, typhoid and influenza have been implicated as causative factors of ME/CFS[31].

Some pharmaceutical companies have taken thimerosal out of vaccines. However, **aluminium oxide**, yet another toxic metal, is used as an adjuvant in many vaccines (a substance that aims to increase the specific immune response towards the antigen). I suppose one can argue that aluminium is a little less poisonous than mercury but the many patients still suffering severe post-vaccination symptoms would disagree. Aluminium has indeed been also shown, like mercury, to exert neurotoxic effects [32]. The good news is that some vaccines are now finally produced without the metal-based preservatives or adjuvants. The preservatives now used are phenol and 2-phenoxyethanol which have both been shown to have toxic side-effects only in **large** quantities[33, 34] So finally patients can have vaccines without the extra risk of immediately worsening their illness. However these preservatives are also used heavily in the cosmetics industry and so, if the lymphatics are not draining as they should, it is plausible that these small amounts of toxins from vaccines and cosmetics over the years can accumulate to dangerous levels of 2-phenoxythanol and phenol being built up in the body with serious consequences. The main advice is to check with your pharmacist and insist on the healthier option if possible. Despite the risks, you need to remember that immunisation is important to reduce the spread of many diseases that threaten global health, especially now as I finish writing this book during the Covid-19 pandemic. Most of the world is in lockdown or practising social distancing and wearing masks in public, waiting for the world's scientists to develop a safe vaccine that will help return us to a more normal existence.

Many other heavy metals have been shown to affect the nervous system and they are probably a major factor in the disease process in some ME/CFS patients[34].

Chelation

If you know that there is a chance of increasing your heavy metal load through vaccines, or amalgam fillings at the dentist or being exposed to petrochemicals which have a high heavy-metal content, then you probably need chelation. Chelation is the chemical process of bonding with metals but is more often used in medicine pertaining to the removal of heavy metals by the intake of specific agents as, discussed in more detail earlier in Chapter 5 (see page 117). So, my advice is definitely to have the vaccines if needed, but, as there is a good chance that your toxic-metal load will increase, you should start taking the supplements detailed in Chapter 5 to aid chelation just before and at least a month after any vaccination.

Pregnancy, birth and breast-feeding

The doses of metal neurotoxins required to produce behavioural and/or sensory dysfunctions are low and may be cumulative, as for example with methylmercury exposure in adults[35]. The nervous system may be particularly vulnerable during foetal development. Some heavy-metal toxicants may exert their greatest effect *in utero* while others, such as lead, produce IQ defects in children, particularly the firstborn, if transferred through breast-feeding[36, 37, 38, 39, 40].

Heavy metals can cross into the mother's milk in breast-feeding, as the milk, even in its first form known as colostrum, given to the newborn in the first few days, is very fatty. Heavy metals, as with many other neurotoxins, are fat soluble and so easily bind to the fat molecules in milk. Breast milk and colostrum have a higher fat concentration than nervous tissue so heavy metals are attracted to them and drain out from lactating mothers. In other words, breast milk is a way of dumping toxins out, unfortunately into the newborn baby[40].

Breast milk is not just a magnet for heavy metals. In a UK government report *Toxic Chemicals in Everyday Life*, published in July 2019, the MPs on the Commons Environmental Audit committee concluded that toxins found in plastics, resins, furniture and electronics such as bisphenols, can reach babies via breast milk or by crossing the placenta in the womb[41].

The report followed three months of evidence from experts and received over 60 written submissions for this inquiry into chemicals in everyday use. It claimed that British women's breast milk had the world's second-highest levels of flame retardants, such as polybrominated diphenyl ethers found in furniture and building materials.

The report warned that the potential impact on health was frightening. The committee called for a ban on the most dangerous chemicals in food packaging and a reduction in the use of flame retardants in domestic furniture.

Breast milk is still better than bottled milk as it contains so many good nutrients that are necessary for the newborn baby. Breast milk also transfers antibodies, also known as immunoglobulins, from mother to child. All five basic forms of immunoglobulins – IgG, IgA, IgM, IgD and IgE – have been found in human milk, but by far the most abundant type is IgA. All these antibodies are essential to the baby's developing immune system. The milk sugar alpha1H found only in breast milk, essential to a baby's development, has also been shown to break tumours into tiny fragments that cancer patients can pass in their urine, without harming healthy tissue. So, I definitely agree with the slogan 'Breast is Best'. However, any female ME/CFS or FMS patient planning on starting a family should begin a chelation programme for six months prior to conception, as detailed in Chapter 5, to remove much of the heavy-metal load. Chelation during pregnancy carries the risk of side effects possibly harming the foetus so is not recommended.

Chemicals used in the home

Many consumers search for environmentally friendly alternatives to lead paints and coatings. The natural mineral zeolite is a volcanic rock with a high silicone content. Zeolite coating is deemed to be wear-resistant, strongly adhesive and compatible with paint. Research has found that zeolite coating can serve as an environmentally friendly, corrosion-resistant coating for aluminium alloys[42].

In addition to environmental impact, chemicals in paints and coatings can also compromise the health of individuals living and working in their vicinity. For instance, sick house syndrome is linked to volatile organic compounds (VOCs), chemicals that have a high vapour pressure at ordinary room temperature. To combat the negative effects of these chemicals, VOC-absorption paint was developed.

Trichloroethane has been used over the years as a general solvent, particularly for degreasing. Exposure to trichloroethane usually occurs by breathing contaminated air. It is found in building materials, cleaning products, paints and metal degreasing agents. Long-term exposure can lead to disease of the liver[43].

Aerosol propellants found in hair spray, deodorants and spray paints contain high levels of methylene chloride, which, when inhaled, affects the brain and liver, causing symptoms such as fatigue, lethargy, headaches and chest pain.

Analysis of the breath in residents in a New Jersey suburb in the USA revealed traces of many toxic compounds, including chloroform, benzene, carbon tetrachloride, trichloroethane and other harmful pollutants[44].

Treating chemical poisoning

Many of the known neurotoxins are chemicals that are widely used and spread throughout the environment. However, toxicity from low-level exposure to chemical substances can be cumulative and eventually cause health problems worse than exposure to large sudden doses of some very noxious poisons.

When you are prescribed a medicine you have to make sure that it does not badly interact with any other medication you may be taking. The same risks of harmful interactions are seen when a combination of different low-level toxins affect the same metabolic pathway, which can lead to damaging certain organs and their connections to the central nervous system. Common examples of many known substances that can interact and cause delayed neurological and psychiatric effects are methyl iodide, which is used in the manufacture of some pharmaceuticals and pesticides, manganese used in the production of industrial alloys and carbon monoxide, to name but a few.

Successful treatment of chemical poisoning requires early diagnosis and cessation of exposure; however, many of my patients are often only alerted to the dangers of neurotoxins when they sit down for their first consultation with me and by then they have been overexposed for many years.

As I have emphasised, one has to look at the long-term history to determine the multifactorial causation that is a feature of all ME/CFS cases. However, in every patient there is a significant aetiological trigger that sends the sympathetic nervous system spiralling out of control. Generally, the onset can be linked to a virus, but it is now accepted by most authorities that the aetiology and trigger can be induced by many different stressors, including exposure to chemicals in the environment[45].

Mobile phone contamination

Radiation exposure can cause the release of a range of toxic compounds in damaged tissue. Most of the problems come from radio frequency (RF) energy. This is the energy source making use of high frequency electromagnetic energy to power all kinds of applications. A survey of 11,000 Norwegians and Swedes found that many were suffering headaches and fatigue from RF from mobile phones. Risk of brain tumours in the temporal lobe has been shown to be increased by the use of analogue cellular mobile phones on the same side as the tumour[46]. Scientists working for the Radiation and Nuclear Safety Authority in Finland have found that exposing humans to one hour of mobile phone radiation affected the integrity of the blood–brain barrier, leading to larger toxic molecules passing into the CSF, with the potential of causing damage to brain tissue[47].

To add further complexity to this issue, damage is done according to the rate at which the body absorbs RF energy. This is known as the specific absorption rate (SAR) and changes in different bands of operation which are all tested differently by each country. Mobile phones are tested to check that they meet the safety standards. However most leading mobile phone companies usually have RF exposure legal warnings hidden away in their general settings, with advice that you should never carry or hold the mobile phone closer than 5 mm to your body, with some authorities advising the safe distance to be as much as 5 cm, or better still use the hands-free option and avoid metal phone casings that increases the SAR. As with other radiation exposure, the inclusion of supplements containing zeolite may help ME/CFS and FMS patients who have been subjected to excess RF energy. To reduce further exposure, patients should buy a blocking device that shields them from the harmful EMF radiation, as discussed in Chapter 6.

Environmental accidents and wars

Major environmental disasters occasionally occur – such as the sinking of an oil tanker, or a pipeline rupture that kills many fish and birds and, sometimes, harms entire ecosystems. However, in recent times one of the worst ecological black spots has been Kuwait during the First Gulf War (1990–1991), where millions of gallons of crude oil were pumped into the sea and part of an entire oil field was set alight. This has been associated with Gulf War syndrome which shares many symptoms with ME/CFS.

Gulf War syndrome

Vaccines have been also associated with Gulf War syndrome[48, 49]. Central as well as peripheral nervous system dysfunction occurred in the veterans of the first Gulf War (GWVs) who were exposed to both chemical and severe psychological war stresses[50, 51]. However, environmental factors could also be responsible for some of the disorders seen in GWVs[52].

Exposure to pesticides (particularly organophosphates), oil and smoke from the oil-well fires, depleted uranium, as well as vaccines, could all have contributed to the many cases of acute and chronic respiratory illnesses reported in GWVs. In fact, as many as 70% of those receiving two or more vaccines, given simultaneously during deployment, showed signs of acute or chronic respiratory illnesses. The war to free Kuwait from the invading forces of Iraq (1990–1991) has been described as the most toxic war in western military history[50] with at least 14% of US GWVs fulfilling the then CDC criteria for chronic fatigue syndrome[53] (see Chapter 2).

The research on GWVs has yielded another important conclusion: post-traumatic stress disorder was not a major factor, and that any soldiers diagnosed with this psychological disorder were mostly ill before deployment – at the time when vaccinations were at their highest level. In fact, occurrences of post-traumatic stress disorder lessened during deployment[54, 55]. This throws doubt on suggestions that GWVs are simply suffering from a psychiatric war syndrome.

Studies at the Neuro-immune Institute at NOVA South-eastern University in Florida revealed high levels of organophosphates in samples taken from Gulf War veterans. This was most probably from pesticides that were impregnated into the kit and uniform of the soldiers serving in the first Gulf War to prevent sandfly disease (also known as leishmaniasis), which is a parasitic infection transmitted by the bites of tiny sandflies indigenous to Kuwait and Iraq.

The US Department of Veteran's Affairs acknowledges that methyl carbamate organochlorine pesticides (lindane) had been used to treat uniforms. DEET was used on the skin as an insect repellent along with the use of other organophosphorus (OP) pesticides and pyrethroid pesticides (primarily permethrin) for specific applications by specially trained individuals.

Excess amounts of the neurotransmitter, acetylcholine, could eventually lead to high levels of choline in the brain. Some toxins irreversibly inhibit the action of enzymes that break down this chemical transmitter, leading to a surplus of acetylcholine, which becomes toxic to the nervous system. This has been seen in the organophosphate-exposed patients who served in the first Gulf War[56]. As discussed in Chapter 5, an increase in choline has been discovered in many patients with ME/CFS[57].

Effects of neurotoxins

As seen in this chapter, toxic chemical exposure can cause many serious conditions, including cardiovascular, kidney and endocrine diseases. The most common organ to be affected by toxins, however, is the brain, leading to fatigue, exhaustion, cognitive impairment, loss of memory, insomnia, depression, psychosis and other disturbing symptoms[58].

There are several specialised regions of the brain's ventricular system, termed circumventricular organs (detailed in Chapter 4). These 'windows' to the brain interact closely with the cerebrospinal fluid. These zones are chemical-sensitive regions that may react with toxins, sending messages to other parts of the brain, especially the hypothalamus.

The hypothalamus controls the hormonal (endocrine) system via a mechanism called biofeedback. Basically, the hypothalamus 'tastes' the blood to check how much hormone needs to be released into the circulation. It then sends messages to endocrine organs around the body to increase or decrease levels of the many different hormones. Since hormones are made up of large protein molecules, the blood–brain barrier (BBB), which normally protects against large toxic molecules, is extremely permeable in the region of the hypothalamus. This allows the passage of specific protein-transport molecules that enable huge molecules to pass through the BBB. Thus, the most permeable region of the BBB is at the hypothalamus, facilitating its ability to monitor hormone levels in the blood. This increased permeability, together with the aforementioned messages from these receptor sites, makes the hypothalamus the most vulnerable region in the brain to suffer a toxic insult from large molecular chemicals, such as cytokines and opioid peptides mentioned in Chapter 4.

Autonomic dysfunction has long been associated with many toxic substances, especially following exposure to organic solvents, with some people exhibiting signs and symptoms of peripheral neuropathy. Under normal conditions, most of the BBB protects the central nervous system from rapid fluctuations in levels of ions, neurotransmitters, bacterial toxins, growth factors and other substances. The permeability of the BBB has been shown to be increased by stress[59].

Each organ or tissue may act as a discrete target for some toxic substances, which may lead to dysfunction of the whole organism. Specific molecules within a particular cell type act as primary targets. Some neurons are less susceptible to toxic damage, leading to regions of the brain that are not as sensitive to toxins.

Diet and toxicity

Exposure to chemicals affects people in different ways depending on several factors. Diet plays a crucial part in the body's ability to withstand toxicity. Toxins can be produced from non-toxic foods that we eat, building up in the central nervous system, liver or kidneys.

Trace elements, which are often used as supplements for good health, may become toxic if ingested in too high a dose. One thinks of selenium, for example, as a promoter of health, but it may be taken up from the soil by certain plants, such as species of the *Astralagus* genus, in sufficient quantities to render those plants toxic. Chronic selenium poisoning in animals, known as alkali disease, leads to cases of livestock with lameness, lack of vitality, hair loss, depressed appetite and emaciation[60].

Healthy food may not be properly digested or absorbed. The person may have a leaky gut due to injury of the intestinal wall, leading to semi-digested food entering the bloodstream[61, 62], causing immune responses, which create further toxicity. Also as discussed in Chapter 5, even fruit and vegetables, especially non-organic ones bought in supermarkets around the world, often contain a cocktail of toxic chemical preservatives and enhancements which will aggravate the situation.

Damage to the lining of the alimentary canal may be caused by a variety of irritants, the most common being alcohol, aspirin, gluten and the yeast *Candida albicans*[63]. Deficiencies in some vitamins, proteins, essential fatty acids and minerals are known to lead to poor intestinal cell growth, causing increased permeability of the gut wall[64].

As discussed in Chapter 4, the gut's microbiome (resident bacterial and other microbes) is essential for the production of most of the chemicals used by the nervous system. Toxins in the gut destroy many of the 'good' bacteria and render the body incapable of producing the essential neuropeptides necessary for a healthy brain. This further exacerbates the toxic soup building up in the central nervous system in ME/CFS and FMS.

Predisposition to toxicity

Previous exposure to toxins will increase an individual's sensitivity to further toxic insult. Some people have a greater genetic ability to detoxify while, unfortunately, others are more likely to experience more severe symptoms from toxic causes due to their individual genetic predisposition. Likewise, one's prior state of health, with the emphasis on the immune system, is a major significant factor to consider when assessing human ability to withstand exposure to poisonous chemicals. Age is important, with children much more susceptible to toxic overload than adults, because of their faster rate of absorption and smaller body weight – hence the smaller dosages of prescribed medicine allowed to children[65].

Several chemicals have the potential to induce autoimmune diseases[66, 67, 68] such as systemic lupus erythematosus, commonly known as 'lupus' or 'SLE'.

Genetic susceptibilities have been discovered in diseases such as autoimmune hepatitis[69]. The immune profile and genetic predisposition in some ME/CFS sufferers is likely to render these individuals more prone to toxic attack. This has been termed 'ecogenetics'[70].

Also, let us not forget epigenetics, mentioned in Chapter 5, where gene expression can change due to external influence, such as increased toxins. As shown earlier in Chapter 3, important genetic research is taking place in the USA on people with neuroimmune disorders and looking at a possible genetic predisposition to ME/CFS. With the largest ever genetic study on 20,000 ME/CFS patients, about to begin in the UK in 2020, scientists hope to learn much more about genetic predisposition to this disease.

The main emphasis of this chapter is to highlight the fact that our bodies are constantly under siege by thousands of poisonous agents, yet many of us remain healthy. The reason for this is that the healthy body is able to drain the toxins away from the brain. If this drainage system is not working properly and pumping the fluid in the wrong direction, problems will arise, and if the neuro-lymphatic system is dysfunctional, neuro-immune illnesses such as ME/CFS, fibromyalgia, and most probably Lyme disease, Gulf War syndrome and Alzheimer's, plus many other unexplained illnesses affecting the central nervous system, will occur.

Case: Mr A

One case I dealt with recently emphasises the serious effect of long-term toxicity. A 43-year-old man came to my Manchester clinic looking more dead than alive. His skin was a greyish yellow and his face was gaunt; he struggled to walk the few metres from his car. He had been forced to stop work due to ill health four years before he came to see me. He suffered multiple symptoms and suspected he had ME/CFS and that is how I came to meet this very brave man who was struggling big time just to exist.

He had worked for 13 years as a process operator in the packaging department at the manufacturing centre of a company which produces pharmaceutical products. He worked for many years as a facilitator without any protective equipment and later insufficient protection when working in an environment with dust from the manufacture of tablets which were known to cause many common side effects that plagued this unfortunate man for many years, such as: abdominal pain; decreased appetite; diarrhoea; nausea; constipation; vomiting; gastrointestinal spasm; glycosuria (sugar in the urine); electrolyte imbalance, epigastric discomfort; pulmonary oedema; renal impairment; respiratory disorders; hives; fever; jaundice; muscle cramps; rash; seizures; tremor; urinary retention; emotional instability; aggression; decreased alertness; anxiety; pain; confusion, delirium and delusions; headache; vision disorders; dizziness; postural hypotension; anaemia; hyperglycaemia; insomnia; weight increase; agranulocytosis; embolism and thrombosis; neuroleptic malignant syndrome; oedema; tachycardia; and severe skin reactions to name just a few.

These symptoms are from just nine of the many drugs produced in the plant.

Other tablets produced or packaged in the plant where he worked included antipsychotics and strong painkillers and at least 10 others with many other side effects.

He initially just had flu-like symptoms after which he repeatedly visited his GP complaining of difficulty breathing, with persistent coughing and fatigue and was eventually diagnosed as being severely anaemic and was given a blood transfusion. His continuing ill health had worsened and affected his lungs, spleen, prostate, liver, skin leading to many symptoms arising from the dysfunction of these organs and eventually his ill health had led to him being forced to stop work.

When I last saw him he was wheelchair-bound and sadly had many more complex severe health problems due to the long-lasting effects from all the toxins he had been exposed to. I am not a miracle worker and this was unfortunately such a severe case that my treatment alone would never be enough.

Chapter 8

The stages leading to ME/CFS and FMS

All truth passes through three stages. First, it is ridiculed.
Second, it is violently opposed. Third, it is accepted as being self-evident.
Arthur Schopenhauer (1788–1860), German philosopher

Case: Nicola's story

I was diagnosed with ME in June 1994, at the age of 26. Previously, I had been highly active. I was doing three jobs at the time, whilst actively involved with my three horses in my leisure time.

In December 1993 I went down with a flu-like bug over Christmas and New Year. On returning to work in January, it was apparent that something was seriously wrong. I had no energy and undertook several trips to the GP to get antibiotics for chronic suspected sinus 'infections'.

Whilst battling on at work, I was feeling more ill with every day that passed. My boss even suggested that I should take some time off but, being determined to 'drag' myself out of it, that fell on deaf ears. I collapsed and fainted one morning at my work from exhaustion. That was the beginning of what was to become many years of Hell.

Fortunately, and unusually for the time, my family GP was fantastic. He knew that I was previously a 'livewire', that I loved life and that I never usually halted. Now I was like a zombie, and he knew there was something seriously amiss.

Each day consisted of sleeping 20 hours out of 24, and barely being able to crawl to the bathroom. I was referred to Edinburgh Royal Infirmary in April 1994, where I was diagnosed with ME in June of that year. I remember the consultant breaking the news and wishing me 'The best of luck' as there was no known cure.

Despite being told that news, I tried every pill, every potion and every alternative therapy I could find in a bid to get well, or even to feel remotely better over the years.

One of the low points that I can remember was having a really bad bout of influenza. Despite being really ill with that, I was horrified to find that I could do more during the two weeks I was bedridden with the flu than I normally could. Three weeks previously, I had been unable to even cut up food and feed myself.

Summarising a very long story, (half of which I don't remember, as there are so many black holes in my memory) I came across the 'Perrin Technique' as a new way to treat ME patients. I Googled the nearest practitioner to me and booked an appointment with Rosalind Stuart-Menteth of Edinburgh and Peebles.

The first consultation with Rosalind was on 3rd August 2012. It was a revelation to me. It mainly consisted of discussion and examination. Towards the end of the session, she was gently probing down my spine when she reached a particular area and struck gold! Suddenly, my numb legs (which always felt like dead fish) started to tingle with the most amazing sensation. It literally felt like water was running down my legs. This was a cause for great excitement on my part! To have some sensation back in my legs after all this time was enough to convince me that I had to pursue this treatment further. I embarked on a 12-week course, keeping notes every day. It was the beginning of a journey to reach light at the end of the tunnel. It soon became apparent that the treatment was having quite some effect.

It has to be noted here (and I'm sure that fellow ME sufferers will agree) that our outward appearance does not always show just how ill we really feel at any given time. What happened next was interesting, and very positive.

Each treatment seemed to generate a delayed reaction. I would start to 'burn up' with extreme heat rashes, I had golf-ball-sized lumps on my lymph glands and even had boils starting to erupt. Whilst this sounds quite extreme, I embraced it all, knowing that it was being caused by the release of toxins which had built up in my body. Bearing in mind that I had suffered from ME for 18 years at this point, I knew that there would be some significant period of re-adjustment as my lymphatic system was in such a poor state. The plus points were very noticeable, however, and this was really exciting. After so many years of having numb, freezing cold legs and feet, sensation started to come back. Soon I started to feel that I had normal human legs again. It felt quite miraculous!

There were many other benefits, too. I've had numerous bizarre symptoms over the years, which I won't list here. Any ME sufferer will have his or her own personal and lengthy list of symptoms. Sometimes it's like watching a kaleidoscope. To my mind, anything that gives relief to a few symptoms is a massive bonus. I had to use a wheelchair frequently over the years. I don't need to do that anymore.

The last few years have been very stressful due to family troubles. I don't want to think what state of health I would be in today had I not had the benefit of this treatment. I'd probably be housebound or even bedridden.

I was fortunate to attend a seminar given by Raymond Perrin. It was extremely informative and helped to explain the reasons behind the various debilitating symptoms that we all suffer with. Having also been diagnosed as gluten- and lactose-intolerant two years ago, I am now pleased to say that I am definitely seeing light at the end of what has been a very long and difficult tunnel.

Thanks to my ever-loyal practitioner Rosalind, and guidance from Raymond Perrin, my health is significantly better than it was. They have not only given treatment in the present, but a clear hope for the future that my health can continue to progress in a positive manner.

Nicola Bower, Scotland
Patient of Rosalind Stuart Menteth, Registered Osteopath and Licensed Perrin Technique Practitioner, Edinburgh, Scotland

To treat ME/CFS and FMS successfully one has to understand the exact nature of the disease and what is going wrong with the body. Once one comprehends the stages (see Table 1 on page 239) that lead to ME/CFS and FMS, one can start to correct the disturbances, otherwise the treatment will be less effective and not as long-lasting.

The problem with my original hypothesis in 1989 was that it was too radical for most scientists and doctors to accept. The concept of lymphatic drainage of the brain and spine was totally in opposition to orthodox medical thinking of the last few centuries. As stated in Chapter 1, the lymphatic drainage of the central nervous system, which I have referred to since 1989 as the neuro-lymphatic drainage system (now also known as the glymphatic system), has now been proven to exist[1, 2, 3, 4].

In fact, there is now further visual evidence of the drainage system into lymphatic vessels which has been discovered in the membranes of the brain in both animal and human studies, and it can be visualised by MRI scanning (see Fig. 17)[5].

The scan in Figure 17, which was the first published visual proof of lymphatic drainage in a human brain, shows drainage in the perivascular spaces in the larger vessels of the brain, such as along the superior sagittal sinus in the centre of the image and then into the lymph vessels in the outer surface of the brain. However, there are many smaller perivascular channels that are too minute to be visualised

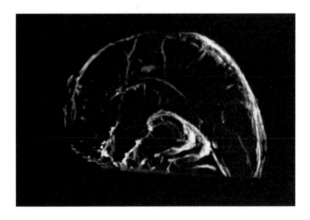

Fig. 17 Magnetic resonance image of lymphatics (shown in green in colour plate 2) in a 47-year-old woman's brain[5].

with this safer technique but were shown in the previous studies on mice.

The discovery that this drainage system exists underpins the basis of my technique and has been a major step in the acceptance of my work by the scientific and medical establishment. However, it amazes me that all the focus of the recent studies on the lymphatic drainage of the central nervous system (CNS) of mice, apes and humans has all been directed on the brain. The CNS includes the spinal cord and so the drainage of the brain via the glymphatic pathway is only part of the process. The perivascular spaces are found next to blood vessels lining the nerve roots that enter and exit throughout the entire length of the spinal cord and this area will hopefully be scanned using the new techniques developed to show the spinal cord's drainage, and scientists in the future will demonstrate how equally important the neuro-lymphatic system in the spine is in the development of ME/CFS, fibromyalgia and many other neuro-immune diseases.

If the drainage in the spine is so important, then the posture of the spine that maintains good flow is equally significant. So it was no surprise when researchers Hedok Lee, Helene Benveniste and colleagues, discovered at Stony Brook University, New York, that a lateral sleeping position is the best position to most efficiently remove waste from the brain. The findings published in the *Journal of Neuroscience* show how important side-lying is in ME/CFS and FMS and many other neurological conditions[6].

It is also no surprise that instinctively, the lateral sleeping position is the most common one in the animal kingdom… nature knows best!

Going back to my earlier studies, three predominant concepts surfaced from the clinical trials on ME/CFS patients carried out during my 11 years of research at the universities of Salford and Manchester. These were:

- The Perrin Technique led to significant improvement in treated patients.
- ME/CFS patients had no detectable gross brain abnormalities using standard MRI scans and that their muscle fatigue was due to functional causes rather than a muscular disease.
- A reduction in patients' symptoms was due to improvements in the neuro-lymphatic drainage system.

The clinical trials 1994 – 2005

I embarked on my clinical research in 1989 following the success of my treatment of the cyclist, Mr E, mentioned at the start of Chapter 1. My first paper was published in the *British Osteopathic Journal* in 1993[7]. The husband of one of my patients was a professor at the University of Salford, a large university in the Greater Manchester region with a major health sciences faculty. He showed my paper to his good friend, Professor Jack Edwards, a world-renowned bioengineer. Professor Edwards invited me to lunch with psychology Reader, Dr Pat Hartley. Over the next three years we conducted the first clinical trial, which eventually led to the paper: 'An evaluation of the effectiveness of osteopathic treatment on symptoms associated with myalgic encephalomyelitis: a preliminary report', published in the *Journal of Medical Engineering and Technology* in 1998[8].

Hardly any research into ME/CFS was being funded by grant bodies in the 1990s, and most of the research trusts that were offering funding stipulated that it had to be paid into another charitable trust. Consequently, the Fund for Osteopathic Research into ME (FORME) was born on 23 February 1995 at the Midland Hotel, Manchester. The FORME trust was set up, together with a group of my patients and friends, to help raise research funds and awareness of the physical nature of ME/CFS. Thanks to donations from grateful patients, and from interested members of the public, and with donations from other trusts, particularly the David and Frederick Barclay Trust, we raised around £250,000 to fund the entire project.

Once you have the funding and the volunteers for a clinical trial, you need official approval from the local health authority research ethics committee. This is even

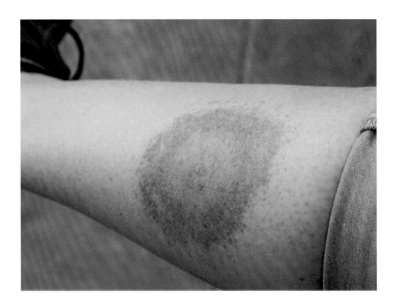

Plate 1: The 'bull's eye' rash (erythema migrans) indicative of a tick bite infected with the Lyme disease bacterium *Borrelia burgdorferi*. (Figure 16, page 183)

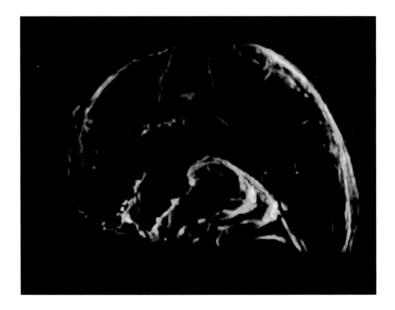

Plate 2: Magnetic resonance image of the lymphatics in a 47-year-old woman's brain.[5] (Figure 17, page 235)

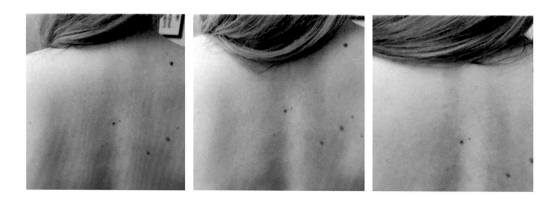

Plate 3: Abnormal flare response following stroking (a) after about 20 seconds following rub of fingers; (b) around 20 seconds later; (c) around a minute after initial strokes showing sustained flaring. (Figure 20, page 245)

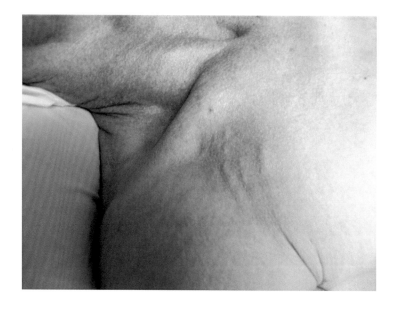

Plate 4: Right subclavicular varicose lymphatics, lacking the blueish hue of varicose veins, in a patient with ME/CFS. (Figure 24, page 249)

more rigorous than a US congressional hearing, with a group of health authority administrators, doctors, scientists and legal representatives. We encountered many complex obstacles, but eventually, by changing the protocol a number of times and by satisfying every question, we were able to start the research projects. Research ethics committees are without doubt necessary (established following the horrors of the experiments conducted by the Nazis during World War II), but one wonders how many research projects, which could improve our knowledge and treatment of disease, do not go ahead due to the exhaustive and detailed process of obtaining the necessary approval.

The efficacy of my manual approach was tested using two separate clinical trials, both with groups matched for gender and age. In the first trial, 33 ME/CFS patients were treated using my technique and a group of matched ME/CFS patients were given any other treatment of their choice. The second trial was a smaller study using three groups of nine subjects each. The first group consisted of ME/CFS patients who received the Perrin Technique. The second group was made up of ME/CFS patients who did not receive my treatment, with the third comprised of nine healthy volunteers. This research was carried out at the Universities of Salford and Manchester between 1994 and 2005 under the guidance of Professor Edwards, Dr Hartley, biomechanics Professor Jim Richards, neurobiologist Dr Vic Pentreath and neuro-radiologist Professor Alan Jackson.

1. The first study examined the change in symptoms following a year of treatment.
2. The second study repeated the first study and examined the possible mechanisms of any improvement.

The studies were designed to develop a greater understanding of the cause, diagnosis and treatment of ME/CFS. Phase 1 of the research trials examined overall symptom change. It included the patient completing a selection of self-report questionnaires, nowadays referred to as 'patient-related outcome measures' (PROMS), which were answered periodically over the course of the year-long treatment. These eight questionnaires related to pain, feelings of depression, anxiety, cognitive function, sleep and overall health. With post-exertion fatigue being a major symptom of ME/CFS, we tested the effects of the treatment by the amount of power the quadriceps muscle in the thigh lost after a specific isometric exercise designed to tire this muscle, in which the subject pushed their right shin against a pressure pad with no actual movement of the leg. The pad was connected to a gauge that measured force.

The second trial, which included the same PROMS assessing symptom change as the initial trial, was divided into two parallel phases, phases 2 and 3. Phase 2 primarily took the form of brain analysis using magnetic resonance imaging (MRI) to confirm if brain abnormalities seen in previous research[9, 10, 11] were found in sufferers of ME/CFS. Central lymph scans were also carried out to see if there was any possible enlargement in the thoracic duct of ME/CFS sufferers. In phase 3, isometric tests were carried out as in phase 1 but with much more accurate computerised equipment[12].

The precise objectives of this research were:

1. To determine whether or not spinal problems were related to the signs and symptoms arising from ME/CFS.

2. To test if my method of osteopathic treatment reduced symptoms associated with ME/CFS compared with those of a matched control group, who received no such treatment.

3. To reveal the sustainability of any improvement by a one-year follow-up study and to investigate the likely replication of the initial study, thus strengthening the argument of a relationship between set osteopathic procedures and the improvement in signs and symptoms associated with ME/CFS.

4. To determine if there is a visible disease process in the brain that may be causing the symptoms of ME/CFS.

5. To determine if there is any intrinsic muscle disorder that may be causing the symptoms of fatigue in ME/CFS.

Conclusions of the research

1. The first stage of the research concluded that the major signs and symptoms associated with ME/CFS showed an average of 40% improvement in the group having the Perrin Technique treatment compared with an average worsening of 1% in the control group. Muscle fatigue was also shown to be significantly reduced in the treated group.

2. In the second stage of the trials it was concluded that muscle fatigue is of a functional nature rather than resulting from any known muscle disease. Secondly, following scanning the brain with magnetic resonance imaging (MRI) to examine the white matter, blood flow and cerebrospinal fluid flow, we discovered that in the ME/CFS patients there was no detectable pathological structural abnormality in the brain. This contradicts other studies that have shown brain anomalies[9, 10, 11]. This conundrum may be explained by there being

severe cases of ME/CFS in which the brain structure may be permanently damaged. However, our research showed that even though a person may have ME/CFS, it does not mean, necessarily, that any damage will be visible on scans. The fact that no major physical abnormality was seen in any of our ME/CFS patients suggests that when employing the standard scanning techniques used in hospitals today, visible structural trauma of the brain is uncommon in ME/CFS rather than the norm.

3. Thirdly, when examining the effects of the treatment programme in both clinical trials, it seemed likely that the improvement in the muscular fatigue together with the overall reduction in all ME/CFS symptoms was a result of increasing toxic drainage from the central nervous system.

The downward spiral

With careful consideration of these clinical findings, I have formulated a theoretical model to explain the cause, signs and symptoms of ME/CFS and the effectiveness of my treatment regime. My belief is that the osteopathic approach does not set out directly to eliminate poisons from the body; rather, it facilitates the patient's own in-built mechanisms responsible for toxin elimination. By reducing the intensity of incoming sympathetic impulses, by means of relaxing the muscles and improving circulation and drainage, the signs and symptoms of ME/CFS gradually diminish.

My theoretical model of the stages of development of ME/CFS (see Table 1) may be applied to all the ME/CFS and FMS patients I have seen since the late 1980s.

Table 1 The stages of development leading to ME/CFS and FMS

Stage 1	Patients with ME/CFS and FMS all seem to have a predisposing history of sympathetic nervous system overload:
a	Physically – by being an overachiever at work, during study, or in sports. Rarely, it may be the opposite by being too sedentary.
b	Chemically – by constant exposure to environmental pollution.
c	Immunologically – by chronic infections or hypersensitivities to multiple allergens.
d	Psychologically/emotionally – by family and/or work-related mental stress.

Stage 2	In Stage 2 either a or b can occur before the other or they can occur concurrently, depending on the causes of the restricted flow of lymphatic drainage in the head and spine.
a	Lymphatic drainage from the brain shows signs of being impaired, mostly in the cribriform plate region of the ethmoid bone above the nasal passages, the neural pathways along the optic nerve behind the eye, the trigeminal pathways in the region of the upper jaw and the drainage along auditory pathways.
b	Lymphatic drainage of the central nervous system is also subject to disturbances in the spine, usually in the cervical or thoracic region, due to either a congenital, hereditary, or postural defect and/or prior trauma.
Stage 3	Toxic effects due to the long-term dysfunction of the central nervous system drainage will compound the chronic hyperactivity of the sympathetic nervous system; this further overloads the hypothalamus and subsequently, the sympathetic nervous system.
Stage 4	A final trigger factor strikes, which usually arises from a viral infection, but may be physical or emotional in nature.
Stage 5	There will be a disturbance in autonomic, as well as hormonal, function, because toxins in the cerebral blood flow and ventricular system directly affect control of the hypothalamus. Hormonal transport within the cerebrospinal fluid may be directly affected by toxic overload.
Stage 6	Dysfunction of sympathetic control of the lymphatics, especially the thoracic duct leads to a reflux of toxins in the resultant retrograde lymph flow, causing varicose lymphatic vessels predominantly in the neck, chest and abdomen. This also further reduces flow of cerebrospinal fluid into the lymphatics.
Stage 7	Further backflow of toxic drainage into the central nervous system, due to the retrograde lymphatics, results in increased hypothalamic dysfunction and an even greater disturbance of lymphatic drainage.
Stage 8	The continuing irritation of the sympathetic nervous system results in further systemic disturbances, leading to chronic adaptive states known as ME/CFS and FMS.

The physical signs of ME/CFS

The concept of ME/CFS being primarily a biophysical rather than a psychological disorder is foreign to most of the medical profession. However, many doctors recognise that ME/CFS causes physical signs and symptoms[13, 14, 15, 16]. Physical components have always been included in the internationally recognised criteria that verify the diagnosis of ME/CFS[14]. These include sore throat, tender lymph nodes in the neck and armpits, and muscle and joint pain. In the 31 years since I started to examine and treat patients with ME/CFS and indeed fibromyalgia, repeated patterns of physical signs have emerged among virtually all the sufferers that cannot be dismissed as pure coincidence. All physical phenomena seen in ME/CFS can be understood when the disease is viewed as the consequence of impaired drainage of the central nervous system coupled with a dysfunction of the sympathetic nervous system. These signs have also been present in the fibromyalgia patients I have seen over the many years in practice, which is another reason I feel the two conditions share a common pathophysiology, the main difference being that FMS patients compared with the ME/CFS have more intense widespread pain in all parts of the body. The main physical signs are shown in Fig. 18.

1. Longstanding thoracic spinal problems (often with flatness, redness, heat or pain in mid-thoracic spine)
2. Varicose lymphatics
3. Perrin's point
4. Coeliac plexus (solar plexus) tenderness
5. Abnormal cranio-sacral rhythm (cranial rhythmic impulse)

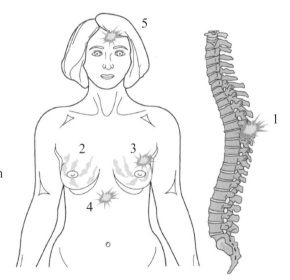

Fig. 18 The observed physical signs of ME/CFS.

These regions of tenderness or dysfunction have been identified in all ME/CFS sufferers seen by the author since 1989 in both the university and clinical settings.

1. Longstanding thoracic spinal problem, sometimes with notable tenderness at T4/T5/T6 segments.
2. Varicose lymphatics.
3. Perrin's Point.
4. Coeliac plexus tenderness.
5. Disturbance in the cranial rhythmic impulse (cranial rhythm).

Postural/structural dysfunction of the thoracic spine

A prevailing observation in the clinical findings of ME/CFS is a mechanical disorder of the thoracic spine, which may be due to bad occupational posture, or related to a congenital event or genetic predisposition.

There is much truth in the famous song *Dry Bones* by the Delta Rhythm Boys, you know the one which has the immortal lines

> 'Your toe bone connected to your foot bone
> Your foot bone connected to your heel bone ...'
> and so on and so on until we get to the top of the body ...
> 'Your back bone connected to your shoulder bone
> Your shoulder bone connected to your neck bone
> Your neck bone connected to your head bone
> I hear the word of the Lord.'

Any physical (genetic or otherwise) defect in one part of the body can have a major influence on another section. For instance if one has one leg slightly shorter than the other it will lead to a compensatory lateral shift in the spinal column causing possible drainage problems in the spinal perivascular pathways and extra strain on the surrounding soft tissue, which includes the muscles, ligaments and fascia. This can then create extra pressure on the the blood and lymph vessel walls, causing disturbed circulation and drainage. Likewise an upper spinal problem can create a disparity in the forces placed on the legs and feet. This actually happened in clinic when a girl came in wearing callipers on her left lower leg. This was due to a weakness in her left ankle that for years had baffled her doctors. I discovered an upper spinal scoliosis (side-bending) that placed too much pressure on her left side leading to eventual pain in the left leg, foot and ankle. Over the years she had compensated for the pain by using her right dominant side much more, resulting in the eventual weakness in her left ankle and foot requiring support.

Another case that illustrates the genetic predisposition to postural related problems was a boy with ME/CFS who was tongue tied at birth which was a familial complaint. The tethered oral tissue when born tongue-tied can lead to the head being tilted low and forward. This stooped posture can affect the neurolymphatic drainage of the spine and surrounding soft tissue with the resultant neurological and circulatory dysfunction.

The most common structural disturbance that I have seen in ME/CFS and FMS patients was a flattening of the curvature in the mid-thoracic spine, usually accompanied by the presence of a kyphotic dorso-lumbar area (an abnormally exaggerated convex curvature in the lower back). An example of this defect is shown in Figure 19a which can be compared with the healthy posture shown in Figure 19b. This postural defect is often caused by a prior condition, spinal osteochondrosis, also known as Scheurmann's disease, which affects spinal development in adolescence, and which may have occurred years before the onset of the characteristic symptoms of ME/CFS and FMS.

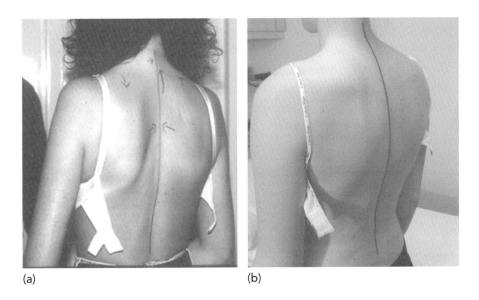

(a)   (b)

Fig. 19 Comparative photographs showing a flattened mid-thoracic spine. Photo (a) shows the familiar flattening of the mid thoracic spine seen in many ME/CFS and FMS patients. This differs from a normal spinal posture in the healthy subject, photo (b).

Also, when one feels the skin lying over the thoracic spine, it is usually hotter (but not always) than other regions of the trunk which may indicate an underlying area of inflammation. Another common finding in this region in ME/CFS and FMS are trophic changes – that is, changes due to interruption of the nerve supply which affects nerve interactions with other cells, such as the skin, leading to molecular changes including dryness, spots and rashes. Scars are also sometimes seen, indicating previous injury or surgery in the region.

The triple response of Lewis

A test to see if the autonomic nervous system and the immune response are overworking in this region is to examine the response to rubbing fingers down the sides of the spine. The practitioner rubs three times with firm pressure which in healthy people elicits what is known as the 'triple response of Lewis'.

This response is due to the neurological reflex that produces a release of histamine from mast cells that are part of the local immune response. First a red line is formed due to blood capillaries swelling, then the redness around the mark flares out due to nervous system control over surrounding blood vessels, and then the fluid leaves the capillaries leading to a loss of colour with small, itching elevation of the skin, known as a wheal.

With ME/CFS and FMS patients, due to the neuro-lymphatic drainage dysfunction in the spine, this stroking action leads to a disturbed response. Most commonly you see the redness and flaring just getting more apparent after the test, as seen in Figures 20 a–c, which are photos of one of my patients taken at intervals over a minute following the three downward rubs of my fingers.

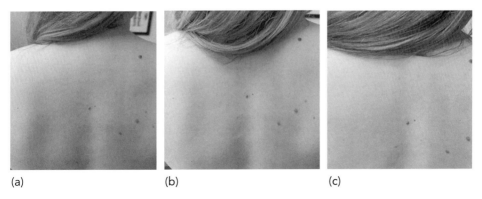

(a)   (b)   (c)

Fig. 20 Abnormal flare response following stroking (a) after about 20 seconds following rub of fingers; (b) around 20 seconds later; (c) around a minute after initial strokes showing sustained flaring. (See colour plate 3.)

Varicose lymphatics and Perrin's Point

In every ME/CFS patient, whether male or female, there is a tender area in the upper lateral region of the breast tissue, roughly 2 cm superior and lateral to the left nipple (see Figures 18 and 21). This finding is significant because the tender area almost always lies on the left side and is level with the position at which the thoracic duct turns to the left. The heart and the main blood vessels are supplied with sympathetic nerves via a bundle of nerves called the cardiac plexus, which has a greater concentration of nerves on the left than the right. Sympathetic nerves run alongside the larger nerves that control movement and sensation in the body (the somatic nerves). As explained in Chapter 3, impulses cross over from sympathetic nerves to somatic sensory nerves and vice versa via contact points known as ephapses between the parallel nerve fibres[17].

When the cardiac rhythm is affected in ME/CFS, the sympathetic nerves send messages to the sensory nerves on the left side of the chest. The thoracic duct travels from the right side to the left side of body above the level of the nipple and so, sympathetic nerves controlling the thoracic duct's pumping action are more left sided above the nipple line. Thus, when these nerves are irritated, they also disturb the adjacent sensory nerves. The resultant pain is at the confluence of these two networks of irritated sensory nerves: This tender spot is now known as 'Perrin's Point' (see Figure 21). In FMS this point is usually extremely tender , much more so than in the normal ME/CFS patient.

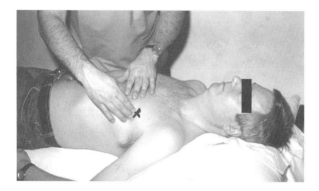

Fig. 21 Examining a male patient for 'Perrin's Point'. Gentle pressure at a point slightly superior and lateral to the left nipple, 'Perrin's Point'(**X**). The amount of sensitivity at this point appears to correspond to the severity of lymphatic engorgement in the breast tissue and also seems to mirror the gravity of the other symptoms

The sensitive region, Perrin's Point, together with congested lymph vessels in the cervical region and breast tissue, was palpated (felt) in the 40 patients chosen for my treatment in the first trial and all of the 18 ME/CFS patients in the second phase of the study. The consistency of these lymphatics can best be described as a 'string of beads' and similar to varicose veins in the leg. Varicosities have previously been described in the lymphatic system[18, 19, 20]. Large incompetent varicose lymphatics, known as megalymphatics, have often been seen when there is a backflow of fluid within the lymphatic vessels, due to a disturbance of the normal pumping mechanism. However, varicosities in the lymphatics are rarely discussed in clinics, due to the misconception that lymph flow can only be unidirectional due to the valvular system in the lymphatic vessels.

Sluggish lymph flow is known to exist in many disease states[21] and is treated by many practitioners world-wide trained in manual lymphatic drainage. However, the concept of a reverse pump causing an actual backflow is not generally recognised clinically. Thus, the possibility of a varicose lymph vessel is rarely considered when a GP or hospital consultant conducts an examination.

Downward pressure due to thoracic duct pump dysfunction caused by sympathetic disequilibrium may lead to a contra-flow within the lymphatics[22], damaging the valves and creating a pooling of lymphatic fluid with exaggerated 'beading' of the vessels. Stasis (fluid not moving) in these varicose lymphatic vessels creates a risk of toxic overload together with additional damage to the lymphatics and surrounding tissue.

Reflux of toxins via lymphatic vessels back into the cerebrospinal fluid will further irritate the central nervous system. Increased toxicity within the central nervous system continues to overload the sympathetic nerves, resulting in a downward spiral of deteriorating health.

From the earliest days of osteopathy, the importance of good lymphatic drainage in the thoracic duct has been seen as paramount to sustain health[23, 24, 25, 26]. It was emphasised that, together with good blood supply, it was equally important to have perfect drainage. This is the pathway I believe to be compromised mechanically as part of the root cause of ME/CFS. Mechanical dysfunction such as this can be detected by palpation and can be released by gentle pressure and massage techniques applied to the cranium and the spine and surrounding soft tissue.

The healthy lymphatic vessel allows only unidirectional flow due to the system of valves illustrated in Figure 22. In ME/CFS and FMS, retrograde flow of the lymphatics is produced by the reverse peristaltic wave of the thoracic duct that arises from dysfunctional sympathetic control of the duct's smooth muscle wall. This causes a reflux of fluid throughout the lymphatic system affecting individual lymph collecting vessels (lymphagia) leading to the formation of varicose mega-lymphatics, initially in the neck and chest, as seen in Fig. 23a–c. Eventually, the lymphatic reflux causes damage to the valves and allows pooling of fluid in between the valves (Figure 23b). This leads to distension of the vessel wall with the characteristic enlarged beaded appearance of a varicose vessel as illustrated in Figure 23c.

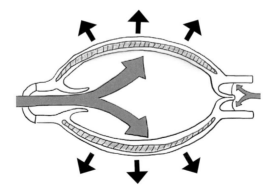

Fig. 22 Schematic illustration showing normal flow within a healthy lymphatic vessel. The valves in this healthy vessel are intact, preventing any backflow, thus maintaining a healthy, unidirectional drainage (note the smooth muscular wall of the lymphangion regulated by sympathetic nerves).

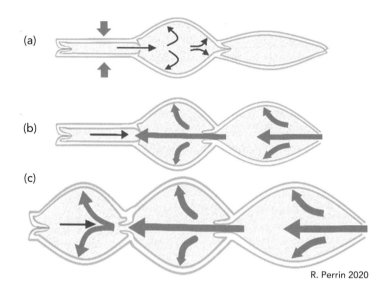

R. Perrin 2020

Fig. 23 The development of varicose megalymphatics (a) The normal lymph flow before the illness. (b) Reversal of the central lymphatic pump forces the colourless lymph fluid back, damaging the valves that separate the adjacent collecting vessels (lymphangia). (c) The lymphangia expand due to the pressure and volume of the backward flowing lymph. This leads to the large beaded vessels (varicose mega-lymphatics) palpated (felt with the fingertips) just beneath the skin in the chest of ME/CFS and FMS patients.

Figure 24 shows the top right section of the chest of a 61-year-old man. One can see the swollen, tortuous beaded vessels just beneath the collar bone adjacent to the right shoulder. The man suffered severely from ME/CFS for four years before being successfully treated with a two-year course of the Perrin Technique. The beaded appearance in Figure 24 is due to damaged valves and subsequent retrograde flow and pooling of lymphatic fluid. This is similar to the formation of varicose veins, although it lacks the darker, bluish hue of superficial varicose veins. The fluid in the lymphatic vessel, known simply as 'lymph', is colourless and so these vessels are definitely lymphatic and not blood vessels as they have the same colour as the overlying skin. These vessels also have a much larger diameter than do healthy superficial lymphatic vessels which are normally extremely difficult to palpate (feel with the finger tips),

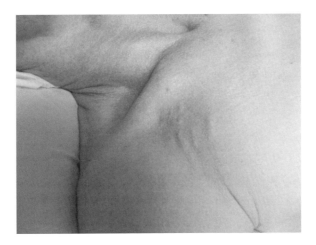

Fig. 24 Right subclavicular varicose megalymphatics, lacking the bluish hue of varicose veins, in patient with ME/CFS (see colour plate 4).

never mind actually see with the naked eye. It is extremely rare to see such pronounced superficial varicose megalymphatics as illustrated here. However, I have been able to feel the presence of varicose lymphatic vessels in the chest of all the ME/CFS and FMS patients I have seen since 1989.

Tenderness at the solar plexus

The largest major autonomic plexus, uniting two large coeliac ganglia, is known as the **coeliac plexus**, more commonly referred to as the 'solar plexus'. This major confluence of nerves is level with the 12th thoracic/1st lumbar segment and is situated posterior to the stomach and in front of tendonous insertions of the diaphragm. Secondary plexuses connected to the coeliac plexus are: phrenic; splenic; hepatic; left gastric; intermesenteric; suprarenal; renal; testicular/ovarian; superior and inferior mesenteric, sending and receiving messages from all the abdominal organs and below.

Through its connections, the solar plexus is excellent as an indicator for any visceral disturbances from the waist down. Tenderness in this abdominal region, known as the epigastrium, seems to be directly related to the severity of any lower extremity fatigue and/or abdominal problem. This, as with Perrin's Point, is due to impulses passing across the ephapses, the connections between adjacent sensory and sympathetic nerves (page 69) and, again, is usually much more tender in FMS patients.

On palpation, the epigastrium is also usually warmer than the rest of the abdomen, possibly due to the back flow of inflammatory toxins pumping down the thoracic duct into the upper regions of the abdomen and also the build-up of neurogenic inflammation from coeliac plexus overload.

Disturbance in the cranio-sacral rhythm

There is a palpable rhythmic pulsation along the spinal cord and around the brain together with that of normal breathing, which is transmitted to the rest of the body and is termed the cranial rhythmic impulse (CRI) or the 'cranio-sacral rhythm'. The rhythm is also known by some osteopaths as the 'involuntary mechanism' and by some as the 'primary respiration' as it is believed by some to be the inherent driver of all other mechanisms and rhythms in the body. Most of the osteopathic profession believe this pulse to be a movement through the tension and continuity of membranes and fascia. The fascia is connective tissue containing many lymphatic vessels that is continuous with the membranes that surround the brain and spinal cord, the meninges, thus allowing the different motions, and tensions, of the body to be transmitted everywhere.

William Garner Sutherland (1873–1954) – see Fig 25 – the founder of cranial osteopathy, proposed that there was a primary respiratory mechanism created within the central nervous system and via the spinal cord, with the bones in the cranium all moving in a rhythmic pattern together with the sacrum at the base of the spine[25].

Sutherland proposed that the primary respiratory mechanism produces a rhythmic alternation of flexion and extension of structures in the midline. This movement occurs simultaneously with rhythmic external and internal rotation of all paired lateral structures[1].

Contractile lymph tissue exists throughout the body, which creates a powerful pumping mechanism[18]. It has been shown that the thoracic duct pump influences the drainage of CSF/lymph from the central nervous system. Together with the pulse rate and the effects of breathing, a separate underlying rhythm may be induced which is very possibly the aforementioned 'involuntary mechanism'. This rhythm echoes along the lymphatic system, resonating throughout the entire body and can be palpated by trained practitioners. In ME/CFS and FMS patients it is often slower, arrhythmic, plus its intensity is shallower than in healthy people, and in very severe cases almost

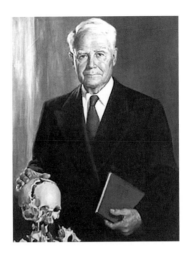

Fig. 25 William Garner Sutherland, DO – founder of cranial osteopathy (1873–1954).

absent. A disturbed CRI was found in all the ME/CFS patients that I have examined clinically and during my research.

To understand the mechanism of the CRI and how it all ties in with what we now know as the neuro-lymphatic/glymphatic system, we just have to look at the basic physiology of cerebrospinal fluid (CSF) production and flow (see Figure 1 in Chapter 1).

CSF is produced in the brain from the blood in a concentration of specialised cells surrounding blood capillaries and connective tissue known as the choroid plexus. It travels through the ventricular system of the brain and along the spinal cord, flowing back to the brain, eventually returning to the blood in the venous sinuses. It is established that the cardiac rhythm continues in the CSF within the brain following the cycle of systole and diastole of 50–100 bpm (beats per minute)[26a, 26b].

Now we know that some of the CSF drains out via the 'glymphatic system' as Iliff and co-workers have referred to it[1]. This neuro-lymphatic system flows into the perivascular spaces down the olfactory, optic, trigeminal and auditory pathways, plus the paravascular drainage from the brain and spinal cord, diffusing into the surrounding lymphatic tissue and eventually into the central lymphatic drainage which possesses smooth muscle walls controlled by the sympathetic nervous system, generating a slow wave with an average rhythm of 4 bpm.

Physics dictates that when two wave patterns meet, they produce an interference wave. The non-physicists among you can understand this phenomenon when watching the waves at a beach. When a large wave comes in to shore it crashes against a smaller wave going out and together, they form a third wave, the interference wave. In the body, due to the neuro-lymphatic/glymphatic drainage from the brain into the central lymphatic drainage, these two wave patterns of 50–100 bpm and 4 bpm meet, producing an interference wave of around 8–12 bpm that osteopaths refer to as the CRI, also known by some as the cranio-sacral rhythm, due to the fact that the wave primarily travels along the central nervous system from the brain down to the base of the spinal cord at the sacrum. Experienced practitioners can feel this rhythm in the rest of the body but it is most palpable at the two poles – that is, the cranium and the sacrum.

Even though my concept of the cranial rhythm is not accepted by all osteopaths, it is based on definite principles of physics and was certainly assessed by scientists at the University of Manchester's Department of Hydrodynamics (formerly in UMIST). Although the physicists could not ascertain the exact beat of rhythm, there was a strong scientific basis to argue that it could be in the region of 8 to 12 bpm, which is the accepted average beat of the CRI among the cranial osteopathic camp.

My hypothesis for the origin of the CRI was published in the same year as my first book, in 2007 in the *Journal of the American Osteopathic Association* and was highlighted on the front page of that edition[27].

My theory is also supported by the fact that CSF drainage into the lymphatics in humans has now been proven and that neuroscientists have shown that breathing and posture affect the movement of CSF and thus aid CSF drainage to the lymphatics, all of which has been discussed in depth earlier in the book[28].

The two minor physical signs

Over the years I have observed two other notable signs that appear in many cases but they are not present in the majority so I call them the minor physical signs. These are stretch marks and pupil dilation.

Stretch marks, known medically as 'striae', are caused by damaged collagen fibres close to the skin surface. As mentioned in Chapter 4, striae are often seen on the thighs and breast tissue of ME/CFS patients and are most probably due to damage to collagenous anchoring ligaments attached to surface lymphatic capillaries. This could occur when there is a major backflow of lymph and is seen in many ME/CFS patients who have never been obese or pregnant, which are the two most common physiological causes of striae.

Pupil dilation: In ME/CFS and FMS, due to dysfunction of the sympathetic nervous system, the size of the patient's pupils can be grossly affected. Some patients, have reduced sympathetic nerve activity leading to pupil constriction but dilated pupils due to sympathetic overload is much more frequent, with the patient needing to avoid bright lights and sunshine. Some ME/CFS and FMS patients need to wear sunglasses all the time, with the worst cases so photophobic that they need to wear blackout eye masks.

The NHS diagnostic study 2015–2016

In 2011, I was travelling to present a poster at the International Association of ME/CFS conference, which in that year was held in Ottawa, and met by chance on the journey, Dr Michael Eshiett, who has been a Consultant Physician in Neurological Rehabilitation at Leigh Infirmary in Lancashire, UK since 1995.

The outcome of our conversation was that Dr Eshiett arranged a meeting between myself and his colleague at Leigh Infirmary who runs a ME/CFS clinic, Dr Tarek Gaber. At the meeting Tarek set me a challenge. If the physical signs are valid, they should be tested as stand-alone signs. In other words, if they are accurate, then one should be able to tell by the signs alone that a person has ME/CFS. I argued that we don't just use the physical signs in clinic. The history and symptoms are also a very important factor in diagnosing ME/CFS and the physical signs are used as a screening tool to confirm the diagnosis.

He counter-argued that he understood that they were an aid but to prove they had any substance to the rest of the medical and scientific community I had to run a blind controlled trial on the physical signs alone without any information about history or symptoms. If the signs in such a research project proved useful in diagnosing ME/CFS, then others would be convinced... and so, the new study was born.

Four years later, after many meetings with doctors, scientists, NHS Trust managers, hours of discussion with research colleagues at the University of Central Lancashire, reams of emails plus the necessary fundraising activities by the charity FORME and the inevitable interrogation at the dreaded ethics committee, the research project was finally ready to begin.

The title of the study was: 'Examining the accuracy of a physical diagnostic technique for chronic fatigue syndrome/myalgic encephalomyelitis'. The research team and co-authors of the study were research assistants Lucy Hives and Alice

Bradley, professor of biomechanics Jim Richards, statistician Dr Chris Sutton, professor of physiotherapy research James Selfe, neuro-rehabilitation consultant Dr Bhaskar Basu, osteopath Kerry Maguire, physiotherapist Gail Sumner, consultant in rehabilitation medicine Dr Tarek Gaber, consultant endocrinologist Dr Annice Mukherjee and Yours Truly.

The objective of the study was to assess five physical signs to see whether or not they could assist in the diagnosis of patients with ME/CFS, and potentially lead to quicker treatment.

I chose two allied health practitioners (AHPs) to work on the study: Gail, a physiotherapist at my Manchester clinic who had actually recovered from severe ME/CFS with my treatment methods (see her story at the beginning of Chapter 5). The other was Kerry, an osteopath who was recruited specifically for the study with no previous knowledge or experience with ME/CFS. I wanted to make things as difficult as possible, so having a practitioner newly trained in my methods would demonstrate to the NHS that we could train allied health practitioners quite quickly and inexpensively to proficiently perform the manual examination as an aid to diagnosis.

An NHS consultant, who had worked in a hospital ME/CFS outpatients clinic, was employed to examine the participants using standard clinical methods and quite simply to see if the participant demonstrated any pattern of illness behaviour that could be a clue to the two AHPs when examining the participants. This study would be successful if it showed that the practitioners using the Perrin Technique to diagnose ME/CFS were significantly more accurate than the consultant using neurological techniques such as testing reflexes with a patella hammer and a rheumatological test such as muscular strength and ability to stand. There were 94 participants recruited from two NHS hospitals and local ME/CFS support groups. The participants were examined for 20 minutes each by the three practitioners on the same day in a randomised order.

Of the 94 participants who were assessed, 52 were ME/CFS patients who had been previously diagnosed by an NHS consultant and were further screened using two separate sets of criteria. To satisfy the NHS we used the NICE guidelines at the time (the guidance for practitioners produced by The UK's National Institute for Health and Care Excellence), and the other screening tool we used was based on the International Consensus Criteria (ICC), in turn based on the Canadian Criteria, which at the time of the research was, and remains, the most recognised criteria within the international community of ME/CFS experts. In addition, 42 non-ME/CFS controls were recruited and screened for being healthy using the same criteria as the patient group. The participants were aged between 18 and 60.

I had to remain climbing the walls of my clinic for the year of the actual study, as I was not allowed within the city limits of the hospital and university locations when the participants were being examined. However, the wait was worth it: when the results were finally analysed, they were better than we could have ever expected.

The physician was able to correctly identify 100% of the healthy controls using the standard clinical neurological and rheumatological examination demonstrating what an excellent doctor he is. However, he was only able to correctly identify 44% of patients with ME/CFS, and the tendency to underdiagnose ME/CFS was highly statistically significant ($p<0.001$). This showed that standard clinical examination was not a useful modality for confirming diagnosis of ME/CFS.

Gail, the experienced AHP, was able to identify the five signs, although breast varicosities and dampened cranial flow did not improve the accuracy of her diagnosis. The results showed that the physical signs can improve the accuracy of diagnosing ME/CFS, but agreement between the AHPs, Gail and Kerry, on the presence of each of the five physical signs varied, which showed that all five physical signs may not be necessary to aid the diagnostic process. Further analysis of all the results found that using only two of the five physical signs (tender coeliac plexus and postural/ mechanical disturbance of the thoracic spine) was the most accurate and efficient method of correctly diagnosing the participants for both the AHPs despite their differing levels of prior experience of ME/CFS and the Perrin Technique.

A previous study by a group of doctors at Hammersmith Hospital, London, had found Perrin's Point to have a diagnostic accuracy of around 80% in patients with ME/CFS[29]. This was very similar to the accuracy we achieved when including Perrin's Point in our research.

So, we concluded that using the physical signs appeared to improve the accuracy of identifying people with ME/CFS and showed agreement with current diagnostic techniques; however, our study concluded that only two of these might be needed. Using physical signs has the advantage of being conducted simply and quickly by AHPs and could be used as a screening tool for ME/CFS.

The main factor to consider in this study is that these results were in a research setting and all without knowledge of the participants' symptoms and history.

In a clinical setting this is obviously completely different, and Perrin Technique licensed practitioners are trained to scrutinise the patient's history and symptoms in detail to build-up a picture of why and how the patient became ill.

The physical signs are used as confirmation of the diagnosis and typically will present at different levels of severity proportional to the illness itself. For example, patients with severe ME/CFS often will have such a tender Perrin's Point that, when pressed, they usually emit an 'Ow!' or grimace. Whereas a patient who has a mild case of ME/CFS might just involuntarily blink when pressed in this region of the chest. Likewise, in severe cases one finds that the thoracic spine is usually more tender, inflamed and restricted, and there are more palpable and often tender varicose lymphatics in the chest, tender and inflamed coeliac plexus and a more disturbed cranial rhythm. However, the research study did not explore the severity of signs but simply if they were present.

Scoring the patient

When calculating the initial score out of 10, with 10/10 being symptom-free (see Outlook chart, Chapter 10), the life of the patient is fully assessed from birth onwards. The clinician will investigate different sources of toxins and, when scrutinising the medical history, make special note of any life traumas and occurrences that increase the neurotoxicity, enabling the practitioner to form a much more accurate diagnosis. Taking into account the number of different symptoms, the practitioner will be able to provide a definitive score once the physical examination has been carried out. This will confirm whether the patient is exaggerating their symptoms, which I must add is very rare with ME/CFS and FMS, or if they are playing down their symptoms and acting as though they are healthier than the five signs indicate. This is much more common with ME/CFS and FMS patients, who hate the fact that they are suffering from such a debilitating illness which most people, including their healthcare practitioners, don't understand. So, they often pretend to all their family and friends that they can do much more than they can actually manage, at a terrible cost to themselves as it inevitably leads to a steady deterioration of the symptoms.

Many patients who I see for the initial consultation fall into this category and there is a massive group of the 'three-and-a-half out of 10' patients acting like a 'seven out of 10'. They are often wives and mothers who need to, or have to, carry on to keep the home as normal as possible for their spouses and children as they feel desperately guilty if they admit how bad their illness is, or try and rest more and pace themselves better.

ME/CFS isn't the worst illness there is, but it is one of the cruellest. It usually affects people with very strong willpowers who are extremely active before and will try and beat the disease with every fibre in their body and with uber determination. However, the more they try and beat the disease, the worse they get. The sympathetic nervous system is the main control mechanism of the neuro-immune system and it is this connection that needs to function properly to enable willpower to beat disease. In ME/CFS, this system is dysfunctional which leads to a more disturbed neuro-immunity, leading to a build-up of pro-inflammatory cytokines with eventual autoimmune problems developing as the body starts to attack itself. This cytokine storm has been shown to occur in numerous patients after suffering from Covid-19, leading to ME/CFS and FMS symptoms. Many leading immunologists, such as Professor Noel Rose from Johns Hopkins University, Baltimore claim that ME/CFS has many of the characteristics of autoimmune disease, and if the disease worsens some patients develop other autoimmune disorders such as rheumatoid arthritis, Sjogren's syndrome, Hashimoto's, psoriasis and lupus.

The diagnostic signs described in this chapter can be easily taught to clinicians. There are plenty of practitioners trained in cranio-sacral techniques who can apply all the above diagnostic procedures that may identify ME/CFS in its earliest stages. In fact, clinically when examining siblings or children of ME/CFS patients, I have discovered that the physical signs often appear long before the symptoms present themselves fully.

This being the case in patients with a familial predisposition, it is possible in these instances to actually diagnose a pre-ME/CFS condition and prevent certain patients from ever succumbing to the full-blown illness. As far as I know I am the only clinician to claim that ME/CFS is preventable.

In May/June 2020 I treated a 42-year-old man from Prestwich, Manchester, who until recently had had no previous history of ME/CFS symptoms. However, since he was infected by Covid-19 in the spring of 2020, he had felt overwhelming physical and mental fatigue with many other symptoms of ME/CFS. He lived near my clinic and knew of my work so made an appointment to see me in May 2020. On examination, his physical signs were prominent and clearly palpable, with mid-thoracic tenderness, huge varicose lymphatics, very tender Perrin's Point and coeliac plexus plus very 'sluggish' CRI. After only three treatments the physical signs began to fade, and his symptoms improved. A couple of months on and he was completely symptom-free and back to full health.

The sooner that a patient receives a physical examination with confirmation of the definitive signs and symptoms of neuro-lymphatic dysfunction, the better. This hopefully will lead to a much quicker initiation of treatment than normal. The earlier the treatment programme begins, the better the chances of recovery and the less likely it is that the patient will start to spiral into the chronic severe state that blights so many ME/CFS and FMS sufferers' lives.

Chapter 9

Osteopathy

It is a perfectly well-established technique, there is no mystery about it.
It ought to be part of the equipment of every doctor in the country.
George Bernard Shaw (1856–1950), Irish playwright,
speaking about osteopathy in 1927

Case: Sue's story

I wanted to briefly share the story of my ME/CFS journey and road
to recovery with Dr Perrin and his team as a celebration of how
far I travelled in just six months. Never would I have thought in a
million years that progress could possibly be so rapid, especially
against adversity with life trauma. I am so tremendously grateful to
Dr Perrin and feel now I have been given my life back with a belief
that full recovery is in reach. I strongly feel that all ME/CFS sufferers
should know about this treatment package. I would love to see GPs,
neurologists etc referring patients for this treatment and it being
funded by the NHS.

I'm not sure how long ME/CFS had been creeping up in my life, but
for sure I had felt ill and struggled for over five years with disturbing
symptoms of physical fatigue and energy loss, loss of

leg/muscle power, reduced concentration, difficulty reading, short-term memory challenges, brain fog, sinusitis, head, neck and back pain, general myalgia, fluctuations in temperature, mood swings, irritable bladder and bowel, sore throats, photophobia, hyperacusis [sound intolerance], tinnitus, dry eyes and mouth, breathlessness, palpitations and feeling much worse after exertion. I had continued to over-exert myself, not realising that I was actually making my health much worse. Following years of GP appointments, referrals to three neurologists, what felt like hundreds of blood tests, MRI scans and almost giving up hope, I stumbled across the work of the Perrin Clinic. What a great day that was! I had truly believed that this was how I was to live my life and with the added concern of year-on-year deterioration in health.

A family tragedy made me even more determined and motivated to get started with treatment and also to fully engage with the programme. I had to get better to support my family, and indeed for myself, to be able to enjoy a full and active life. Brilliantly, Dr Perrin has the evidence-based knowledge to diagnose ME/CFS by looking at five physiological markers. I had all five markers. Dr Perrin assessed my health score at 3.5, with very weak cranial flow. Treatment started at the Prestwich clinic to improve my neuro-lymphatic system and remove toxins from my body. I supported this weekly treatment with daily home treatment, a focus on nutrition, supplements as recommended by Dr Perrin, pacing and resting. I also took long-term sick leave from work to be able to fully focus and optimise my chances of recovery.

Three months later my score was 4.5, and two months later my score was 6. One month later my score was 7. Absolutely incredible – I was really feeling different, better, energised. You do forget what 'normal' feels like!

I have to give a shout out to my therapist Elisa who has been just amazing. She has been so kind, professional, and respectful offering a huge amount of knowledge and compassion around ME/CFS. Her sessions are always friendly, caring and with dignity and respect. To Elisa and the team, I am so thankful. Words cannot express the admiration I have for their knowledge, passion and skill. They are incredible.

Now, seven months into treatment I have just started to attend monthly and I am very disciplined about the home treatments. I have so much more energy, can walk much further without after effects, my head is clearing, tinnitus and sinusitis much improved, I have power back in my legs (they no longer just stop working), and I feel refreshed in the morning! I am back in work (phasing my return slowly) and helping myself by pacing and being mindful of how my body feels. Overall, I am much stronger than pre-treatment. I know I still have further to go, but I honestly believe now that it is possible that I will make a full recovery from what has been a very hard and worrying few years.

My top tips for other patients on this journey would include:
- Attend your appointments regularly as advised. Don't drive. Have someone with you for support if you possibly can. Pace and plan your journey.
- Be disciplined with your home treatments – don't miss any. Check you have understood what you need to do.
- Rest, rest, rest, rest… and more rest.
- Remember the 50% rule – do only half of what you think you can manage. It's so easy to do too much. Listen to your body.
- As you start to improve, keep resting, keep pacing.

This treatment is life changing. I am no longer thinking about very early retirement, I can enjoy once again my midwifery career. I no longer need to worry about taking my grandchildren for a walk (in case I can't make it back) – I can trust my legs and energy levels. If I have done a little too much, I have confidence that rest, and sleep, will sort me out – feeling refreshed again the next day. I can look forward to a family holiday knowing that I will be able to walk down the beach and feel the sea on my feet. It's the simple things in life that give us pleasure. Why should ME/CFS take that away from us when there is a way to feel well again? I feel myself growing stronger each week and love it when other people notice my new-found energy. It's been a while…but I'm getting back to the person I was. Where washing my hair was too much effort sometimes, now I can walk up the lane near my home to the 'top of the world'. Maybe the 'three peaks' one day, who knows.

Sue Henry, Darwen, Lancashire, UK
Patient of Elisa Dispenza Registered Osteopath and Licensed Perrin Technique Practitioner, Cheshire, UK

Sue's story… epilogue

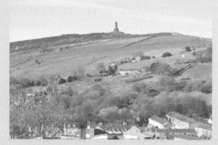

Fig. 26 Postcard of Darwen Tower

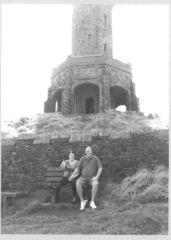

Fig. 27 Sue having reached Darwen Tower

Hi Raymond,

I haven't been able to walk to Darwen Tower for over 5 years. Last year I could only walk for 5 minutes on a good day. Thanks to your treatment programme over the last 15 months, today I did the uphill walk to Darwen Tower. It felt exhilarating. I wanted to share this as it was one of my personal goals and I knew you'd love to see. Please share with Elisa. She has been incredibly brilliant with me

Thank you

Sue Henry

Osteopathic treatment

Many of you reading this book may be more familiar with ME/CFS and FMS than with osteopathy. By now you may have a clearer understanding of the biophysical processes leading to ME/CFS and FMS, but you may still wonder how osteopathy can help.

As detailed in this book, the treatment available for ME/CFS and FMS includes dietary regimes[1, 2, 3], with evidence to suggest that essential fatty acid intake must be normalised in the management of the disease[4]. Psychotherapy, physiotherapy, exercise programmes, pain-killing drugs and antidepressants have all been advocated. The different treatment programmes – whether chemical, hormonal, environmental or psychological – all focus on palliative treatment that improves the symptoms but does not address the overall underlying causative problem.

As stated in Chapter 6, the effect on the body from long-term stress, known as allostatic load, can lead to many different disease states. The osteopathic techniques in this book aim to treat ME/CFS and FMS through stabilising the body's structure and function in the face of these stressors – that is allostasis. This reduces the irritation of the autonomic nervous system, thus allowing a return to a healthy homeostatic state. My hypothesis is that this can be achieved by increasing the drainage of toxins from the cerebrospinal fluid via the lymphatics using cranial techniques and manual lymphatic drainage techniques on the head, neck and thorax. The treatment also reduces autonomic tone by improving structure and overall quality of movement of the spine, together with relaxation of surrounding musculature, especially the thoracic and upper lumbar spine regions.

The two trunks of the sympathetic nervous system are paired chains of sympathetic nerves that run the entire length of the spinal cord and attach to nerve roots from the thoracic and upper lumbar spine and are integrally related to the overall structure of this area. By reducing mechanical irritation, disturbed sympathetic afferent impulses may be minimised, further helping to stabilise blood and lymph flow. Working on the suboccipital region at the top of the neck also will help stabilise messages along the vagus nerve, one of the major nerves of the parasympathetic nervous system, which when functioning correctly helps calm the body's internal systems, especially the cardiovascular system. So, the treatment advocated is basically to balance the body's control mechanism.

This approach, by the way, is in total agreement with the latest draft guidelines for ME/CFS from the UK's National Institute of Health and Care Excellence (NICE) which were published while I was completing this book. Section 1.11.11 of the guidance states that practitioners should include physical maintenance in the management plan for people with ME/CFS and consider techniques that aim to improve overall joint mobility; muscle flexibility; postural and positional support; muscle strength and endurance; plus cardiovascular health[4a]. The Perrin Technique addresses all these issues plus the all-important neuro-lymphatic health.

History and principles of osteopathy

Dr Andrew Taylor Still (1828–1917) of Kirksville, Missouri, founded osteopathy in the latter part of the nineteenth century as an alternative to the poor quality of medicine practised at the time. Taylor Still called his new system of medicine 'osteopathy' from the Greek words for bone *osteon* and disease *pathos*. His basic tenet for viewing the body as a machine was based upon his religious beliefs and, at the same time, his despair, due to the futility of most medication at the time. He formulated his original hypothesis from a Biblical text: 'Let us make man in our image' (*Genesis*, Chapter 1, Verse 26). Taylor Still, who was the son of a minister, took this verse literally. He postulated that if the Creator is perfect, man must have been made perfect. As he stated, 'The principles of osteopathy give us an understanding of the perfect plans and specifications followed in man's construction'. Osteopathy teaches that structure governs function. Thus illness, Taylor Still maintained, develops when the perfect structure is out of balance.

Osteopathy became popular in the American mid-west and there are now 20 established osteopathic medical schools in the USA, with an enrolment of nearly 10,000 students. The first osteopathic college in the UK was the British School of Osteopathy, now the University College of Osteopathy, founded in 1915 by John Martin Littlejohn, a student of Still, but was not incorporated until 1917 due to the First World War. Today, there are over 5000 osteopaths in the UK registered with the General Osteopathic Council, formed by Act of Parliament in 1998. The profession is now accepted in Britain to some extent by other mainstream medical disciplines.

According to the General Osteopathic Council, 'osteopathy is an established recognised system of diagnosis and treatment, which lays its main emphasis on the structural and functional integrity of the body. It is distinguished by the fact that it recognises that much of the pain and disability we suffer stems from abnormalities in the function of the body structure as well as damage caused by disease'.

How osteopathy helps

As mentioned, one of the major concepts of osteopathy is that the structure of the body governs the function of the organs within. Osteopaths work on the principle that a patient's history of illnesses and physical traumas is written into the body's structure. It is the osteopath's developed palpatory sense that enables the practitioner manually to diagnose while treating the patient. The osteopath's job is to restore a healthy structure of the body and thus its function. The osteopath gently applies manual techniques of massage and manipulation to encourage movement of the bodily fluids, eliminate dysfunction in the motion of the tissues, relax muscular tension and release compressed bones and joints. The areas being treated require proper positioning to assist the body's ability to regain normal tissue function.

Another of Taylor Still's students, William Garner Sutherland, noticed that when the bones of a dis-articulated skull were viewed in a certain way, they resembled the gills of a fish. Accordingly, he hypothesised, in 1898, that their shape was designed to allow for movement and as explained previously, cranial osteopathy was born (see Chapter 8)[5].

Drainage of toxins

The main lymphatic vessels are now known to be under sympathetic nerve control. The smooth muscle wall of the thoracic duct, when stimulated, produces a wave of contraction – peristalsis – aiding lymph drainage into the subclavian vein. This produces a negative pressure along the lymphatics and aids further lymphatic drainage.

Sutherland emphasised the importance of the choroid plexus in the chemical exchange between cerebrospinal fluid and the blood (see Chapter 1, Figure 1), but stressed the part played by the lymphatics in the drainage of toxins from the central nervous system. Sutherland said, 'When you tap the waters of the brain by compressing the fourth ventricle, see what happens in the lymphatic system. Visualise the lymph node that is holding some poison that has gathered there, changing the constituency before the lymph is moved along into the venous system'[5].

Andrew Taylor Still discussed the importance of examining disturbed fluid motion in the head, in the pathogenesis of many signs and symptoms, such as headaches, enlarged tonsils, dizziness and loss of memory, all associated with ME/CFS. He said,

'We strike at the source of life and death when we go into the lymphatics'[6]. Taylor Still emphasised that it was equally important to have perfect drainage as well as good blood supply.

Sutherland postulated that each facial sinus has one or more bones that help drain the mucus produced in the goblet cells of the sinus epithelial lining, by a gentle pumping action. This facilitates a wafting action that forces the mucus into the nasopharynx. When mechanical or other forces damage this mechanism, the sinus is less able to drain the mucus. As a result, the mucus pools, thickens and makes the subject prone to infection. The nasal mucosa becomes continually inflamed with an abundance of purulent mucus and associated enlargement of adenoids and tonsils. Lymphatic vessels in the submucosa of the nasal sinuses are the initial recipients of the drainage of CSF through the cribriform plate (see Fact 6 in Chapter 1). As osteopathy's founder stated over a century ago, 'Harmony only dwells where obstructions do not exist'[6].

Mechanical dysfunction such as this can be detected by palpation and can be released by gentle pressure techniques applied to the cranium and the spine. As early as the1890s, Still noted, 'The lymphatics are closely and universally connected with the spinal cord and all other nerves, and all drink from the waters of the brain'[7]. From the earliest days of osteopathy, the importance of good lymphatic drainage in the thoracic duct has been seen as paramount to sustain health. Still himself wrote: 'At this point I will draw your attention to what I consider is the cause of a whole list of hitherto unexplained diseases, which are only effects of the blood and other fluids being prohibited from doing normal service by constrictions at the various openings of the diaphragm. Thus, prohibition of the free action of the thoracic duct would produce congestion'[7].

The average pulsation of the cranial mechanism was believed by Sutherland to be between 7 and 12 beats per minute in health[5, 8], although in more modern times authorities have calculated the average rate to be 12.47 impulses per minute with the rate for normal adults being 10–14 cycles per minute (cpm)[9, 10, 11, 12], although other studies relying on manual palpation of the CRI have recorded values of between 3 and 9 cpm[13, 14, 15, 16].

As detailed in the previous chapter, one can comprehend the mechanism of the cranial rhythmic impulse (CRI) by understanding that its production is a result of the interference wave produced when the rhythm of the cerebrospinal fluid and of the lymphatic pump of the thoracic duct, clash. This was the theoretical basis of my techniques and was published in the *Journal of the American Osteopathic Association* and is now based on factual evidence due to the now discovered neuro-lymphatic/glymphatic system, as described in earlier chapters[17].

Examination of my patients in three separate studies[18, 19, 20], totalling over 100 patients, and in clinical assessment of over 2000 more sufferers since 1989, has revealed an arrhythmic, disturbed cranial flow in patients with ME/CFS[21] compared with any of the average healthy rates mentioned above. These findings coincided with postural and mechanical problems in the thoracic spine, lymphatic pump reversal leading to palpable engorged varicose lymphatics and disturbed sympathetic neural pathways leading to specific tender regions in the chest and abdomen.

As osteopathy's founder stated over a century ago: 'Harmony only dwells where obstructions do not exist'[6]. The Perrin Technique, based on traditional, classical osteopathic principles coupled with methods supported by the latest scientific breakthroughs, seeks to reduce the obstructions and restore harmony and thus has a very significant part to play in the effective treatment of people with ME/CFS and fibromyalgia.

Chapter 10

Treating the patient

I am dying from the treatment of too many physicians.
Alexander the Great (356 BC – 323 BC)

Case: Jade's story

I developed ME after a nasty bout of glandular fever at age 6. I was eventually diagnosed after my first 'crash' at 11 years old, shortly after starting secondary school. Over the next seven years my condition got progressively worse, seeing many 'crashes' and meaning that I couldn't be educated in mainstream school because of the severity of my condition. By the time I reached my 18th birthday, I was extremely unwell.

I was wheelchair-bound, unable to stand for more than a few seconds, light sensitive, noise sensitive, very nauseous and in constant severe pain and fatigue. After so many years of being severely ill my body was giving up, and at 18, so was I. I had to rely on my parents as carers, couldn't leave the house and had no quality of life, with no end in sight.

We heard about the Perrin Technique from a family friend who also had ME. Her mum had been told about the treatment by a hospital nurse whilst receiving treatment for cancer, and my friend thought the information was worth passing on. As I was too unwell, my mum did some research on the Perrin Technique and agreed it was worth a go. Until this point no other treatment had helped me, including seven years under a paediatric consultant, a referral to the head of paediatric ME for the country, graded exercise, pacing, allergy testing, diets and several alternative therapies. We felt that this was my last chance to get better as I was deteriorating every week (see Figure 28).

We met with Dr Perrin on 17th February 2010 and he, and the treatment, made immediate sense to us. He explained ME in a way nobody else ever had, all the symptoms that other doctors had brushed off, looked confused at, or had made me feel like they were 'all in my head' suddenly had a real medical explanation, and thankfully – an answer. I was examined by Dr Perrin and officially and positively diagnosed with ME, I was graded at 2/10 on the Perrin scale, which is severe, but I was still able to be helped. I came away from the clinic feeling hopeful for the first time in many years. I knew I had a long way to go but was stubbornly determined that I could get there. I started a programme of treatment soon after with my weekly treatment being done in nearby Longridge and overseen by Dr Perrin due to my severity.

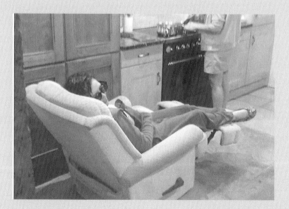

Fig. 28 Jade at home before starting the Perrin Technique, desperately ill, housebound for many years, wheelchair bound for two years, being cared for by her devoted mother, Barbara Hodgkinson.

As expected, I got worse before I got better, and my condition deteriorated quickly. After one particular treatment with Dr Perrin in around April 2010, I reacted very severely and was partially paralysed for 24 hours. This reaction, although rare and frightening at the time, was the best thing that could have happened to me as once I got through it, my recovery accelerated and I was soon seeing vast improvements in my condition. I took my first steps shortly after this reaction and dumped the wheelchair for good in June 2010, a mere four and a half months after starting my Perrin journey. By September, I was working part-time, had enrolled in college and was practising for my driving test which I passed the next month. I was starting to finally lead a normal life for the first time in 11 years.

A year after I ditched the wheelchair, I challenged myself and did a sponsored climb up Scafell Pike, the tallest peak in England, in aid of the charity which backs the Perrin Technique, accompanied by Dr Perrin, my parents and several friends (see Figure 29a). On reaching the top and looking out over the Lake District I knew I had done it and my life would never be the same. I was never going back to being that ill shell of a person thanks to Dr Perrin and the Perrin Technique.

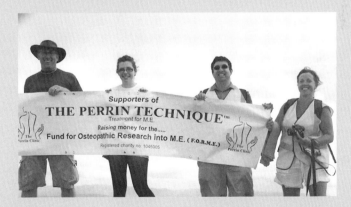

Fig. 29(a) Jade well enough after 18 months of treatment to climb with her parents Barbara and Andrew, and myself, plus a group of friends (not pictured) to the top of the highest mountain in England, Scarfell Pike, to raise funds for my research.

Nine years on and although I still have treatment every couple of months to ensure I stay well, I am largely symptom free. I am now married (see Figure 29(b)), have a 3-year-old son and am expecting my second child. I have a normal, happy, healthy life now. Without the treatment, there's no way I would have the life I have today, and I am forever grateful for the second chance at life that it gave me.

Jade Benson, Lancashire, UK

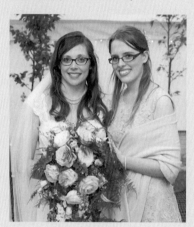

Fig. 29(b) Former severe ME/CFS patients Jade Benson and Jen Turner at Jade's wedding. See Jen's recovery story in her own words at the beginning of the Introduction (page 3).

The osteopathic techniques that I have developed to treat ME/CFS and fibromyalgia syndrome (FMS) patients are based on some new procedures that I have developed but mainly on standard procedures used by many trained osteopathic practitioners and some physiotherapists and chiropractors[1,2].

Reducing inflammation

The first task is to reduce any possible inflammation present at the damaged segments of the spine. This can be achieved in various ways. Some practitioners would prescribe anti-inflammatory drugs. However, contrast bathing (warm alternating with cold) is deemed preferable, as it has no toxic side effects. The warm compress usually consists of a warm (not hot) water bottle. Too hot a compress could scald the patient's skin. The 'cold' is as cold as the patient can tolerate and this is sometimes just cool, i.e. fridge temperature; it is safer if a frozen pack is wrapped with a cover, especially as ME/CFS patients often cannot tolerate extremes of temperature. Frozen peas, which easily mould around the back, can be a used, although special cold compress packs, which remain soft even when frozen, are preferable and less messy, especially if the peas fall out of the bag!

My clinical experience has shown that the sequence of contrast bathing that gives the best results in reducing the inflammation in ME/CFS is as follows:

```
COLD –    3 minutes  }
WARM –    1 minute   }
COLD –    1 minute   } Total 10 minutes
WARM –    1 minute   }
COLD –    1 minute   }
WARM –    3 minutes  }
```

This process has no adverse side effects, and so it is safe to be used as many times as required. Application of at least three times a day to the upper thoracic region is recommended if there is inflammation in the neck and shoulders (or there are cerebral symptoms) and the lower thoracic area when the abdominal or lower extremities are affected. The main advantage of contrast bathing over anti-inflammatory drugs is that it works quickly and directly on the affected area. Even when there is no palpable or visible inflammation, shown by heat and redness, contrast bathing to improve circulation in the thoracic region is still advised as it will aid circulation in the region which will, in turn, help the lymphatic drainage of the spine and help improve the health of the tissue lying alongside the spine.

With FMS, patients respond better to cold only on the spine for 5 minutes followed by, or at the same time, placing warm compresses or a warm water bottle on the surrounding muscles. For example, if there is much pain in the shoulders, arms and hands then the patient should apply warm to these areas and the cold (not freezing) compress on the very bottom of the neck and upper back.

Likewise, if the pain is in the legs and feet, then warm these areas and at the same time place cool packs on the upper lumbar spine, around the waist level. This is the level supplying the bottom of the sympathetic nerve chains mentioned earlier and will hopefully reduce the overstimulation of the sympathetic nerves of the abdomen, legs and feet.

Perrin Technique protocol for fibromyalgia syndrome (FMS)

Note that the treatment of FMS is virtually the same as with ME/CFS with two exceptions. I advise far less effleurage (stroking massage, explained below) as most patients with FMS can only cope with a little effleurage before the skin becomes painful. It is essential with FMS to use more oil or cream to avoid any friction. Leon Chaitow, ND, DO (1937–2018), a world-renowned author and practising naturopath, osteopath, and acupuncturist, advocated more long-lever stretches for fibromyalgia, which I have found to be most useful. So, with FMS I reduce the effleurage and gently stretch the spine with the long-lever technique mentioned below[3].

The other major difference between the treatment of ME/CFS and of FMS is that although I always advise against over-treating with ME/CFS, I am doubly cautious with FMS concerning the whole treatment session. Besides effleurage that should be minimal, the use of direct manipulation, and high velocity-low amplitude manipulation should be restricted to the bare minimum in FMS.

Post-traumatic FMS

The condition known as post-traumatic fibromyalgia, which is a very severe form of fibromyalgia that occurs as a result of a traumatic injury, usually to the neck, such as a whiplash injury sustained in a car crash, remains very difficult to treat. I have found in these cases that the most gentle cranial stimulation, together with a multi-discipline approach such as hypnosis, mindfulness, or psychotherapy to advise on coping strategies plus acupuncture may help. Sometimes the pain is too much for even the slightest touch, and then I have to hope there will be some improvement from the other approaches before I can try and help.

A physician who suffered from this disease was Dr Mark Pellegrino, who shares the theory of fibromyalgia researchers such as Dr Muhammad B Yunus, at the University of Illinois College of Medicine. They maintain that the disease bears all the hallmarks of hypersensitisation of the central nervous system together with neuro-hormonal dysfunction, as seen in ME/CFS due to hypothalamic and sympathetic nervous system overload[4, 5].

Stages of treatment: The 10 steps of the Perrin Technique

The manual treatment of each ME/CFS patient consists of a number of stages:
1. Effleurage to aid drainage in the breast tissue lymphatics.
2. Effleurage to aid drainage in the cervical lymphatic vessels.
3. Gentle articulation of the thoracic region and soft tissue techniques with upward effleurage.
4. Effleurage to aid drainage in the cervical lymphatic vessels.
5. Soft tissue massage to relax muscles and encourage lymph drainage of the cervicothoracic region.
6. Further cervical effleurage towards the subclavian region.
7. Functional and inhibition techniques to the suboccipital region.
8. Further cervical effleurage towards the subclavian region.
9. Stimulation of the cranio-sacral rhythm by cranial and sacral techniques.
10. Final cervical effleurage towards the subclavian region.

As Rudyard Kipling (1865–1936) once said: 'The cure for this ill is not to sit still'. Movement is an essential part of the healing process. So gentle exercises are prescribed to improve the quality of thoracic spine mobility and the coordination of the patient.

The treatment schedule listed above and detailed below is almost the same as the protocol followed throughout the clinical trials in the years 1996–1997 and 2000–2001. It has altered slightly over the years as I have found that certain techniques further improve the neuro-lymphatic drainage. The amount of time spent, and the pressure exerted on to the patient whilst using the following techniques depends on the physical state of the patient and on the symptom picture at that particular stage in their therapy. So, as always with ME/CFS and FMS, with every patient the techniques are distinct, and each individual treatment session is marginally different to the other consultations with the patient. The exact nature, content, intensity and timing of each treatment is determined by the trained and experienced practitioner.

Lubrication for effleurage

Congested and varicose lymphatics throughout the body are relieved by effleurage, a method of massage that requires stroking motions along the surface of the head, neck and trunk. To avoid any friction, which will aggravate any inflammatory condition, you must use plenty of lubrication when carrying out the effleurage.

The type of oil or cream is very important. It should be hypo-allergenic and unscented. The oils that I use are coconut oil and sweet almond oil, although some practitioners prefer using an aqueous cream. Baby oil is not suitable, as it is a perfumed mineral oil, a by-product of refining crude oil to make gasoline and other petroleum products. It is composed mainly of alkanes and cycloalkanes which, like other hydrocarbons, benzene and formaldehyde, can cause damage to the nervous system.

In a retrospective study on over a quarter of a million people in China, a research team in Taiwan showed that long-term exposure to airborne hydrocarbons increased the risk of a stroke[6]. Although topical exposure is not the same as airborne toxicity, this finding illustrates the danger to the nervous system from long-term exposure to hydrocarbons.

Stage 1: Effleurage to aid drainage in the breast tissue lymphatics

The gentle strokes are carried out rhythmically towards the subclavian region, at the level of the left and right subclavian veins, which drain all the lymph fluid into the bloodstream. Effleurage stimulates the lymphatic drainage through direct routes into the thoracic duct and the right lymphatic duct and hence into the venous return (see Figure 30). Care is taken to avoid stimulating drainage into the axillary lymph nodes in the armpit, which are prone to swelling and congestion in ME/CFS sufferers due to the backflow. It is hypothesised that the more direct route forces a high pressure within the smaller parasternal vessels, which creates enough force within the thoracic duct to alleviate the backpressure and restore a healthy drainage of toxins into the venous return.

When male practitioners are treating female patients, effleurage to the breast tissue should be carried out in the presence of a chaperone, if one is available, after explaining the exact nature of the treatment and using consent forms usually supplied by the practitioner's governing body. The gentle stroking is applied upwards covering the entire breast tissue towards the clavicle (collarbone) using the back of the hands so not to be too heavy-handed. Also, the back of the hand offers a less invasive approach.

Stage 2: Effleurage to aid drainage in the cervical lymphatic vessels

After pushing the lymph upward in the chest, it is followed by further effleurage down the front and sides of the neck towards the clavicle (collar bone) remembering to use lots of oil to reduce friction.

The black arrows in Figure 30 show the direction of the massage technique, which

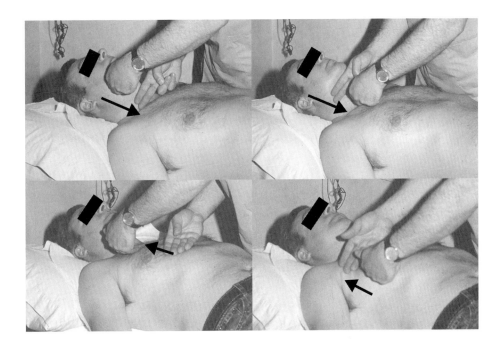

Fig. 30 Effleurage down neck and up chest to clavicle.

is always towards either clavicle on both sides. This is the region above the drainage of lymphatic fluid from the right lymphatic duct and the thoracic duct into the right and left subclavian veins respectively.

The concertina and siphon effect

This continual massage towards the subclavian region creates what I call 'the concertina effect'. As in a concertina or an accordion, where putting pressure on the ends of the bellows forces air through the instrument to produce the desired musical effect (see Figure 31), so effleurage performed towards either clavicle (collarbone) on both sides creates a pressure that forces the lymph to drain out through the central drainage into the subclavian veins (see Figure 32).

This increased pressure of lymphatic fluid produced within the thoracic and right lymphatic ducts creates a negative pressure in the lymphatic vessels above and below, which then produces what is known as the siphon effect which is familiar to anyone who has ever cleaned out the bottom of a fish tank – sucking on a tube creates a pressure gradient. Fluid will always flow from an area under higher pressure to an area of lower pressure. So, lymph will continue to drain from the entire system, eventually including the lymphatic system of the brain and spinal cord. Toxins stuck in the central nervous system, some for many years, will slowly and surely drain away after being sucked up, just like the siphon tube in the fish tank, into the main trunks and ducts of the lymphatic system.

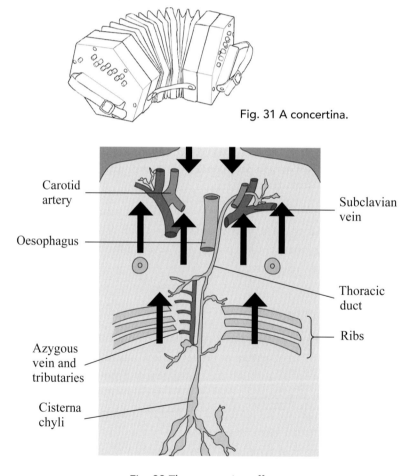

Fig. 31 A concertina.

Fig. 32 The concertina effect.

Stage 3: Gentle articulation of the thoracic region and soft tissue techniques with upward effleurage

The next stage is gentle articulation of the thoracic and upper lumbar spine, plus long-lever stretching and articulation of the ribs along with longitudinal soft tissue stretching plus effleurage of the paraspinal lymphatic vessels – the lymphatics that run up either side of the spine.

This combination of gentle articulation and soft tissue techniques improves movement of the thoracic and upper lumbar spine plus the ribs and relaxes the paravertebral muscles, trapezii, levator scapulae, rhomboids and muscles of respiration. This is achieved together with the upward effleurage from the waist to the level of the collarbone to increase the lymphatic drainage of the spine.

The main objective of the articulatory, soft tissue techniques and occasional high velocity manipulation is to improve the structure and overall quality of movement of the dorsal and upper lumbar spine.

All the articulatory techniques are slowly and gently applied with minimal force in order to avoid irritating spinal inflammation and to reduce any reactive spasm from the surrounding muscles.

The two sympathetic nerve trunks are integrally related to the overall structure of the area. By reducing mechanical irritation at this region, as well as relaxing disturbed afferent impulses, the dysfunction of the sympathetic nervous system can be corrected. There are perivascular spaces along the nerves that enter and leave the spinal cord. Improving the biomechanics of the spine and lymphatic flow in this region aids overall neuro-lymphatic drainage. This is all helped by the very rhythmic and gentle nature of this technique, which, when combined together with stretching and movement of the ribs, creates an extremely relaxing yet powerful treatment, not just for ME/CFS, but also for many upper body mechanical dysfunctions and general back pain.

This technique will also help relax the crura of the diaphragm – the muscular wall between the abdomen and thorax. The crura are the two tendinous structures that join the diaphragm to the upper lumbar vertebrae. The thoracic duct, the central 'drainage pipe' of the lymphatics, passes through the diaphragm alongside the largest artery, the aorta. Helping reduce diaphragmatic tension will aid lymphatic drainage. To quote the founder of osteopathy Andrew Taylor Still: 'At this point I will draw your attention to what I consider is the cause of a whole list of hitherto unexplained diseases, which are only effects of the blood and other fluids being prohibited from doing normal service by constrictions at the various openings of the diaphragm. Thus, prohibition of the free action of the thoracic duct would produce congestion'[7].

In cases of hypermobility, which is rarely found in a patient's thoracic spine, mobility of the adjoining areas of the spine is improved by articulation and manipulation. This takes the strain off the hypermobile segments. What is predominantly found in patients with ME/CFS, as I have said repeatedly, is a restricted dorsal spine. Frequently, the entire thoracic region is stiff, while occasionally just a few segments are affected. However, one of the most common mechanical disturbances seen in ME/CFS and FMS is a mid-thoracic spine that is flatter and more rigid than normal. Together with the mid-thoracic problem that most commonly affects T4, T5 and T6 segments, is the hypermobility of the upper cervical and the lower lumbar regions – in other words, the very top and bottom of the mobile spinal column. Paediatrician Professor Peter Rowe, who runs a specialist clinic for young ME/CFS patients in Baltimore, USA, has seen hypermobility in the cervical and lumbar spines of most of his patients, as discussed in Chapter 6. More significantly, he also observed a flattened restricted mid-thoracic region in these patients, similar to my findings.

Professor Rowe and his team at Johns Hopkins Children's Center Chronic Fatigue Clinic also found restrictions of limb movement in ME/CFS patients due to abnormal tension or tightness within the nerves and soft tissues, which can lead to abnormal pulling that makes the nerves hypersensitive. This neural tension leads to an abnormal increase in muscular tone which further restricts movement and contributes to the myalgia and fatigue in ME/CFS and FMS. Further tension is set up in the surrounding fascia and lymphatics, which also affects the neighbouring autonomic nerves. So, together with the other stages of the Perrin Technique, the combination of gentle articulatory and soft tissue techniques will reduce this neural tension and improve the overall symptoms of ME/CFS.

This stage of the treatment is carried out with the patient lying on their side to allow a gentle stretch of periscapular and paravertebral muscles together with gentle massage upwards along the spine to improve lymphatic flow. This is combined with a gentle stretch of the ribs, which is performed by holding the patient's arm with one hand whilst massaging up the angles of the ribs near the vertebrae with the other, and gently moving the held arm upwards, stretching the diaphragm and thorax. Combined stretch and massage, using the patient's arm as a long-lever, produces excellent results, with movement of the ribs increased by articulatory stretch techniques (see Figure 33).

Generally, the massage technique for the relaxation of all the paraspinal muscles groups takes the form of gentle but deep longitudinal upward strokes with the

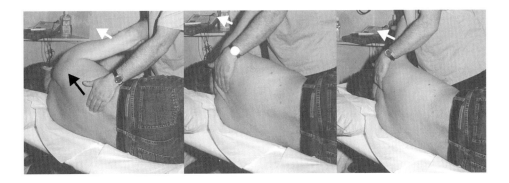

Fig. 33 Combined articulation, soft tissue stretches and paraspinal effleurage.

hypothenar eminence of the practitioner's hand. This is the bulge of the palm formed by the three muscles that help control the little finger. With the massaging hand slightly cupped, the practitioner should use a tad more pressure from the pads of their fingers to drain the paraspinal lymphatics up towards the central drainage into the blood at the level of the first thoracic vertebra. Care should be taken to carry out this effleurage technique without pressing on the spinous processes to avoid irritating the inflamed spine. As mentioned previously, when treating patients with fibromyalgia one should do less soft tissue massage and carry out more of the long-lever stretching techniques.

Besides stretching, I occasionally use more specialised osteopathic methods known as inhibition or functional techniques, which involve gentle pressure or positional holds. These are used to reduce the tone of the tightened musculature, especially the diaphragm itself.

Figure 33 shows the combination of three soft tissue techniques: long lever stretches of the intercostal muscles, using the patient's arm as a lever; direct longitudinal stretch of the dorsal erector spinae with the cupped hand, and effleurage to the paravertebral lymphatics using the fingertips. The black arrow illustrates the direction of the massage and the white arrows show the direction of movement of the patient's arm.

I try to avoid lying the patient in a prone position to avoid unnecessary pressure on the breast tissue. However, if the practitioner finds it necessary for the patient to lie prone, their face should be placed into a breathing hole in the treatment plinth to avoid unnecessary strain on the neck. The patient should be positioned on to their side as soon as possible, in order to carry out the paravertebral soft tissue work in this healthier position, while keeping the head horizontal and level with the knees apart with the aid of pillows.

After increasing the movement of the restricted spine and relaxing the surrounding musculature, an attempt to improve the respiratory mechanics is undertaken. This is important in ME/CFS patients, since the amount of oxygen in the body affects the chemical content of the body and this has a direct effect on the functioning of the body's tissues. Reduced oxygen produces greater fatigue in the patient and will aggravate the symptoms. By improving the mechanics of respiration in the rib cage, the patient's lung capacity is increased during inspiration (breathing in), thus raising the patient's oxygen intake.

Inspiration has been shown to aid cerebrospinal fluid motion, which in turn aids the cranial rhythmic impulse which I believe drives neuro-lymphatic drainage[8].

Although increasing spinal mobility and relaxing paravertebral muscles will enhance movement of the ribs, the specific respiratory muscles should also be treated in order to improve respiratory mechanics. These include the intercostal muscles, serratus anterior and posterior, pectorals, abdominals and, most importantly, the diaphragm. As stated above, gentle inhibition to the edge of the diaphragm dome will usually reduce the tone of the muscle and aid breathing. This technique is known as 'diaphragmatic release'.

After increasing the mobility of the thorax by articulation and stretching, as well as relaxing the musculature, the patient usually feels more comfortable and can lie in a supine position with knees slightly bent in readiness for the next stage of therapy.

Stage 4: Effleurage to aid drainage in the cervical lymphatic vessels

After pushing the lymph upwards in the back, it is again followed by further effleurage down the front and sides of the neck towards the clavicle, again creating the concertina effect, remembering to use lots of oil/aqueous cream to reduce friction.

Stage 5: Soft tissue massage to relax muscles and encourage lymph drainage of the cervicothoracic region

The next stage of the treatment is to relax the trapezii levator scapulae and periscapular muscles – for example, the rhomboids, as well as any other hypertonic back, shoulder and lower neck muscles (see Figure 34).

As with the other muscular stretching techniques, this 'kneading' of the trapezii and associated shoulder and cervical muscles should always be towards the sub-clavicular region in the front, level with the first thoracic vertebra in the back (see Figure 3,

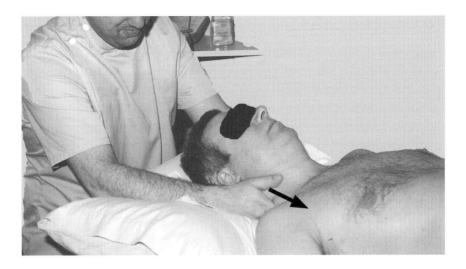

Fig. 34 Longitudinal and cross fibre stretching of lower neck and shoulders
(trapezii and levator scapulae muscles).

Chapter 1). This is combined with a kneading technique that also incorporates gentle effleurage of the surface lymphatics towards the clavicles.

Many practitioners find this stage of the technique challenging since many physios and osteopaths are originally taught to massage the muscles of the neck upwards when carrying out kneading techniques of the trapezii. This is plainly wrong as it ignores the direction of lymph towards the sub-clavicular veins beneath the collar bones.

This technique involves a slow rhythmic kneading action applied across the fibres of the lower cervical erector spinae, trapezii and levator scapulae with gentle downward effleurage with the thumbs superficially along the border of the sternocleidomastoid muscles using plenty of oil to avoid any friction.

Stage 6: Further cervical effleurage towards the subclavian region

After pushing the lymph downwards in the front, it is again followed by further effleurage down the front and sides of the neck using the backs of your fingers downwards towards the clavicle, remembering to use lots of oil to reduce friction.

Stage 7: Functional and inhibition techniques to the suboccipital region

Two major regions that often require attention when dealing with spinal problems are the suboccipital region, where the upper neck meets the cranium, and the lumbosacral area which is the where the lumbar spine joins to the wedge-shaped bone at its base, the sacrum. It is important when one treats posturo-mechanical strain of the spine to balance the suboccipital and lumbosacral segments. Any abnormal curvature will alter muscular tone along the spinal column and thus place extra load on the uppermost section and base of the spine. Similarly, positional alterations at the top and bottom of the spinal column will affect the overall mechanics of the entire spine.

Osteopaths and chiropractors may use an effective procedure in these regions known as the functional technique (see Figure 35). If, during subtle movement of the spine, a restriction is detected, however slight, the back is held at the point of restriction until a release of muscle tension occurs. In practice, osteopaths rely on finely developed palpatory skills. The main principle of any osteopathic treatment is that structure governs function (see Chapter 9). The principle of the functional technique is that by placing a joint or a group of muscles in a certain position that is

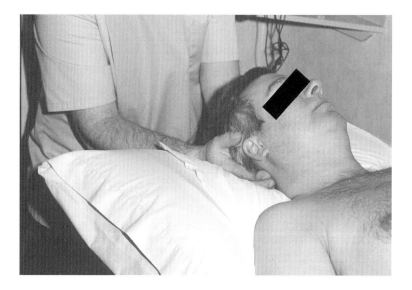

Fig. 35 Functional technique to the suboccipital region.

functionally suited for that particular bodily part, the result is a relaxation of tissues and an overall improvement in muscular and fascial tone in the region.

The suboccipital muscles can be relaxed efficiently and painlessly using this technique. With the patient lying supine (on their back), the osteopath's hands are placed at each side cradling the occiput, which is then lifted slightly off the pillow. The cervical spine is then gently extended and slowly rotated and bent towards the right or left. Traction or compression is applied and by asking the patient to breathe deeply, one is able to utilise exhalation as a relaxation tool.

A further technique that I often employ to reduce the tone in the suboccipital muscles is known as 'inhibition'. This involves the patient lying supine with the practitioner cradling the back of the patient's head. Gentle pressure is then exerted through the practitioner's finger tips just below the base of the skull and held in a fixed position, and as the pressure increases to a certain level specific to each individual case, the skilled practitioner should feel the tightness in the tone of the muscles slowly and surely 'melt' away. This technique can lead to a significant relaxation of the offending musculature.

The occipito-atlantial joint is the joint between the top vertebra of the neck, the atlas, and the back of the skull, the occiput. This joint is extremely important for the integrity of the autonomic nervous system as is the atlanto-axial joint (the joint below the atlas with the second cervical vertebra, the axis). In fact, if there is any problem with this region of the spine, many severe symptoms can arise. This is because of two main factors:

1. The Xth cranial nerve, the vagus, leaves the cranium and travels out of the spine in this region. If it were to be irritated, as has been discussed in Chapter 3, it could affect many of the body's functions, especially the heart rate and the digestive system. As we now know from the work of Dr Steven Porges, there are two distinct parts of the vagus: the ventral vagus at the front and the dorsal vagus at the back. Trauma and irritation in the cranio-vertebral region could overstimulate the dorsal vagus which can lead to worsening of some symptoms, slowing down the metabolism to a pathological level, leading to symptoms such as slow heart rate (bradycardia) and sleep apnoea when one can stop breathing while asleep.

2. The vertebral arteries. There are two major arteries travelling up each side of cervical spine. These vertebral arteries enter the cranium alongside the spinal cord and if there is a mechanical problem this can affect the flow to the brain.

Major injury to either of the vertebral arteries is rare; however, if the flow along the artery is impaired by possible arthritic changes in the cervical spine or postural and mechanical strain to the neck, it may lead to a condition known as vertebral artery insufficiency which can cause dizziness and other neurological injury, but often the symptom is head and suboccipital (uppermost region of the neck) pain. It can occur following severe trauma, but it is more common due to wear and tear of the region.

One of the leading pioneers of integrative medicine, Dr Mosaraf Ali, stresses the importance of a good flow of the vertebral arteries in his book *The Neck Connection*. As Dr Ali maintains, the carotid arteries at the front of the neck are only found in mammals and supply blood to the conscious brain. The vertebral arteries found in all vertebrates supply blood to the subconscious part of the brain, including the hypothalamus and the other centres of the autonomic nervous system. Dr Ali, although not an osteopath or chiropractor, holds by osteopathic and chiropractic principles that problems around the spine can lead to many disorders. In the neck, mechanical problems can lead to psychological and emotional as well as physical symptoms. By improving the structure and function of the cervical vertebrae one can help the cerebral blood flow, restoring overall health to the central nervous system and the whole body[9].

As mentioned previously, many patients who develop ME/CFS have injured their heads in the past. A trauma to the cranium, especially the top of the head, may result in a compression injury causing restriction of the suboccipital region. However, as discussed in Chapter 6, hypermobility in this region is common in some serious cases where patients may also have Ehlers-Danlos hypermobility type syndrome. There is a group of ME/CFS patients who also exhibit extreme symptoms, which worsen on extension of this region, which could very well be due to a Chiari malformation, as discussed in Chapter 6. The most serious cases of cranio-cervical instability require surgery to fuse the bones and stabilise the joint. However, most can be helped with the correct gentle strengthening exercises detailed in the self-help section found later in this chapter.

Stage 8: Further cervical effleurage towards the subclavian region

After working on the suboccipital region, once again the practitioner should carry out further effleurage down the front and sides of the neck towards the clavicle.

Stage 9: Stimulation of the cranio-sacral rhythm by cranial and sacral techniques

Cranial stimulation commences near the end of each consultation (see Figure 36). This technique is the most important and powerful part of the treatment as it directly affects the fluctuating, slow-wave previously described by Sutherland[10, 11], known as the cranial rhythmic impulse (CRI), which, as explained in Chapter 8, is, according to my hypothesis, the pulse of neuro-lymphatic drainage. Cranial techniques have been shown to be effective in helping all aspects of the patient's health.

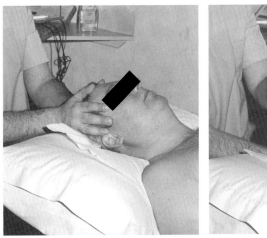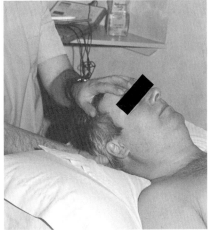

Fig. 36 Cranial treatment.

In this technique, the osteopath's hand is placed in two different positions, cradling the head laterally and antero-posteriorly. The cranial procedure involves very gentle pressure and minimal movements. The CRI has a flexion (inspiration) phase and an extension (expiration) phase, faintly changing the shape of the ventricles. Similar to the effects of the thoracic duct pump influencing the entire lymphatic system, the CRI can, by skilled practitioners, be palpated throughout the body as the lymph spreads throughout the organs and limbs[8].

The main cranial technique I use is a procedure similar to what is known in the osteopathic world as a CV4 (the compression of the fourth ventricle), although I believe it does effect a compression to the ventricular system as a whole. This compression is achieved by gentle force applied with both hands, pressing medially at the lateral angles of the occiput and around the side of the head. This is followed by rhythmically expanding the cranium by gently opening the hands and lifting the pressure of the cranium. The direction of force through the hands and arms of the practitioner when applying this technique resembles the mechanism of pumping and sucking the air in and out of blacksmith's bellows but with far less pressure and amplitude (see Figure 37).

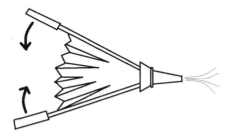

Fig. 37 A blacksmith's bellows.

During the compression phase of this gentle technique, the volume within the ventricular system is reduced, forcing the cerebrospinal fluid out and thus drainage through the olfactory, optic, trigeminal and auditory pathways plus down the spine is enhanced and accordingly, by directly improving the neuro-lymphatic drainage, it plays an important part in overall treatment.

The other main cranial hold which achieves a similar effect is known as the occipito-frontal hold, again cradling the occiput, but this time in the centre of the rear of the skull, with one hand underneath the cranium and the other hand gently pressing down in the centre of the patient's forehead.

Although to the observer, and indeed from the patient's point of view, cranial techniques may look very gentle, they are extremely powerful and often produce major changes with only a little application There are more specialised cranial techniques that I sometimes use and this is all about the individuality of the treatment, palpating the patient's specific needs at the time of each treatment, so the holds may vary at each treatment, regarding how long and how much pressure one uses. Generally, it is very gentle, with the patient feeling very little going on until the cranial treatment is over. Cranial techniques, however, should always be done after the previous eight stages of the technique mentioned above.

Some practitioners refer to the CRI as the cranio-sacral rhythm. This is due to the fact that the rhythm can be palpated easily at the sacrum at the base of the spine as the cerebrospinal fluid moves down the spine from the cranium to the sacrum and then turns back and up towards the brain. The practitioner can palpate and further stimulate the CRI at this level by cradling the sacral bones when the patient lies supine (face up) (see Figure 38).

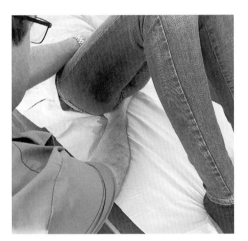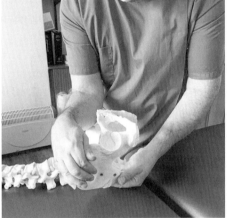

Fig. 38 Sacral treatment.

One of the osteopath's hands is held under the sacrum while the other hand balances the pelvic girdle from the front making very slight postural changes to the region. These minute changes due to altered direction of pressure from both hands allow subtle changes in the cerebrospinal fluid mechanism that can have major effects on the neuro-lymphatics and the overall spinal neural pathways.

Stage 10: Final cervical effleurage towards the subclavian region

The treatment is completed by a final few seconds of effleurage down the front and sides of the neck towards the clavicle.

After treatment

Immediately after treatment the patient may feel slightly giddy and possibly even nauseous. To avoid the patient fainting or being too disorientated they should first lie on their side, gently swing their legs over the edge of the treatment table and slowly sit up from the side lying position. They should then have a slight rest just sitting at the side of the treatment table with their feet on the floor for a minimum of 10 seconds before trying to get up from the treatment plinth. Before the patient stands up, I often apply a little alcohol-based cooling gel along his/her spine. This is to counteract any flare up of inflammation or overstimulation of the sympathetic nerves that may occur during some treatments, especially if I have manipulated any joints. I often joke to the recipient that 'this is the closest you are getting to alcohol at the moment'. Make sure the patient is not sensitive or allergic to the contents of the gel and that they are happy for you to apply it. Some patients love the effect of the cooling gel and look forward to it after their treatment, but others find it irritating and feel more of a burning sensation. This is obviously not the effect you desire so, in these cases, wash it off immediately with a damp towel and add a warning to their notes that cooling gel is not to be used in the future. In these cases, advise patients to place a cool pack (not freezing) on their spine when they get home.

Sometimes it may be a few minutes before the patient can stand up following their treatment session, and some need a drink of water to help their nausea and dizziness. This is due to the fact that this treatment 'does what it says on the tin'. Real poisons and nasty toxins are being released from the central nervous system during the half hour or so of the treatment session. The body has to be able to cope and we help the detox programme with a few choice supplements that should relieve many of the nasty side effects to this process. As the French artist Paul Cézanne and the animated character Shrek famously said, 'Better out than in'.

However, another adage, 'Less is More', originally from a poem by Robert Browning and made famous by architect Ludwig Miles van der Rohe, encompasses my golden rule for treatment of ME/CFS and FMS. When doing the Perrin Technique, always apply this rule, especially concerning cranio-sacral treatment. Particularly in the early stages of treatment, care should be taken not to over-stimulate the drainage, especially the cranial rhythm, with too long or forceful a treatment as one might drain off excess toxins at one session, causing too much of a severe reaction. As the therapeutic programme progresses and the patient improves one can gradually increase the treatment and, if necessary, use additional techniques.

Additional techniques

On top of the 10-stage treatment protocol, the practitioner will occasionally need to employ other techniques that are useful for some patients in certain circumstances. These include high velocity-low amplitude manipulation of the thoracic and upper lumbar spinal segments using supine and side-lying combined leverage and thrust techniques. Also, sometimes the diaphragm is very tight under the ribs and requires direct techniques to relax this important muscle.

The sequence, strength and duration of all the above techniques are based on each individual case, but care should be taken not to over-manipulate, especially in the lower cervical region, as this can severely exacerbate the symptoms… remember: 'Less is more'.

High velocity–low amplitude manipulation ('clicketypops')

If any of the joints are severely immobile, it may prove necessary to increase movement (see Figures 40, 41 and 42). In osteopathy, this technique is called high velocity-low amplitude (HVLA) or simply the high velocity thrust (HVT). In chiropractic, this manoeuvre is called an 'adjustment' and is commonly known as a manipulation. Physiotherapists call it Maitland mobilisation grade 5.

This manoeuvre is the best-known technique in the osteopath's armoury and involves a short, sharp motion usually applied to the spine. This procedure is designed to release structures with a restricted range of movement. There are various methods of delivering a high velocity thrust. Chiropractors are more likely to push on vertebrae with their hands, whereas osteopaths tend to use the limbs to make levered thrusts. That said, osteopathy, hands-on physiotherapy and chiropractic techniques are converging, and much of their therapeutic repertoire is shared. This technique may produce a 'cracking' sound. For my younger patients, I reduce the anxiety concerning this technique by referring to it as **'clicketypops'** treatment which usually brings a smile to the young patient's and their parent's faces.

The HVTs of the thoracic spine can be achieved with the patient lying prone (on their front), but it is preferable and safer to turn the patient on to their back and manipulate them in a supine position. Vertebral joints in some patients may appear slightly fused, and therefore strong manipulation should be avoided in order to prevent any damage to the bone.

In Figure 39, my left hand is positioned in a loose fist around the spinous process of the vertebra. As pressure is exerted from my right hand downwards, the force directed along the plane of the facet joints at the side of adjacent vertebrae will cause this joint between the vertebra to gap. When the tension has built up by positioning the patient's upper spine in a flexed and rotated position, a fast but gentle pressure is applied through the direction of force as illustrated by the arrow which further gaps the joint and brings about a long-lasting increase in mobility.

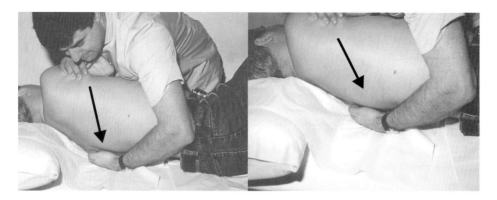

Fig. 39 Combined leverage and thrust of mid-thoracic vertebrae.

In Figure 40, the upper lumbar vertebrae are gently rotated, creating a tension at a restricted joint. By applying a further quick thrust with my hands across the joint it opens and creates more overall movement.

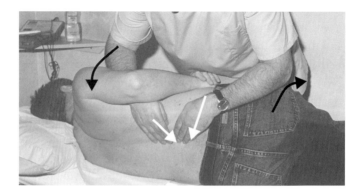

Fig. 40 Combined leverage and thrust on the upper lumbar spine.

Figure 41 shows this manipulative procedure, which involves bending the patient's neck to the left while rotating the cervical spine towards the right. Gentle pressure is placed towards the direction of the arrow, gapping the joints at the side of the restricted vertebrae, creating more movement.

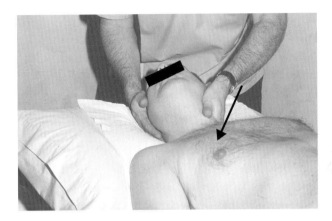

Fig. 41 Gentle combined leverage and thrust on the lower cervical spine.

Diaphragm release

As well as relaxing the crura of the diaphragm, I generally reduce tension within the diaphragm by inhibition methods similar to the inhibition of the suboccipital region mentioned earlier in this chapter. Gentle increase in pressure on the soft tissue underneath the rib cage on both sides in the upper abdomen will relax the diaphragm and aid central drainage.

Functional techniques on the sacrum and the pelvic and lower lumbar spine

Similar to the functional technique to the suboccipital region of the neck, with the patient lying supine, gentle movements are applied to the pelvic and lower lumbar region by cradling one hand under the patient's sacrum and palpating the muscular tone in the lumbar-sacral region. Traction or compression is applied and by asking the patient to breathe deeply, one is able to utilise exhalation as a relaxation tool. There is a fixed position whereby palpating the muscular tone in the lower lumbar region just

293

above the sacrum, one is able to feel the point of maximum relaxation for the pelvic and lumbar erector spinae muscles. As with other functional techniques, this position is held for a short period, resulting in a reduction of tone in this muscle group.

Inhibition and functional techniques only take a few minutes to achieve their effects, so are excellent extra tools to use alongside the standard treatment protocol of the Perrin Technique.

This chapter has touched upon the osteopathic techniques used in the treatment of ME/CFS and FMS. Some of the excellent books written about the entire spectrum of osteopathic techniques are listed in the bibliography at the end of the book.

There are a few other manual techniques that I sometimes employ when necessary, depending on the individual case. One such technique is abdominal massage. Many ME/CFS and FMS patients complain of irritable bowel syndrome, therefore, if the patient is suffering from severe bowel symptoms such as pain and bloating, or the surface abdominal lymphatic vessels feel congested and varicose, then I may use the following mild abdominal massage technique: using plenty of lubricating oil or cream, I will gently massage the tummy following the pathway of the large intestine, first going up on the right side of the patient then across the top of the abdomen to the left and then down. This slow clock-wise motion is repeated for a minute or two, usually in conjunction with the effleurage treatment of the chest.

Further down the line as the patient progresses, an experienced practitioner may wish to add other manual techniques of their own to the sessions with the patient. They may possibly be techniques specific for the patient's requirements or some procedures that have helped others. As long as they promote improved drainage of the lymphatics as well as blood flow and do not encourage any backflow of the central lymph they can be gradually added to the Perrin Technique protocol, but with caution to avoid too quick a detoxification or overloading the sympathetic nervous system by too vigorous a technique.

Self-help advice

Osteopathic treatment is not synonymous with manipulation. Many treatments of numerous conditions would be found to be insufficient if they relied on manual therapy alone[2]. As in standard osteopathic practice, advice is given to the patient to help improve their general health. Over the years, it is the patients who have followed my instructions to the letter that have done the best with the Perrin Technique.

I do realise that my exercises and advice are not always easy to follow but patients should try their best and hopefully see the benefit of being strict with the regime. The golden rule regarding exercises for ME/CFS and FMS is the same as with the treatment:

'PAIN = NO GAIN'.

You are doing nobody any favours if you push yourself through the pain barrier. Pain is the body's natural protection telling you to stop and not to push on, especially as the pain control mechanisms of the brain in the basal ganglia and thalamus are disturbed in ME/CFS and especially in FMS. This leads to a reduction in the amount of the pain-suppressing neurotransmitter GABA and increased production of the pain stimulant neuropeptide P, which have both been shown to be disturbed when the neuro-lymphatic system becomes dysfunctional (see Chapter 2).

Dorsal rotation and shrugging exercises

Manual treatment of the patient improves the function of the thorax and the spine especially, when enhanced by routine mobility exercises. Some effective exercises to improve and maintain the quality of movement of the dorsal spine areas follows. I have written them in easy-to-understand English in the second person as these instructions are important for patients to follow as accurately as possible. (Thanks to Dr Lisa Riste for helping with the plain language version.)

Sitting down (see Figure 42), facing ahead, place your hands around both sides of your neck with thumbs nearest your shoulders, elbows facing forward and down. Slowly rotate your upper body first to the right (from the waist up) keeping your head and neck facing the same direction as your upper body. This gentle rotation is designed not to stretch muscles and joints, but gradually and subtly to increase movement of your upper back. You should only rotate or twist about 45 degrees in total from right to left. Now twist gently and slowly, without stopping in the middle, to the left side. The movement must be rhythmic and as relaxed as possible during the entire process. This should be repeated five times each way.

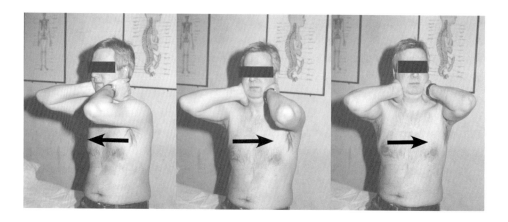

Fig. 42 Upper thoracic rotation exercise.

In the next exercise (see Figure 43), cross your arms and hug your shoulders with your hands. Repeat the movement five times each way, making sure that your head, neck and shoulders all stay in line with each other. This exercise encourages movement in the middle section of the thoracic spine.

Finally, in the third exercise (see Figure 44), fold your arms at the waist. Repeat the movement five times each way, again keeping your head, neck and shoulders in line. This exercise improves mobility of the lower thoracic spine.

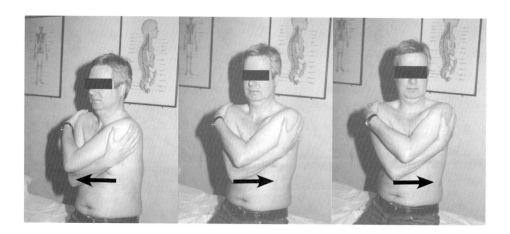

Fig. 43 Mid-thoracic rotation exercise

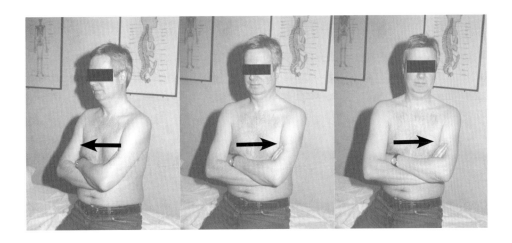

Fig. 44 Lower thoracic rotation exercise

Following the above three exercises, stand up if you are able, and gently roll your shoulders slowly forward five times and then slowly backwards repeating the rolls five times (see Figure 45).

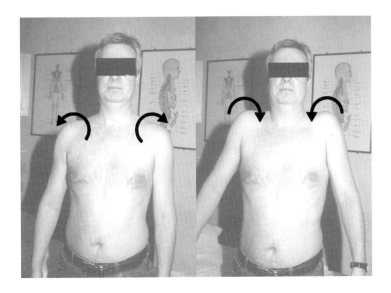

Fig. 45 Shoulder rolling exercise

The 3-stage trunk rotations together with shoulder rolls will take about one minute, if done at the correct speed.

You should carry out the entire sequence of rotation and shoulder rolling three times a day. Since it is a very gentle exercise, even if your ME/CFS is severe, this should not prevent you from carrying out these exercises. However, you are advised to cease exercises if pain develops at any time during or following the routine.

Cross-crawl

One can stimulate both halves of the brain to work together in harmony with the whole body by the following simple exercise, known as the cross-crawl. The cross-crawl exercise is basically marching on the spot crossing one limb over to the opposite side. The marching action should be slow and deliberate, with your right arm moving in unison with your left leg with best results touching your flexed left knee with your right hand.

This action is repeated moving your left arm forward together with your right leg touching your right knee with your left hand. ME/CFS patients sometimes find this simple task difficult to perform at the beginning of therapy, since their bodies are so un-coordinated. It is very important not to move the arm and leg of the same side together, as this will succeed in throwing your body (and mind) further out of balance. After practising for a while, patients are able to carry out the cross-crawl exercise without too much difficulty. The marching routine is to be done up to five minutes during an entire day, a minute or so at a time. Remember that it shouldn't exhaust you as any exercises that over-exert you will worsen your condition and are always to be avoided.

This technique can be adapted by very severe patients who are wheelchair bound or even bedridden. This can take the form of the patient gently moving their left hand slowly up and down together with their right foot followed by their right hand together with their left foot, and flexing and extending each hand and foot five times at a time. This can be repeated every day, or more frequently if the patient feels that they are still following the half rule, without ever exhausting themselves.

Strengthening exercises for hypermobile spinal joints

Suboccipital hypermobility

If patients suffer from suboccipital hypermobility/cranio-cervical instability, I advise the following isometric exercise routine (i.e. with only pressure but no actual movement). It is essential that no movement of the neck takes place. Repeat the six different stages of the exercises five to 10 times as long as it is not too taxing for you. The whole routine should be completed three times a day as long as you can cope with the exercises and feel that it is not too strenuous. In other words, keeping with the tenet of the half rule, you should feel that you are easily able to do double the amount of exercise without aggravating your symptoms.

1. Lying down or sitting upright, gently hold one or both hands on your forehead. Try to slightly flex your neck, i.e. face looking downwards, but stop any movement with your hand/s pressed on your forehead so that your head remains at all times facing forward. This attempt to bend your head downwards should be maintained for three seconds and then you should gently relax the pressure before repeating the exercise five to 10 times in total (see Figure 46a).

2. Next try to slightly extend your neck (i.e. bending head back), again without any actual movement, stopping the extension with your hand/s pressed on the back of your head (occiput). This attempt to bend your head backwards should be maintained for three seconds and then you should gently relax the pressure before repeating the exercise five to 10 times in total (see Figure 46b).

3. Try to slightly tilt your head to the right stopping any movement with your

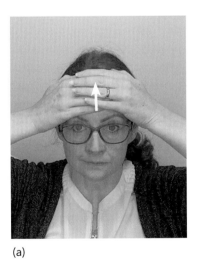
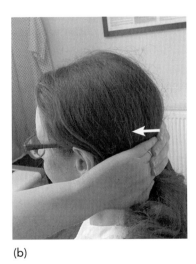

(a)   (b)

Fig. 46 Cervical isometrics (a) Attempting to bend head forward, prevented by gentle backwards pressure of hands. (b) Attempting to bend head back, prevented by gentle forward pressure of hands.

right hand on the side of your head. This attempt to bend your head sideways should be maintained for three seconds and then you should gently relax the pressure before repeating the exercise five to 10 times in total (see Figure 46c).

4. Repeat the same exercise in stage 3 for the left side (see Figure 46d).

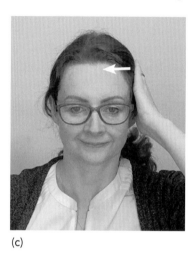 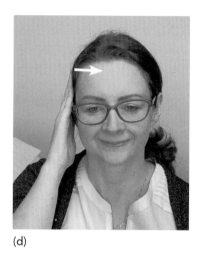

(c)   (d)

Fig. 46 Cervical isometrics (c) Attempting to bend head to the left, prevented by gentle counter-pressure of left hand. (d) Attempting to bend head to the right, prevented by gentle counter-pressure of right hand.

The first four stages gently strengthen the whole neck; however, the next two exercises are specifically designed to remedy the suboccipital instability.

5. Now try to slightly flex the very top of your neck by trying to tuck in your chin, stopping any movement with both your thumbs pressed into the inside of your chin. This attempt to tuck in your chin should be maintained for three seconds and then you should gently relax the pressure before repeating the exercise five to 10 times in total. For the exercise to be successful it is important that little or no movement of your chin or neck takes place (see Figure 46e).

6. Try to slightly extend the very top of your neck by trying to poke out your chin stopping any movement with one or both hands pressed against the front of your jaw. This attempt to push out your chin should be maintained for three seconds and then you should gently relax the pressure before repeating the exercise again five to 10 times in total. As with stage 5, it is essential that little or no movement of your chin or neck takes place (see Figure 46f).

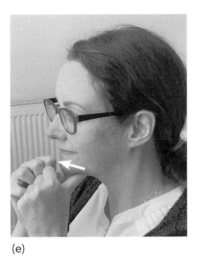
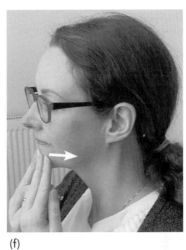

(e)   (f)

Fig. 46 Cervical isometrics (e) Attempting to tuck in chin, prevented by gentle forward counter-pressure of thumbs. (f) Attempting to push chin forward, prevented by gentle backwards counter-pressure of fingers.

Hypermobility of the lower lumbar region

In cases of hypermobility of the lower lumbar region, I advise patients to carry out the following exercise routine. You should repeat the different stages of the exercises up to 10 times, three times a day, as long as it is not too taxing for you.

1. First, lie on your back, preferably on a firm surface such as a yoga mat, with knees bent. Lying on the bed will be okay if you find it difficult to lie on the floor.
2. Next, lift your bottom and lower back gently up a few centimetres from the floor and hold for three seconds.
3. Slowly lower your bottom and gently relax the muscles before repeating the exercise. For those familiar with yoga, this exercise is similar to 'the bridge' position but without lifting the bottom so high.

Home-massage routine

Patients are advised to aid the lymphatic drainage of their head and spine through a self-massage routine carried out at home which further aids lymphatic drainage from the central nervous system into the blood. As we now know, the main bulk of toxins are drained from the brain into the lymphatics during delta-wave sleep, which is why it is so restorative. However, as discussed in Chapter 3, ME/CFS and FMS patients unfortunately don't get much delta-wave sleep but too much alpha-wave sleep, which is non-restorative.

Therefore, stimulating neuro-lymphatic drainage at night will hopefully mimic what is meant to happen naturally and you will wake up more refreshed as the toxins drain out of your central nervous system. So, the full routine as shown below should be done once at night, preferably just before bed.

Nasal release

Sitting down, rest your elbows on a table in front of you and apply gentle pressure with the pads of both index fingers to just below where the upper and lower eyelids meet (in the corner of your eyes). Push slightly upwards, or if more comfortable, pull slightly downwards just above the bridge of the nose. Choose the position that feels most comfortable and lets you breathe the easiest. If neither method is more effective at aiding breathing, then you should always choose downward pressure as the default method. For the first 10 days of this self-treatment, apply this pressure for seven minutes. After this you should reduce this to one minute in order to maintain the improvement.

After the first 10 days, you should continue with nasal release for a one-minute period each day in order to maintain the improvement (see Figure 47).

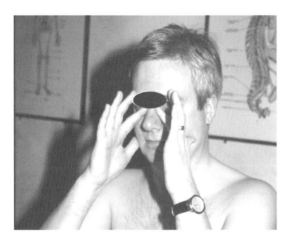

Fig. 47 Nasal release.

Facial massage

Spread the fingers of one hand across your face, as if trying to span your forehead, and slowly stroke your fingertips down your face to your chin (see Figure 48). Repeat this gentle facial stroking for 20 seconds with one downwards stroke roughly every four seconds.

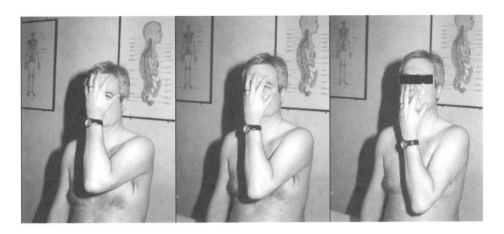

Fig. 48 Facial self-massage.

Head massage

You should now gently massage the sides and the back of your head:

(a) For the sides of your head: repeat the strokes used in the facial massage above, using your hands to gently stroke downwards on both sides of your head at once from the top of your head to your chin with the same slow rhythm again for 20 seconds.

(b) For the back of your head, repeat again with gentle downward stroking using both hands at the back of your head working down to your neck for a further 20 seconds (see Figure 49).

For the remainder of the self-massage, you should use some massage oil. This can be sweet almond, coconut oil or similar depending on any allergies or sensitivities you may have). NB: Avoid baby oil or any other petrochemical-based cream.

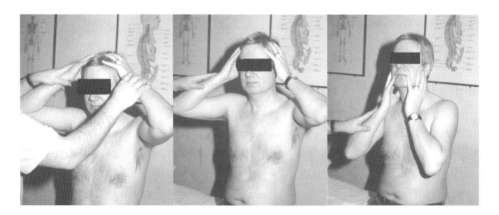

Fig. 49 Self-massage to head.

Self-massage to front of neck

Lie down and using the oil, massage gently from the top of your neck just under your ear, down towards your collarbone using the fingertips of one hand and the back of your other hand for 20 seconds on each side (see Figure 50).

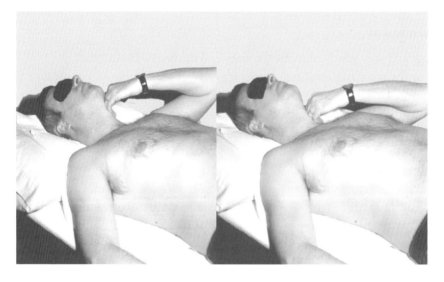

Fig. 50 Self-massage to front of neck.

Breast massage

The breast/chest massage is easiest done in three sections (outer, centre and inner), using massage oil for 20 seconds in each area so the right and left areas are massaged for one minute each. The massage must always be towards the clavicles, thus directing the lymph away from the axillary lymph nodes to avoid risk of glandular swelling in the armpit (see Figure 51).

> **Outer:** Massage the side of your chest with a slow rhythmic stroking movement, with the flat fingertips of one hand and rubbing upwards with the other hand in a loose fist position. Start just underneath the breast area and work upwards towards the collarbone (not towards armpits).

> **Centre:** Repeat the massage movements but working over the centre of the breast so the massage is up over the nipple area, again up to the collarbone.

> **Inner:** This is the same movement but using the backs of the fingers with both hands flat on the inside area of the chest.

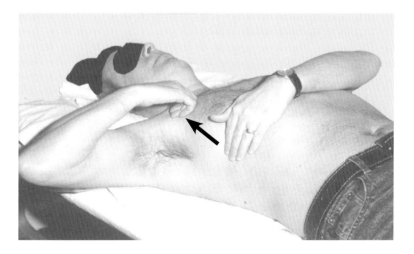

Fig. 51 Self-massage of the breast.

In Figure 51 the black arrow shows the direction of the self-massage technique. The pressure applied by the patient should be much less than during a treatment session, concentrating only on the superficial lymphatics.

Back massage

Having adopted a prone position, the patient receives back massage from a family member or friend. The massage routine comprises of one minute of gentle upward effleurage to the sides of the spine, finishing in the shoulder region level with the clavicles. If no help is available, patients should use back brushes to accomplish the back massage. There are specific back massagers made out of wood with rubber heads, or other metal ones which are extendable and rubber rollers. Both these massage hammers are easy to use and are available to buy online. One useful tool to do the back massage oneself is a small fluffy paint roller with a long handle used to paint behind wall radiators. Just move the roller upwards each side of the thoracic spine to the level of the collar bones just below the base of the neck.

Back of neck massage

The self-massage routine ends with slow downwards rhythmic massage of the back of the neck towards the level of collarbone carried out for 20 seconds on each side of the spine.

The full routine is summarised in Table 10.1.

Table 10.1 The full routine

(To be completed at night, before bed, by the patient or with help from a carer)

Nasal release	Rest elbows on table; place tips of index fingers on either side of nose (above the bridge); gently pull down/press up for 7 minutes for the first 10 days, followed by 1 minute thereafter
Facial massage	With fingers spread out apply a little pressure and gently stroke down the face for 20 seconds (five times taking 4 seconds each)
Head massage	a. Gently stroke down the side of the head for 20 seconds each side b. Gently stroke down the back of the head for 20 seconds
Neck massage (use oil)	Down for 20 seconds each side simultaneously or one after the other, whichever you find best

Breast massage (use oil)	Up for one minute each side (NB Divide breast into three sections; outer, middle and inner and massage for 20 seconds each towards the collar bone and not the armpit)
Back massage (use oil)	Up for 1 minute each side of the spine (careful not to touch spinal column)
Neck massage – back (use oil)	Down for 20 seconds each side (simultaneously or one and then the other, whichever you find best)

Some patients whose symptoms are not too severe may find that a more regular self-massage routine speeds up the healing process. In the following extra top-up routine, only the head and neck are targeted, and it starts with the nasal release for only 1 minute. The shorter self-massage routine is completed with downward massage of the face and head followed by gently stroking down the front and back of the neck. This can be done anywhere as it is achieved without oil and without having to remove any clothing (see Table 10.2).

Table 10.2 The head and neck drainage routine
(To be completed up to three times a day)

Nasal release	For 1 minute
Facial massage	Down for 20 seconds at a time
Head massage	Down for 20 seconds at a time
Neck massage	Down for 20 seconds at a time each side, front and back

Active head rest

This is a do-it-yourself technique that I recommend for patients if I feel that the cranial flow could do with a little extra help, usually in the later stages of the treatment programme, as initially it may be too much too soon. It should only be done by patients at the beginning of therapy if they cannot access the actual Perrin Technique treatment. It is a simple exercise that is taught by practitioners of the Alexander technique (see Chapter 5).

In the early days of osteopathy in the late nineteenth century, Dr Andrew Tayler Still, the founder of osteopathy, developed a similar exercise when he suffered from a severe headache. The story goes that he lay down and balanced his head on a swing. In those days in Missouri standing swings that rested just above the ground were all the rage, and Taylor Still found that by positioning his head at a certain angle he felt comfortable and in a short time his headache disappeared. This probably was the first cranial treatment ever performed.

One of the principles taught to me as a student osteopath was 'comfort governs function', which basically means that if the body is in the most comfortable position it will function better. So, if the head is positioned in the most comfortable position then the cranial flow AKA the neuro-lymphatic drainage from the brain will improve.

Nowadays we don't use planks of wood or swings. You, the patient, should experiment with a paperback book or books placed under the occiput, which is the bone at the back of the head, until the most comfortable angle is achieved (see Figure 52). You should lie on a yoga mat or a duvet placed on the floor, so the ground is firm but not too hard, in a semi-supine position (on your back with knees bent) for about 10–15 minutes at night, preferably after the self-massage routine summarised in Table 10.1, just before going to sleep.

If you do not find any suitable book that you feel comfortable with, then this exercise should not be carried out as it will probably worsen the condition…it only works if it feels comfortable…remember: 'comfort governs function'.

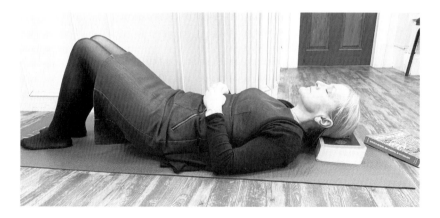

Fig. 52 Head rest exercise

Returning to good health

Patients are advised to avoid any stress, whether physical, mental or emotional, whenever possible. It isn't always easy and sometimes it's impossible, but you should try as hard as possible to reduce stress.

Activities that exert strain on the body are to be avoided. If your occupation involves too much physical or mental activity, you are advised to stop work temporarily or reduce your workload. This especially applies to tasks that put extra mechanical strain on your thoracic spine.

Physical and mental tasks that exert too much strain on you are, if possible, to be done by a helpful colleague. Members of your family are advised to share the workload at home, including any paperwork, to make life as bearable as possible, until treatment has restored you to better health.

If you usually spend time in front of a computer, or VDU, or if you are desk-bound at work, you are advised to stand up every half-hour for a minute or two and walk around the office. You should also take a 15-minute break, every two hours.

You are instructed to avoid slumping into a soft chair. When relaxing, you are advised to sit in a supportive chair and if your case is severe, to lie on your side as much as possible on a couch or a bed with your head well supported and a pillow between your knees. Lying on your side puts minimal strain on to your spine. It has also been shown that the neuro-lymphatic drainage occurs more when lying on the side. As mentioned already in Chapters 1 and 5, scientists have discovered that a lateral sleeping position is the best position to most efficiently remove waste from the brain[12].

Diet and nutrition

In Chapter 5 there is a comprehensive section on advice often given to ME/CFS and fibromyalgia patients by nutritionists and dieticians. Although there are specific needs for many patients with allergies and sensitivities, generally I advise most patients to vary their diet with as much diversity as possible. This reduces the possibility of placing strain on any particular region of the gastro-intestinal system. Patients should all reduce their intake of sugar and yeast, dairy products and foods containing gluten. Processed foods should be avoided as much as possible and brown flour and brown sugar should replace the white variety. Stimulants such as caffeine are to be reduced and avoided if possible. Decaffeinated coffee and decaffeinated tea or herbal tea can be drunk instead, but, because decaffeinated coffee has been shown to increase cholesterol levels, this should be taken only in moderation. Naturally caffeine-free tea such as Rooibos/Red Bush tea is preferable.

Patients should eat regular, healthy meals and drink plenty of healthy fluids, such as filtered or bottled mineral water – 2 litres a day for an adult should be enough.

I am totally against smoking as it has so many proven detrimental effects on health; however, the stress of trying to stop smoking may be too much for some patients and place excess strain on the sympathetic nervous system so, as much as I hate saying this, for some patients it is better to continue smoking than trying to quit while they are trying to recover from ME/CFS and FMS.

Alcohol is an absolute NO! NO! for ME/CFS. This is for two fundamental reasons. The detrimental effects alcohol has on the liver are well documented and it is known that alcohol is the main cause of cirrhosis and liver disease. The main aim of the Perrin Technique is to drain toxins out of the central nervous system into the lymphatic system. The lymphatics will eventually drain the toxins into the bloodstream with most ending up in the liver, which will need support rather than a further toxic load provided by alcohol.

However, the main reason why even a small amount of alcohol aggravates ME/CFS, and FMS, is due to its effect on the brain. We now know which one the main areas affected by a backflow of the neuro-lymphatics into the brain. As discussed earlier in Chapters 2 and 5, research has shown that when the drainage through the perivascular spaces was stopped there was a build-up of toxins in the thalamus and basal ganglia of the brain. The thalamus contains high levels of N-methyl-D-aspartate (NMDA). The methyl in the name is the clue, as this neurochemical is affected when one drinks any alcohol and it is this neurotransmitter that causes many of the symptoms of drunkenness. In ME/CFS and FMS, NMDA overstimulation leads to increased pain and more sleep disturbance as well as reduced cognitive function. So, alcohol, even a tiny drop, will usually worsen a patients' symptoms and indeed many patients find they cannot tolerate much alcohol anyway, with a small amount making them feel drunk.

This brings us to the next part of the advice to patients to aid their return to better health – supplements. Many supplements come in tinctures in little bottles which allow droplets of the remedy to be taken easily into the body rather than in pill or capsule form. The liquid medium of the tincture is usually alcohol-based and so if one takes tinctures of supplements with alcohol then drop it into boiling water first which will evaporate the alcohol, wait until the water has cooled down and drink the safe mixture.

Supplements

As well as a healthy diet, a supplement of vitamins C and B complex is advised. The former increases the patient's resistance to infection, while B complex improves energy production and general functioning of the nervous system. A daily dose of 500 mg of vitamin C and a strong, or whole B complex tablet are recommended. Vitamins B and C are both water-soluble so that any excess is excreted from the body. However, one of the functions of vitamin C is to aid the absorption of calcium, so there is a risk of developing kidney stones if the vitamin C intake is too high. I always try to err to the side of caution and so advise patients to take only 500 mg a day.

Beware of taking so many different supplements that any possible benefit is likely to be outweighed by undesired side effects. In addition, many supplements can have an adverse reaction with other medications and may exert a strain on the gut as well as the liver and thus the lymphatics and the sympathetic nervous system. This will undoubtedly worsen the symptoms of ME/CFS and FMS.

One of my patients was taking so many supplements and prescribed medications that the first instruction I gave to her was to reduce all these supplements and go back to her doctor and check which medications she could stop or reduce the dose of (see Figure 53). It took quite a while for her body to pick up after reducing this overload of

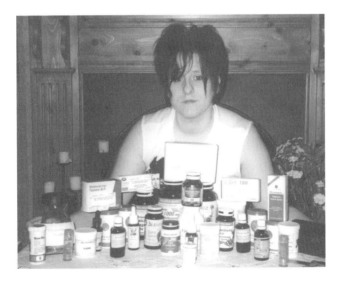

Fig. 53 An ME/CFS patient and her daily medication

supplementation and medication. However, together with the treatment she received from myself and one of my colleagues, she began to recover as is clearly demonstrated in the photo of her taken a few years on (see Figure 54). It is always best to seek expert professional advice when taking any medicinal treatments, whether pharmaceutical or herbal. So, speak to your doctor, pharmacist, naturopath, nutritionist or herbalist to find out what is best for you.

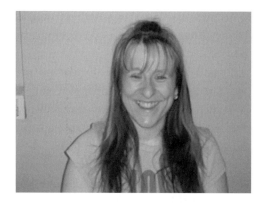

Fig. 54 The same patient after receiving the Perrin Technique and reducing her supplements and medication intake

Even though excessive use is harmful, occasionally supplements may be needed. After a patient has received a good few treatments, and when the overall symptoms of ME/CFS or FMS, start to lessen, many patients begin to develop a full blown cold or suffer from flu for maybe the first time in years. This may sound crazy, but this is usually a very positive sign. It means that the immune system is starting to work properly after a very long time. In many cases of ME/CFS, initially there is an upward regulation of the immune response, so in the early stages patients with ME/CFS rarely experience colds or flu, they just feel constantly ill with their general ME/CFS and FMS symptoms worsening. It is akin to a troop of marine commandos attacking a country which responds by dropping a nuclear bomb on the commandos, killing them but destroying a large part of the country in the process. The immune system of a ME/CFS patient will initially over-react to a virus, bacterium or fungus and kill the offending pathogen, but at the same time use up their energy reserve, exhausting the patient and aggravating all the other symptoms.

This overactive immune response has been demonstrated in recent research at Kings College London. The research team demonstrated that in the early stages of the disease, the immune system is 'primed' to give exaggerated responses to infections which exhausts the patient and leads to chronic fatigue. However, this hyper-immunity didn't seem to last for more than six months. They concluded that in ME/CFS there is an abnormal immune mechanism[13].

Eventually, in time the immune system starts to try and balance, there is more and more chance of developing colds and other infections like normal individuals. However, some severely ill patients eventually suffer from a depleted immune system where the whole immune process has become exhausted and these very debilitated patients become susceptible to infection after infection which ultimately leads to disastrous effects on their overall health. In the very worst cases this eventually can cause organ or system failure. It is in this terrible state that a few individuals over the years have succumbed to the illness, such as Sophia Mirza and Merryn Crofts mentioned in Chapter 6.

Getting worse before getting better

One proof that the Perrin Technique is not a placebo is the fact that most patients feel a great deal worse at the beginning of their treatment. Placebo treatments generally do not make you feel worse. The reason for this initial exacerbation in the symptoms is due to the fact that, for the first time, the toxins embedded (possibly for years) in the central nervous system are being released into the rest of the body.

Headaches and pain are due to excess toxicity. As the treatment encourages the toxins to leave the brain, they will initially affect the superficial tissues in the head and, as they drain down to the rest of the body, pain may follow. We know from the earlier studies of the glymphatic system by the research team at Rochester University in New York, that the first points of toxic build-up when the drainage stops are the thalamus and the basal ganglia, which control pain perception around the body[14]. So, any pain felt by the patient due to stimulation of any nociceptor (pain receptor) outside the brain is exaggerated. However, the toxins within the brain do not cause actual pain since there are no nociceptors within the brain itself. Nevertheless, toxins do affect the *function* of the brain and spinal cord, and this accounts for most of the symptoms of ME/CFS and FMS.

Another unpleasant sign that occurs when the body's drainage is improving is the appearance of spots, boils and other skin eruptions. Until the lymphatic channels are working properly, the toxins have to go somewhere and the quickest way out of the body is often through the skin. These normally clear up as the treatment progresses. Some patients in the past have suffered from severe acne which occurs when the oil from sebaceous glands block hair follicles in the skin. Bacteria which infect the plugged follicles, causing the pustules seen in acne, may resurface with treatment and re-infect the hair follicles leading to a resurgence of the acne.

The first few weeks, or sometimes months in severe cases, are always the most trying for the patient. In clinic I have often noticed that the worse the patient is in the early stages of treatment, the better, usually, it bodes for their prognosis as the toxins flow out of the central nervous system. However, we need the patient to cope with the side effects and if the reaction is too unpleasant and the patient suffers too much it can be counterproductive.

The Perrin Technique is patient-centred at all times. It is important that the practitioner listens to the patient and initially goes very softly, softly with the treatment. If the patient is in too much pain with the initial treatment, or other symptoms become unbearable, the practitioner should lessen the treatment intensity and sometimes space out the treatment sessions to a level where the patient can cope. Occasionally, patients respond better when the treatment is more intense and more frequent. As I have stressed throughout the book, every ME/CFS patient is different.

In the early days of my treatments, when I was developing my techniques, some patients dropped out of therapy as they could not cope with the side effects. I realised that every patient needs a different amount of treatment and by listening to the symptoms of the patient at the early stages both patient and practitioner can work out the routine that suits the patient's condition and achieve the best results in the longer term.

The main aspects for ME/CFS and FMS sufferers to focus upon are the changes occurring with the treatment. (If change has not occurred in any way during the first 12 weeks of treatment, the patient may have to take an alternative route in their search for a cure.) My treatment often hugely improves the patient's health, but most will need other treatments in tandem in order to alleviate all symptoms. I have noticed that other treatments – whether they be based on nutrition or pharmaceuticals – work better after the patient's neuro-lymphatic pathways have improved. Patients who have tried supplements before treatment, to no avail, are advised to try some of the supplements again after undergoing the Perrin Technique, as they may now prove more effective.

For colds and flu

When patients do start to develop full blown colds and other infections, some are really excited, as they remember me telling them in their initial consultation that this is sometimes a sign of the immune over-activation lessening and a good symptom. Some have come into the clinic with a big smile across their faces telling me with glee that they had a proper cold complete with coughing, sneezing and red nose and it lasted a few days but they have mostly recovered without any major effect on their ME/CFS or FMS symptoms. However, we don't want the patient to continue with repetitive infections, so to help avoid the immune system going into free fall when infection strikes, I recommend a number of supplements to help.

- **Garlic** is known for its antimicrobial properties. I usually advise patients with infections to take the highest dose possible of allicin. This is one of the active ingredients of garlic and has been shown to exhibit antibacterial activity against a wide range of gram-negative and gram-positive bacteria which won't directly help viruses but reduces the chance of secondary bacterial infection that could lead to pneumonia; allicin has also been shown to promote antifungal activity, particularly against *Candida albicans*; antiparasitic activity, including against some major human intestinal protozoan parasites, and antiviral activity[15].

- **Phytosterols (plant sterols)** have been shown to target specific lymphocytes – Th1 and Th2 cells – improving immune activity. I regularly advise patients to take a small dose of plant sterols as preventative supplements when there may be an outbreak of flu in their neighbourhood, and if they are suffering symptoms of colds and flu then maximum dose helps balance the immune system as the patient fights off the infection[16].

- If the allicin and phytosterols don't help I would advise the patient to next try *Echinacea* – a good natural immune system stimulant. Echinacea, also known as coneflower, is a native of central North America and used by native American tribes for sore throats, snake bites and sepsis. *Echinacea purpurea* is the most commonly used form. It seems to help the immune activity rather than target specific viruses. The recommended dose is usually in the region of 500 mg taken three times a day. However, Echinacea shouldn't be used for more than a few weeks at a time and it is often recommended only for short-term use.

- One of nature's natural antibiotics, **bee propolis**, is also a useful tool when fighting infections.

- Another very effective, but probably the most hideous-tasting natural remedy, is **grapefruit seed extract** which enhances the immune system and can be used to help with all manner of infections, whether parasitic, viral, bacterial or fungal. Grapefruit seed extract has been shown to be effective at very low concentrations to reduce candida, and bacterial loads[17].

Flu jabs are at the patient's discretion. Most stockpiled vaccines used to contain thimerosal (which is a mercury-based preservative, as described earlier – page 219). However, most flu vaccines are now made differently, so patients should be okay. It is still important to check with your doctor and pharmacist that the vaccine is toxin-free.

Patients with heavy-metal poisoning struggle to respond to treatment since the heavy metals lie ingrained deep within the glial cells of the brain. Therefore, the standard lymph drainage techniques are simply not powerful enough to drain the heavy metals away. Detoxing with chelation agents as mentioned earlier in Chapter 5 (page 117) is necessary in these cases to help with overall treatment process.

Frequency of treatment

At the beginning of treatment, it is important that the patient is treated once a week and that the treatment remains regular and weekly. This usually carries on for at least the first 12 weeks and, slowly, as the symptom picture improves, there is a gradual increase in the time between consultations. With very severe cases, weekly treatments may be necessary for much longer than three months. Eventually, when patients remain symptom-free between their six-monthly check-ups and are able to perform all reasonable activities, doing all they could do before they were ill with no side effects, I will score them 10 out of 10. This is difficult to achieve, but it does happen every so often and is a wonderful feeling for both sufferer and practitioner. When I discharge the 10/10 patients it gives me the motivation and strength to carry on my clinical work treating some very severe bed-ridden patients and continue my research into ME/CFS and FMS.

While acknowledging that every patient is different, I have devised a chart based on the general severity of the illness that is a guide to both the patient and practitioner when calculating the overall prognosis – see Table 10.3.

Table 10.3 The outlook

Score	Description	Prognosis
1	Extreme symptoms and signs for more than a year. Totally bed-ridden or sitting all day, little cranial flow palpable.	3 years +
2	Severe symptoms and signs for more than a year. Bed-ridden or sitting all day, little cranial flow palpable.	2 years+
3	Severe symptoms and signs for more than a year, resting most of the day, little cranial flow palpable.	2 years
4	Severe symptoms and signs for 6–12 months, resting most of the day, little cranial flow palpable.	18 months+
5	Severe symptoms and signs for at least 6 months; able to carry out light tasks but requires regular rest periods.	12–18 months
6	Moderate symptoms and signs for at least 6 months; able to work part-time with a struggle.	8–12 months
7	Moderate symptoms and signs for at least 6 months; able to work full-time with difficulty.	8 months
8	Moderate symptoms and signs for at least 6 months; daily life slightly limited. Symptoms worsen on activity.	6 months
9	No symptoms but still signs of slight lymphatic engorgement and experiences mild symptoms following over-exertion	3 months
10	Symptom-free for at least 6 months. Able to live a full active life …within reason.	Discharged

Table 10.3 is a sliding scale and should be used as a general guide. In other words, if a patient initially scores 5/10 on ME/CFS alone, and is also suffering from another disorder, the overall score may be 4/10 or lower. If the physical findings during the examination are very evident and apparent, the overall score is lowered. As I have said, I often find that the patient is trying to appear healthier than they really are. This fits the profile of average ME/CFS sufferers who try as hard as they can to keep going until, eventually, they have to admit they cannot go on or they just collapse.

In 2014, Dr John Juhl, DO, an osteopathic physician in New York, who attended my workshop on the Perrin Technique, posed the following challenge. He argued that the score 0–10 should accurately correlate with the patient's history and overall condition rather than just rely on a score based on my experience, and should also focus mainly on the patient's quality of life.

I agreed wholeheartedly with him. He said, 'it seems important both to give the patient a sense of whether they have the diagnosis at their initial office visit, and how long they should expect the treatment to last'. This is important and I could see it being difficult for a practitioner new to my techniques to make an accurate score that was reliable.

So in 2014 I set to work for a few months analysing dozens of initial scores that I had given in prior cases. I devised a weighted scoring system that I adapted to reflect the different factors that led me to a reasonably accurate initial score for most patients; I further updated this in 2019. This new four-part scoring system delivers an objective method of determining a more precise overall prognosis that can be used by all trained practitioners.

The Perrin-Juhl ME/CFS scoring system

A. ME/CFS symptoms

The first score we calculate is the number of common symptoms of ME/CFS and FMS that a patient has. This is achieved by using the general health questionnaire devised for my initial clinical trial, the 50-symptom Perrin Questionnaire for chronic fatigue syndrome/ME (PQ-CFS)[18] (see Appendices, page 422, for a copy of the questionnaire).

Note that the PQ-CFS maximum scores are:

Adult female = 49

Adult male = 47 (as no symptoms would be reported related to menses).

The maximum scores are not 50 and 48 since ME/CFS does not cause joint swelling (question 16 on the questionnaire), so patients with only ME/CFS will not place a tick for this symptom. If they do, it means that there is a comorbidity (another condition) that is some form of arthritic condition, and thus they would add the score for that comorbidity to the PQ-CFS score – see part B.

B. Comorbidities

The next part of the Perrin-Juhl scoring system reflects the impact of other conditions that may be present together with the ME/CFS or FMS.

For **each** comorbidity add the following to the PQ-CFS score in part A:

if minor impact + 5

if moderate impact +10

if severely affected +20.

C. Quality of life

One should then analyse how the patient's life has been affected by their various symptoms/comorbidities and factor that into the overall calculation, as follows.

Add the following to the total scores from Part A and Part B:

Able to continue as normal + 0

Only able to work part-time/struggling to cope with work + 5

Unable to work but not housebound + 10

Housebound + 20

Totally bedridden +40.

D. Longevity of symptoms

Add the following score to reflect the time the patient has suffered from their symptom(s):

Under 12 months + 0

1–5 years + 5

5–10 years + 10

More than 10 years + 20.

Calculate a total score by working through parts A–D, then convert this to a score out of 10 using Table 10.4.

Table 10.4 Conversion chart

Total score	Severity of ME/CFS
125+	1/10
101–124	1.5/10
81–100	2/10
71–80	2.5/10
61–70	3/10
51–60	3.5/10
46–50	4/10
41–45	4.5/10
36–40	5/10
31–35	5.5/10
26–30	6/10
21–25	6.5/10
16–20	7/10

As patients show a significant change in their symptoms or their quality of life improves, then it will change the scores. Equally, if they recover from their comorbidity then the ME/CFS score will improve.

I and other practitioners can expect to see very few new patients over 7/10 as they are just about coping and usually do not see the reason to seek medical help.

Later on in the treatment, as the patient improves, a score above 7 represents the patient's ability to do more normal things without feeling worsening symptoms, which is reflected in my original Table 10.3 on the overall prognosis for the illness.

Also, most important: if using the new Perrin-Juhl ME/CFS scoring system, and you find the patient hasn't scored too high (e.g. 39) but is clearly suffering more severely than the converted 5/10 score suggests, then a physical examination usually helps to produce a more accurate score. For example, if the physical signs are very noticeable and palpable, then the ME/CFS severity score should be reduced by 1, so in this example the patient would score a 4/10 rather than 5/10 which should give a more accurate prognosis. Some more examples are shown in Table 10.5.

Table 10.5 Actual patient examples

	WT, 27-year-old student	AB, 28-year-old director	JR, 34-year-old civil servant
PQ-CFS score	25	18	19
Comorbidities	None	Growth on adrenal gland but minor impact + 5	Migraine minor impact on ME/CFS +5
Quality of life	Able to attend university for full-time masters course	Unable to work but not housebound +10	
Longevity of symptoms	9 months	Ill for 6 years +10	3 years + 5
Initial PJ-CFS score before physical exam	25 6.5/10	43 4.5/10	29 6/10
Physical exam results	Flat spine; many varicose lymph and very tender Perrin's point; tender coeliac plexus and sluggish CRI	Severe tender points and spine plus very sluggish cranial rhythm	All signs mild
Adjusted PJ-CFS score after exam	5.5/10	3.5/10	No change: 6/10
Notes	The adjusted score still gave him a good prognosis aiming to get him back to good health about a year after the start of treatment.	Due to the severity of the physical symptoms which were much worse than a usual 4.5, I then reduced the score.	Good prognosis 8–12 months

As we have noted earlier in the book, ME/CFS patients often try to appear healthier than they actually are. So, after the consultation you may find that the patient might actually be a 3/10 but is trying to act as a 7/10. Practitioners can now use the history, QoL, comorbidity, symptoms and most importantly the physical signs to give a much more accurate score.

Once an accurate score has been established, then refer back to Table 10.3 as a guide to the recovery time.

The body cannot lie and, after physically examining the patient together with taking a detailed history, the trained practitioner should be able give a reasonably accurate score that informs the patient of the overall prognosis and how long the treatment programme may take. As the treatment progresses and the symptoms improve, a periodic reassessment of the score based on the change in the initial symptoms and the physical signs is useful. For example, if a patient scored 5/10 at their first consultation and after the initial worsening they began to improve by around the 12th weekly treatment showing a reduction in symptoms and some palpable improvement in the physical signs, I would most probably increase the score to a 6/10.

With a more severe case of say 3/10 it may be months before there is any improvement and it may be over a year before they reach a score of 6 or more out of 10. However, the score is only a guide and is based on averages, so some patients do much better than anticipated and improve their scores much more quickly than expected. Unfortunately, the opposite can occur, and sometimes it seems forever before there is a change for the better.

Many of my patients constantly want to know what score they are, and I find it very helpful to reinforce the benefit of treatment by informing them of the changing score's relevance regarding the overall prognosis.

Patient compliance

The one factor that is most important affecting the outcome and treatment recovery time is compliance with the instructions that I give to patients. The self-massage and exercise routines have to be done according to the instructions in this chapter. Of all the thousands of patients who have now tried the Perrin Technique, the ones that improved the most usually followed the advice to the letter.

The hardest part to follow is the instruction on pacing. I constantly amuse my patients by confessing that I would probably be my worst patient ever. If a clinician had told me to do only half of what I feel capable of, I would be climbing the walls.

Most ME/CFS and FMS patients were pushers and doers before they became ill so it is against their nature to pace, but without pacing the condition will worsen, no matter what treatment protocol is followed. So, I empathise with patients but the advice and instructions in this chapter will speed up the therapeutic process and most certainly help the majority of ME/CFS and FMS patients on their road to recovery.

Annual check-up

Whether the treatment proves to bring about a permanent remedy or just a remission depends on many factors that will affect the patient after being discharged. If the patient habitually overstrains their body, s/he may experience the return of symptoms. S/he should seek treatment as soon as the symptoms reappear in order to avoid a long-lasting relapse. The predisposition to developing ME/CFS and FMS takes the form of a disturbed neuro-lymphatic drainage system. Consequently, the patient should continue for life with the dorsal rotation exercises after being discharged, and occasionally, maybe once a week, do the self-massage routine in the shower. Annual check-ups are a good idea even though some patients unsurprisingly prefer to put the whole episode behind them.

ME/CFS in children

There are thousands of childhood cases of ME/CFS and FMS a year recorded in the UK. Juvenile FMS affects mostly young teenage girls following puberty. This also seems to be the case with ME/CFS, although I have also seen many young boys over the years suffering from the most terrible symptoms.

You rarely see children younger than five with ME/CFS and FMS, due to the fact that the disorder takes time to develop and is usually linked to postural problems in the spine, affecting the body's drainage of toxins. A child starts to walk at about one year and it takes a few years to develop a painful, bad posture. A major spinal trauma may precipitate the onset of ME/CFS and FMS in the very young, but this is extremely rare.

There are also cases that I have seen in clinic starting very early in life following major infection affecting the central nervous system, such as meningitis. I have recently seen a 13-year-old boy who has almost certainly had ME/CFS since birth, with nasal drip and 20 symptoms of the disease throughout his short life, plus he has had sleep apnoea diagnosed which could be due to trauma of the upper cervical region affecting the vagus nerve, as mentioned in Chapters 3 and 10.

Babies are normally born head-first with their chin tucked in. This child was a tenth baby, whose mother, due to the nine previous pregnancies, had a very weakened pelvic floor. The baby was lying very low in a potentially dangerous face presentation for four weeks before he was delivered by an emergency Caesarean section. In a face presentation the chin is not tucked and the neck will be hyperextended. This poor baby had a whole month of the most immense pressure on his facial bones with potential damage to his upper spine before birth. This highly unusual case demonstrates the impact that birth and even prenatal trauma can have in the build-up of ME/CFS.

The problem with children becoming ill with a condition that many paediatricians do not understand is that the parents are often forced into treatment modalities that are clearly worsening the child's health. If they refuse, the parents or guardians often become the subject of controversial investigation by social services and sometimes the police. I have over the years been involved in some very distressing cases supporting families where the mother is accused of fabricating the illness and the diagnosis of fictitious illness syndrome is banded about. (Fictitious illness syndrome used to be called Munchausen's disease by proxy.)

In the early years of my work in 1990s I tried, together with a local GP, to stop a psychiatrist forcing a young eight-year-old ME/CFS patient into in-patient psychiatric care. She was wheelchair bound and unable to straighten her legs due to the long-term spasticity in her muscles that presents in some severe ME/CFS patients, and yet with all her physical symptoms the paediatrician was convinced it was all hysterical, i.e. due to psychological stress. The consultant at the conference was more senior in the health service to the GP and I was ignored as a total quack, so sadly the girl was forcibly taken away from her parents and put into hospital care. She was forbidden by law to have any further contact with myself or the GP. Thankfully, she was given some physiotherapy to stretch the tightened tendons and muscles in her legs, so she was able to sit and lie down with straighter legs; however, the illness that had caused her problems was never addressed. Figure 55 is a copy of her letter smuggled out of hospital to me that I have kept filed for around a quarter of a century. Sadly, many years later she remained in psychiatric hospital care, her life ruined by ignorance and misconceived ideas of this illness that woefully still remain in some quarters of the health, educational and social services.

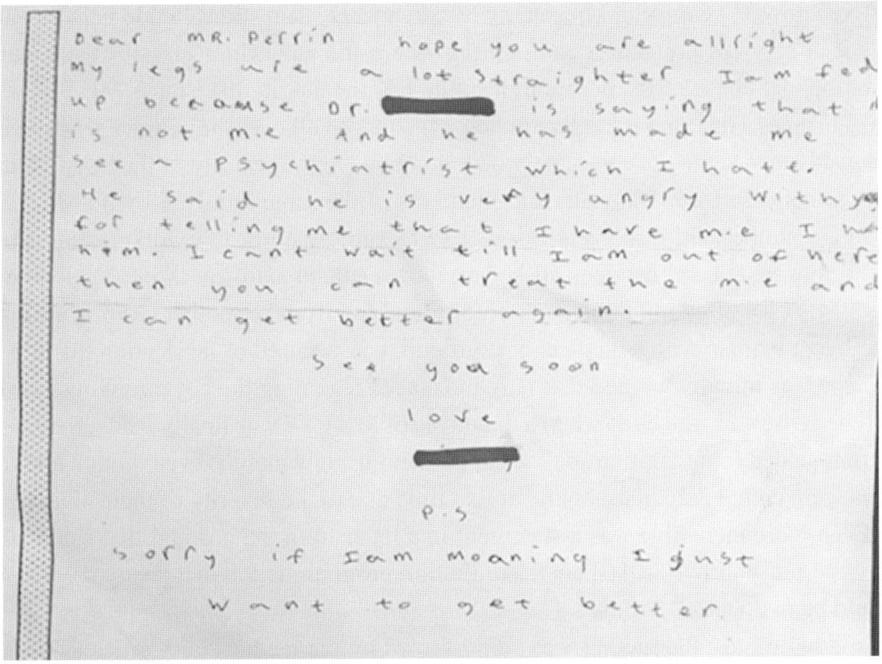

Fig. 55 Letter from a child. (Transcribed below.)

Dear Mr Perrin

Hope you are all right. My legs are a lot straighter. I am fed up because Dr XXXXX is saying that it is not ME and he has made me see a psychiatrist which I hate.

He said he is very angry with you for telling me that I have ME. I hate him. I can't wait till I am out of here then you can treat the ME and I can get better again.

See you soon

Love

Xxxxx

P.S.　Sorry if I'm moaning. I just want to get better.

Even now 31 years after I began my research work, I am still called to help families in social services protection conferences where the authorities classify these cases as emotional abuse of the poor child. In the UK the charity the Young ME Sufferers Trust (Tymes Trust) is very active in helping children all over the country who are not believed when some are completely bedbound due to the severity of their symptoms.

Another case I had was with four members of the same family, all with ME/CFS. A single mother and three young sons had to battle with health workers, education authorities and social services all because a consultant said it was inconceivable to have ME/CFS affecting three sons in the same family. The mother, who is a highly intelligent woman with a medical background, was accused of fabricating this illness and she was initially warned that 'any blockages regarding the boys moving forward will be addressed' and even when a diagnosis of ME/CFS was finally made, they were recommended re-integration back to school within a few months even though all three boys were completely housebound at that time due to the severity of their illness.

Even more incredible was a statement in a letter from the hospital that said that if they did not improve with their rehabilitation programme the diagnosis of ME/CFS would be in doubt!

In other words, the mother was being forced by the medical authorities to subject her poor children to a programme of graded exercise and CBT when they needed to pace themselves from the outset. The forced activity regime would inevitably worsen their condition. The outcome of this would most probably lead to a diagnosis of a psychiatric condition and they would be removed to in-patient care. In this case the diagnosis of fictitious illness syndrome was banded about by the social services. However, the authorities finally realised that in some cases many in the same family can develop ME/CFS and FMS and there is a genetic component in many cases, as explained earlier in the book (page 75).

The fact is that ME/CFS does quite often run in families. I have already discussed in Chapter 3 that ME/CFS can be familial[19], and I have personally seen many patients of the same family affected due to genetic factors.

Whilst I understand the importance of education and social integration with other children, forcing a child back to school before they are ready to return will severely aggravate the condition. Often it is this constant pressure to get the child back into full-time education that can do permanent damage and lead to some children becoming totally bedridden as they force themselves to follow the advice of authorities that are oblivious to the fact that post-exertion malaise is the main symptom of ME/CFS.

Pacing children

When the child has sufficiently recovered and only complains of mild symptoms, it is then that they should gradually build-up their hours at school, but still following a paced approach doing only half of the activity that they feel capable of.

It is difficult to persuade children to reduce activity when they want to do so much. At the same time, it is hard to help the parents maintain a positive attitude when, initially, they may see their child becoming more ill. Some patients do improve immediately and do not necessarily worsen before starting to recover. One patient improved so quickly that within weeks he was able to take up football and tennis; I think it was lucky that I treated him at just the right time for his body to quickly and safely to return to normal. However, most patients are not that lucky and may suffer to begin with during treatment. Often, the parent looks at me, as if to say, 'What are you doing to my child?'

I have a great deal of sympathy with the parents of any sick child. ME/CFS affects the whole family, so I often try to have as many members of the family as possible at the initial consultation so that they can understand what is going on.

Our son, Max

I empathise with parents who see their lovely child go from a healthy, active boy or girl to a wheelchair-bound invalid. When my son Max was only five, he started exhibiting signs and symptoms of fatigue. My wife Julie and I began to be concerned when Max complained of constant headaches. We became very worried when Max started projectile vomiting every morning and so we took him to our GP who referred him to the hospital. There he was examined by a paediatrician and a trainee doctor who refused to scan his brain, saying that it was a virus. I told them that I had spent years studying the brain and that Max's signs bore the hallmarks of increased intracranial pressure. Max had banged his head a week before and I was concerned that this was the reason. They took a chest X-ray but refused to do a brain scan and sent us home. Another two trips to the doctor's and we were again told that it was a virus. One doctor said, remarkably, to me that Max, who by then had to be carried into the surgery, was suffering from 'sibling rivalry': Josh, my youngest son, was born the year that Max fell ill, so, maintained the doctor, Max was seeking attention.

A week later Max was undergoing surgery to remove a pilocytic astrocytoma from his cerebellum or, to put it into lay terms, a tumour from the back of his brain.

The pressure caused by the tumour had damaged the ventricular system in the brain, affecting the drainage of cerebrospinal fluid. Max therefore required a further operation in which the surgeons implanted a ventricular peritoneal shunt. This is a tube with a valve, placed under the skin, which drains the CSF from the brain to the abdomen where it is absorbed back into the blood.

Watching a child suffer, even when the techniques and operations save life, is an experience that no parent should have to endure. I fully understand the anxieties of young patients' parents and the long wait for the child to start to recover. Seeing the child re-emerge from ME/CFS and FMS is an exhilarating experience, both for parents and the practitioner, and helps maintain the practitioner's enthusiasm during the long and sometimes arduous treatment programme.

It *will* get better

What has kept me going over the years is the fact that most of my patients do improve and we haven't just seen this in our research projects and in the licensed clinics around the world practising the Perrin Technique. Other independent bodies have also seen that my technique helps many who don't seem to get much relief from all the varied medications and treatment approaches out there.

This is why the NHS-run ME/CFS hospital clinic closest to my practice in Manchester are interested in integrating the Perrin Technique into the UK's National Health Service, as we are improving some of the most severe bedridden patients whom they cannot help.

If patients don't respond to the treatment in the usual way, we usually find some other disorder aggravating the ME/CFS or FMS and we may need to treat two or three conditions at the same time. It is very rarely that we have to give up and throw in the towel. What I hope by reading this book is that you now understand that the neuro-lymphatic system disturbance is a fundamental problem that needs to be addressed in ME/CFS, FMS and possibly many other neurological and neuro-immune diseases. Once resolved, and the toxins are flowing out of the central nervous system via the correct physiological pathway, the brain and body work better. This then allows the other approaches to treatment mentioned in this book to be more successful.

As you come close to finishing this book you will also appreciate that I do not just use manual techniques. Advice to patients regarding pacing their activities and learning how to relax and cope better with life's stressful challenges are equally important in my overall treatment programme.

As already mentioned in Chapter 5, a nationwide survey by the ME Association of the UK in 2010 entitled *Managing my ME* which examined the approaches that were most recommended by British patients with ME/CFS placed pacing first, second was relaxation/meditation and third was the Perrin Technique, which I am quite proud of considering this was a survey by an independent body.

I have personally examined and treated or overseen treatment in thousands of patients over the past three decades. An earlier clinical audit carried out on 240 of my patients seen between 1989 and 2009 is shown below.

TOTAL NUMBER OF PATIENTS SEEN = 240

Female patients = 165 (68.75%)

Male patients = 75 (31.25%)

Patients improved after 1 year = 217 (90.42%)

Patients whose symptoms overall unchanged after 1 year = 21 (8.75%)

Patients worse after 1 year = 2 (0.83%)

Patients who suffered a relapse after initial improvement: = 31 (12.92%)

Patients eventually completely symptom free* = 37 (15.41%)

Average score* at beginning of treatment = 4.33

Average score* after 1 year = 7.06 (63% improvement)

Average score* with further treatment after 1 year = 7.83 (81% overall improvement)

* SCORE: 0–10 where 10 = symptom free

As we can see from the above audit, ME/CFS affects many more female patients than male. The reasons are basically two-fold. More lymphatic congestion in breast tissue, which is much more developed in women, and the complex hormonal interactions in women, play major parts in the disease. Changes in hormone levels will affect the hypothalamus and with female hormones subject to monthly changes it comes as no surprise that ME/CFS often starts in girls around puberty, with another very common trigger being the menopause. An epidemiological analysis by Stanford University's

Beth Unger showed that some studies showed three or even four times more women suffer from ME/CFS than men, with a higher number of 40- to 50-year-olds than other age groups in the female population.

Despite a number of unpleasant signs and symptoms initially, it is only a matter of time for most ME/CFS and FMS sufferers before my treatment begins to work and the characteristics of these debilitating diseases start to recede.

If you are a healthcare practitioner or scientist, after reading this book you hopefully now understand why so many people around the world suffer from ME/CFS and FMS and what goes wrong in the body of these unfortunate patients. You should now have a much better idea how to confirm the diagnosis of these two conditions and what treatments are required to help.

If you are a patient with either ME/CFS or FMS or are worried about these and other related illnesses, you hopefully now have a much better understanding about the processes leading to these disorders, what can be done to help you and – most importantly – how you (and your family) can help yourself.

This book has shown many different approaches that can be used in conjunction with my treatment. The analogy I like to use to explain the importance of treating the neuro-lymphatic dysfunction in ME/CFS and FMS is that of a jigsaw puzzle. When one tries to complete a jigsaw, it is best to start with the corners and edge pieces first. The four corners of the recovery jigsaw in ME/CFS and FMS are pacing, relaxation, meditation, and rest. The edge pieces are the treatment protocol that is the Perrin Technique, correcting the biomechanics and improving the neuro-lymphatic drainage and thus creating a framework for the rest of the picture to be filled in. Sometimes the jigsaw puzzle of recovery is made up of only corners and edges which makes the task much more straightforward and represents a patient making a complete recovery with just my standard advice and treatment. Most are much more complex, with many difficult sections to be filled in. The supplements, medications, diets and talk therapies all form part of the sea and sky in the jigsaw puzzle picture of health. One can of course start with the centre of a challenging jigsaw puzzle first, but it will make the task much more difficult and one could give up before the picture is complete. So, start with the corners and edges to bring about the best result.

In the first edition of this book I laid out my theory of how ME/CFS can develop, be diagnosed and treated. As I have shown throughout this second edition, science has caught up and explains in much more detail how ME/CFS and FMS develop and can be overcome. I hope this knowledge can help thousands join the many patients around the world who have already benefited from the Perrin Technique.

Chapter 11

ME/CFS and FMS: your questions answered

*We learn more by looking for the answer to a question and
not finding it than we do from learning the answer itself.*
                    Lloyd Alexander (1924 – 2007), American writer

---

Case: Mike's story

It is 14 December 2018, the day after my latest treatment with
Raymond. Tomorrow I will be doing my favourite Peak District walk –
Alport Castle. This will be the fourth time I've done this six-mile walk
in the last 10 days. It is one of the highest points in the area and is a
hidden gem.

The Peak District and hill-walking feature prominently in my ME story.

In September 2010 I walked with a friend from Hayfield to Kinder
Scout – nothing unusual in this but a week or so later I began to feel
really ill and had what I thought was a bad case of 'flu'. I just couldn't
get better and was unable to work, I spent most of the time in bed.
After a couple of months, I had a blood test and the results came
back – Q fever... me neither.

It's not a very common virus – about 70 cases a year in the UK, and was identified following analysis at Porton Down, the government facility which opened in 1916 to test chemical weapons in WW1. I was then referred to the Department of Infectious Diseases at the Royal Hallamshire Hospital in Sheffield… getting worried now.

After being monitored for several months and not recovering I was diagnosed with ME/CFS. What that actually meant was, – 'We really don't know what it is, so by elimination, it must be ME'.

I was referred to the Sheffield CFS clinic. I had a course of cognitive behavioural therapy (CBT) and an introduction to pacing. Marginal improvements followed but nothing sustainable. I tried acupuncture but that didn't do it either. I was prescribed gabapentin and amitriptyline during this time – they helped with the pain, but I stopped taking them as I didn't like the side-effects.

I had varying periods of absence from work – three months, six months and from September 2013 I was absent from work for 12 months. Most of 2010–2013 was spent horizontal – a horrible existence; the crushing feeling of exhaustion is hard to describe.

Two low points stick in my mind: firstly, being in a car park in Cornwall not knowing which side of the road to drive on; and secondly, in February 2014 when my wife broke her back in a walking accident in the Peak District and my elderly mother was in and out of hospital for many weeks. Trying to cope with these events and the care I had to try to give to them whilst really struggling with ME almost pushed me over the edge. I couldn't see a way out.

In May 2014 I was in bed reading an article in a magazine about the Perrin Technique which my sister-in-law's mother had sent me. I thought about it for a few days before I made an appointment with Raymond – everything was such an effort then.

I had my initial consultation and commenced my treatment. He estimated that he would get me back to 80% of what I used to be like within two years. That sounded great to me and for the first time in years I had real hope of a pathway to recovery and an acceptable quality of life.

I'm a perfectionist/finisher – I was determined to do whatever Raymond asked of me – weekly appointments in the first instance, no tea and coffee, no alcohol ...eek!

I took the vitamins and supplements he recommended for me and completed the exercise and self-massage routine every day.

Raymond explained that my symptoms would worsen in the early stages of treatment and I imagine that most patients would be apprehensive about this, but you have to trust in the process. I did feel worse, but I was determined to stick with it.

I began to improve after about three to four months and I began a phased return to work in September 2014. I took early retirement in August 2017 and in the three years I was back at work I did not have a further ME-related absence from work.

Over the years I have built up my fitness and I do a lot of hill walking – Raymond would say too much. I still have a tendency to overdo it, but I am better at managing myself these day; my wife still uses the refrain 'What would Raymond say?'

I now see Raymond quarterly. I could go to six-monthly appointments, but I prefer the current schedule: it helps my self-management and curbs my natural instinct to keep pushing myself.

I still self-massage every day, I don't drink tea or coffee but happily enjoy an alcoholic drink ... or two.

> I don't really think about whether I'm 80–90% there, I just know
> I've got ME (that is, myself) back and I'm just so grateful for what
> Raymond has done for me and so many others. Thank you, Raymond.
>
> **Michael Hodgkinson**, Sheffield, Yorkshire, UK

Chapter 1 was designed to help patients and others without bioscience knowledge understand the basic theory behind the Perrin Technique. I hope it achieved that aim. To help the same group of readers – ME/CFS and fibromyalgia syndrome (FMS) patients, their families and friends – understand my approach to management, treatment and recovery without having to read the whole book. I have included this chapter in an easy to follow question-and-answer format. It is basically a summary of the main features in the book with simple advice for patients to follow. This will hopefully guide each patient along their own individual road to recovery. Further on in this chapter is a quick guide to the dos and don'ts in the protocol that is 'the Perrin Technique'.

What are the causes of ME/CFS and FMS?

There are many factors involved in the process leading to chronic fatigue syndrome/ myalgic encephalomyelitis (ME/CFS) and fibromyalgia syndrome (FMS). The head may be traumatised at birth and this occurs more in first-born children as they are the first babies to pass through their mother's birth canal; alternatively, there may be a forceps or ventouse delivery, which places even more pressure on the baby's head. The first labour is usually the longest, but sometimes a very quick birth in younger siblings can also be traumatic for the small vulnerable cranium of the newborn.

There may be a genetic predisposition affecting the normal development of the head or back and I see quite a few families with more than one member with ME/CFS and FMS.

Years before the onset of symptoms, perhaps even in early childhood, the patient might have suffered from trauma to the head or spine. Teenage years bring with them problems of their own and the spine of a very active teenager is vulnerable to postural disturbance. The majority of ME/CFS and FMS patients were very sporty or high-achieving people who pushed themselves to the very limit. However, there are a few sufferers who have tended to be 'couch potatoes' with a tendency to slouch and are more into reading and sedentary activities than sports during their teenage years but are still prone to developmental problems of the spine.

In the brain and spinal cord there is a fluid known as cerebrospinal fluid. One of the functions of the cerebrospinal fluid is drainage. Some poisons caused by infection, inflammation or toxins from a polluted environment enter the brain and spine and flow out through perforations in the skull and minute channels in the spine, entering the lymphatic system[1]. Certain structural problems affecting both the head and the spine together can result in no (or very little) drainage pathway for the cerebrospinal fluid to take. In a ME/CFS and/or FMS sufferer, these normal drainage points have initially become congested, leading to a build-up of poisons within the central nervous system[2].

The main organ in the brain to be affected by poisons is the hypothalamus, which is the control centre for the hormones and the sympathetic nervous system. The latter helps the body cope in times of stress. In ME/CFS and FMS, the toxic cocktail brewing in the hypothalamus leads to an overload of the sympathetic nervous system, which will have been affected by other stress factors – physical, allergic, emotional or infection – in the years leading up to the illness.

One final trigger, which is usually a viral, bacterial or fungal infection, will lead to a breakdown in the normal functioning of the sympathetic nervous system[3]. Furthermore, the lymphatic system, which is meant to aid drainage, is under the control of the sympathetic nervous system[4]. When this system is functioning poorly, toxins may be pumped in the reverse direction, which adds further poisons to the central nervous system. As the toxicity builds up, brain function worsens, leading to further sympathetic nerve disarray and increased toxicity in the brain and spinal cord. The vicious circle that ensues leads to the myriad of symptoms affecting the patient. With ME/CFS and more so in FMS, the toxins affect the pain centres in the brain making the patient even more sensitive to any pain stimulus around the body.

Is fibromyalgia syndrome (FMS) a different disease to ME/CFS?

Yes and no. Although there is some argument about this, I look at both of them within the same spectrum of disease, with ME/CFS producing post-exertion malaise as the principal complaint and FMS's main symptom being widespread severe pain throughout the body.

It is also very important to realise that *post-exertion* malaise is not the same as post-exercise malaise. Often patients can exercise a little without suffering the consequences. It is exertion that precipitates the many symptoms of ME/CFS – in other words, doing more than the patient feels happy doing or capable of, and it doesn't have to be physical exertion. Mental, emotional or immunological exertion can trigger a worsening of symptoms. I have seen some patients who were often very fit before they were ill with ME/CFS or FMS who feel much better exercising, but when they have a cold or are under emotional or mental stress they crash and may spend the next few weeks bedridden following perhaps an innocuous virus or extra stress at work.

The reason for the different clinical presentations of FMS and ME/CFS is that the toxins in FMS predominantly affect the nuclei of the brain that control pain. This is why widespread pain is the most prominent feature in FMS rather than in ME/CFS where the toxins mainly affect areas of the brain responsible for coping with change and preventing many other physical, emotional and cognitive problems. However, FMS and ME/CFS share the same common physical findings that we in clinic use as an aid to the diagnosis of both disorders.

Which type of people suffer from these diseases?

ME/CFS and FMS can affect all ages and all ethnic groups and social backgrounds and do affect men as well as women. I have recently seen a boy who has suffered the symptoms from birth, though this is extremely rare. The youngest patient with ME/CFS I have actually treated was five years old and the oldest, 85.

However, many more women suffer from ME/CFS and FMS than men. This is because:
1. Women's hormone systems are so much more complex than men's and those hormonal changes affect the hypothalamus which is the central controller of hormones in the brain and is affected by toxins in ME/CFS and FMS.
2. Levels of the cytokine leptin, which is a hormone affecting satiety and hunger and appetite or loss of it, and is found more in females, has been shown to be directly linked with the symptom severity of ME/CFS.
3. There is much more lymphatic tissue in the female breast and thus there is much more potential for congestion of the tissue in the chest, creating more toxic build-up, irritating more of the sympathetic nerves in this important area.

It is interesting that at the time of writing the last stages of the book in August 2020, we are seeing in clinic a rising number of new patients with post-Covid-19 syndrome also known as 'long Covid' and that most of these post-Covid-19 patients are women. This seems to be puzzling as it has been reported worldwide that men suffer worse symptoms with Covid-19 than women and more deaths in men have been recorded due to the illness. The solution to this conundrum is the same as the reason why women develop ME/CFS and FMS much more than men as explained above.

What does the Perrin Technique treatment involve?

The Perrin Technique stimulates the motion of fluid around the brain and spinal cord via cranial techniques. In normal circumstances this fluid carries toxins away from the brain and spinal cord to areas of the body where they can be processed and disposed of. Treatment to the spine, as well as certain exercises, further aids drainage of these toxins out of the cerebrospinal fluid. A specific lymphatic drainage technique and massage of the soft tissues in the head, neck, back and chest direct all the poisons out of the lymphatic system and into the blood, and eventually to the liver where they are broken down and readily detoxified. Some of the drainage travels out of the body via the bowels and genitourinary tract or through the skin.

Eventually, with no poisons affecting the central nervous system, the brain starts to work better, gradually stimulating improved lymphatic drainage. Thus, the body starts to function correctly, and, providing patients do not overstrain themselves as the nervous system is recovering, their symptoms should gradually improve.

'The rule of the artery reigns supreme.' This tenet was formulated by the founder of osteopathy, Dr Andrew Taylor Still, who stated that illness is mainly due to stagnation of body fluids and that if you can stimulate blood flow and other fluid motion, including cerebrospinal fluid and lymphatic drainage, the body will recover.

My method of treating ME/CFS, using the principle above, is analogous to mending a blocked main drain in your home. By increasing pressure into the main drain, one pumps out the blockage and reverses any backflow.

It is obviously more complex in the body, and by cranial treatment, articulation of the spine and specific manual lymphatic drainage massage techniques, one stimulates the movement of cerebrospinal fluid from the brain and the spine to the lymphatics. This increases pressure in the correct direction and thus improves the central drainage of lymph fluid from the lymphatic ducts into the blood.

What responses to treatment should I expect?

One proof that the Perrin Technique is not a placebo is the fact that most patients feel somewhat worse at the beginning of the treatment. Placebo treatments do not generally make you feel worse. The reason for this initial exacerbation in symptoms is because, for the first time, the toxins embedded – for years, possibly – in the central nervous system are being released into the rest of the body.

The most common symptoms in the early stages of treatment include nausea, headaches, general pain and the appearance of spots, boils and other skin problems. However, one should always remember the old adage 'Better out than in'!

The worse the patient is in the early stage of treatment, the better the overall prognosis is usually likely to be. The main aspect to focus upon is the change that occurs with the treatment. If change has not occurred in any way in the first 12 weeks, it does not mean that the patient has no hope of recovery, but it might be a much slower process than they had envisaged. It may also mean that they have to seek an alternative/additional therapy on top of this technique in their search for a remedy. Some fortunate patients do improve immediately, so it is not necessarily the case that a ME/CFS patient's condition worsens before improvement[5].

How quickly will I recover?

Every patient is different, and some recover much more quickly than others. The majority of patients improve significantly in the first year (see the audit on page 329). Some mild cases can be resolved in a few months and the very severe bedridden patients may take years to achieve a much better quality of life, but my methods have helped some patients who had virtually given up but now are on the road to recovery, with many leading a completely normal life after the treatment programme. (Please see the outlook Table 10.3 in Chapter 10, page 317). Some of those recovered patients' stories feature at the beginning of each chapter.

Once the patient has noticed a reduction in their symptoms, they can begin the uphill battle to improve health and stamina. One has first to convalesce, which for those younger readers who have never heard of the word, means to rest in order to get better after an illness. Convalescence is no longer a fashionable concept. People having some operations nowadays tend to be discharged from hospital within a day and may be at work within the week. Convalescent rest, however, is a must during the recovery process from ME/CFS and FMS.

In order to turn the remission period in ME/CFS and FMS into a permanent state of health, as well as convalescence one has to keep to the 'half rule' until one has been symptom-free for at least six months, that is doing only half of what one feels capable of doing safely. As I tell my patients, 'Remember that half of more is still more'. In other words, as one recovers and can do more before fatigue and other symptoms begin, one should only gradually increase activity, while still taking care to avoid too much exertion.

How often should I receive the treatment?

At the beginning of treatment, the patient is usually treated once a week. As the symptom picture improves, there should be a gradual increase in the period between consultations.

A patient with moderate symptoms with a score of 5/10 on my scale usually adheres to the following treatment schedule.

Treatment schedule

Weeks 1–12: weekly

Weeks 13–24: every 2 weeks

Weeks 25–36: every 3 weeks

Weeks 37–52: every 4 weeks

Months 12–18: every 3 months

Month 24: Final check-up (if symptom-free for six months, patient is discharged).

However, the lower the score at the beginning, the longer it takes before recovery starts and so it may be over six months before the practitioner spaces out the weekly sessions in cases who initially score 3/10, which represents 30% of what one would call good health.

What are the dos and don'ts for patients with ME/CFS and FMS?

The answer to this question is difficult as every patient has different presentations and what is good for one is often bad for another. However, the best way of giving a constructive response is to go through an ideal 24 hours in the life of a patient and what I have found is best advice for most.

Waking up

Let us start with getting up in the morning. It should be morning, not after midday. This is very important, as getting into a reasonably normal sleep pattern is essential. One should aim at getting up every day, and even in severe cases one should try to wake up at the same time, preferably in the morning.

The sleep-awake cycle is controlled by the hypothalamus, with the pineal gland in the brain which produces the hormone melatonin stimulated by the dark and supressed by how much light passes through the eyes, which is why some people refer to the pineal gland as the third eye. Dark and light stimulate the production of melatonin and serotonin respectively. The melatonin/serotonin balance is crucial in maintaining a good diurnal rhythm and helping us stay awake during the day and sleep at night.

In the winter the darker days aggravate the rhythm and some people suffer a drop in serotonin and become more depressed, leading to what is known as SAD (seasonal affective disorder). Also, many ME/CFS and FMS patients sleep much worse in the summer as they have too little melatonin and too much in the winter. To help the balance in winter, a SAD light which mimics daylight hours does often help. So, if you have this problem, a SAD light is important first thing in the morning at dawn for an hour, and another hour later on in the evening at twilight/dusk is also recommended.

Getting out of bed

If this is possible (and unfortunately I have seen many patients who are unable to lift their heads off a pillow, never mind get out of bed), always alight from the bed in stages; never jump up as the control over blood pressure is often disturbed and experiencing dizziness when getting out of bed is common. So, before sitting up make sure you are lying on your side and slowly swing your legs over the edge of the bed and gradually sit up at the side of your bed where you should remain for a minute or so before slowly standing up. If you suffer from POTS (see Chapter 5, page 172) you should stay seated for at least three minutes before trying to stand up.

Shower in morning

This should never be too hot or too cold as the hypothalamus is the thermostat of the body and too extreme temperatures will stress an already overloaded part of the brain. Make sure any soaps, shampoos and shower-gels are not too perfumed. It is worth buying the least allergenic products recommended by your local pharmacist even if they are more expensive.

Try to avoid hot baths at any time. They are worse than showers as besides overheating the body, the muscles will relax while the spine is in an unhealthy position unless you are able to float in the bath. It always amazes me as an osteopath how many people take a hot bath when they have lower back pain. Sitting in the bath places extra strain on the lower back and can aggravate any postural problem. With ME/CFS and FMS it is double trouble as the heat and the postural strain together exacerbate any inflammatory changes in the spine, which creates more toxicity within the central nervous system.

Comfortably cool baths that you can lie in are healthier for ME/CFS and FMS patients and sometimes relieve many of the symptoms, but if the water is too cold it will aggravate the condition by increasing tone in already tightened muscles. If you are going to try cool baths, make sure that when you are lying there you are not shivering and that you are comfortable. I recommend about 10 minutes at a time.

Showers are usually better for ME/CFS but if the patient feels dizzy or weak standing and does not have a bath then they should use a shower chair. If a patient constantly feels faint or actually faints in a hot shower and the heart rate frequently races, then again suspect possible POTS (see Chapter 5).

Having frequent short cold showers of around 16–23°C may also be of benefit to some ME/CFS and FMS patients. As with cool baths, moderately cold showers have been shown to reduce pain by stimulating the production of endorphins which reduce pain without causing any harm.

Cool showers and baths have been shown to stimulate the locus coeruleus in the brain stem which forms a major axis, together with the hypothalamus, in the control mechanism of the neuro-lymphatic drainage system. In health this axis switches off during the night in deep restorative delta-wave sleep. It has been shown that in ME/CFS, delta waves are produced in the brain throughout the day with the axis switching off at the wrong time leading to the patient feeling sick and exhausted as the toxins drain out of the brain. To reverse this problem, we need to stimulate the locus coeruleus during the day. So brief, comfortably cool hydrotherapy in the morning will greatly help some patients.

Exposure to cold typically causes activation of the sympathetic nervous system (SNS) which can cause problems with ME/CFS and FMS since the sympathetic nerves are usually overloaded. However, small amounts of stressful or harmful agents can sometimes be beneficial. This phenomenon is known as hormesis. Similar to the body's immune response needing to first be exposed to an infectious agent before it builds an immunity, as seen in vaccination, it is believed by some that exposure to cold can temporarily reverse autonomic dysfunction and therefore improve symptoms.

If your symptoms are improving with the manual therapy in this book but you wish to boost your energy, try the hydrotherapy once in the morning for just a few minutes, either lying in a cool bath or having bursts of a cold shower for a few seconds at a time over a couple of minutes. If it brings any relief, continue each morning as long as you always feel well afterwards. If it worsens your condition in any way, then immediately stop as it isn't for you. Remember that every ME/CFS and FMS patient is different, and unfortunately people respond differently to any stimulus[6].

On that note, there is a completely different form of hydrotherapy developed in Japan that has shown to relieve mental fatigue. This is known as 'mild stream bathing' which involves a mild stream of warm water continuously passing from the sole to the calf, thigh, waist and back, providing a massage function[7]. This form of therapy would stimulate lymphatic drainage, working against any backflow, so it may help ME/CFS and FMS as long as the water isn't too hot. It should only be attempted in the later stages of treatment as full body massage could easily overload the drainage of toxins and be too much for your body to cope with when embarking on the Perrin Technique.

Getting dressed

Loose clothes that are easy to slip on and off are recommended as clothes that are too tight may restrict circulation of blood and lymph and lots of buttons etc can place strain on the hands that do get fatigued and sometimes become very painful, especially in FMS. For women, tight bras are a definite no-no, especially tight underwired bras, which do place extra pressure on the breast lymphatics. Sports bras tend to be better, but the main issue is finding a properly fitted bra; bra-fitting services should be used and are available at good quality shops around the world.

Deodorants, antiperspirants and cosmetics

Most should be avoided as much as possible, especially heavily perfumed products as they usually contain high levels of petrochemicals and other neurotoxins. There are safer products that are less toxic, but one has to shop around. In the same vein, many of my patients relax by lighting scented candles at home. Unfortunately, aromatic candles are nearly all highly toxic with the wax usually having a high petrochemical content and the wicks usually containing heavy metals. If you enjoy candles to relax please try and use beeswax candles with natural, non-metallic wicks.

Mealtimes

Diets have been discussed at length in Chapter 5, but the basic advice I give is not to eat anything in excess and generally 'Variety is the spice of life'. Eating a large variety of food generally places less strain on a particular part of the gastrointestinal system, which is often disturbed in ME/CFS and FMS patients, with many having irritable bowel syndrome and gut dysbiosis.

Dietary intake of sugar should be low as it stimulates the production of yeast. Patients with ME/CFS and FMS should eat less casein (found in milk-based products), less gluten, as well as less yeast, as these are all composed of large molecules and therefore require the lymphatics to drain the excess away from the gut.

Small meals eaten regularly are best and I often advise patients to divide each meal into two, eating frequently but less at a time. Adults should drink around 2 litres a day of water and healthy drinks such as herbal non-caffeinated teas. Patients should reduce the intake of caffeinated coffee and tea as caffeine can over-stimulate the nervous system. Alcohol should be avoided at all costs as, besides it obviously placing extra strain on the liver, it has been shown that patients with ME/CFS and FMS have overactive receptors in the brain that are stimulated by NMDA, the neurochemical activated by alcohol intake. Most of my patients do not find this advice difficult to follow as they feel worse after a little sip and almost drunk following the smallest amount of alcohol.

Chillax (chill and relax)

During the day and especially at night the patient has to learn how to relax and possibly meditate. A new word has been coined that embodies both relaxing and remaining chilled and calm: 'Chillax'. There are plenty of different strategies mentioned in Chapter 5 to do this, including mindfulness (page 47).

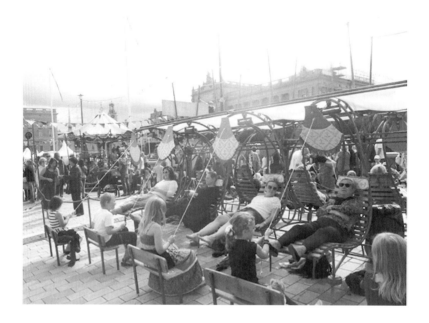

Fig. 56 These parents and grandparents in Stockholm know the meaning of 'chillax' with these rocking chairs and fans controlled by the children!

Bedtime

Difficulty falling asleep and staying asleep, known as insomnia, and hypersomnia, when the patient sleeps too much, and other sleep disturbances are very common symptoms of ME/CFS and FMS. Leading sleep experts including Dr Jason Ellis, who is a Professor of Sleep Science and Director of the Northumbria Sleep Research Laboratory in the UK, advocate cognitive behavioural therapy for insomnia, often called CBT-I.

CBT-I is an approved method for treating insomnia aimed at changing sleep habits and includes regular, often weekly, visits to a clinician and completing a sleep diary to work out the best way of tackling the specific disorder.

Sleep clinics around the world offer many ways of analysing the sleep problem and for those patients with severe sleep disorders a polysomnography test is essential. Also known as a sleep study test, polysomnography records your brain waves, the oxygen level in your blood, heart rate and breathing, as well as eye and leg movements.

Exercises to help you to fall asleep should be attempted, such as counting backwards from a thousand …in sevens – i.e. 1000, 993, 986, 979 etc. It isn't easy and that is the main point. By taking your mind off everything else your brain will be calmer and you will gently fall asleep. At the same time it can also help if you think 'I am not going to sleep…I am not going to sleep' and repeat this over and over again in your mind while counting down from 1000 in 7s.

It is best to have a set bedtime and stick to it as closely as possible. Use blackout curtains and switch off all lights in the room. It's best to take all the electronic gadgets away from the bed. Avoid tea, coffee and any other drinks with caffeine before bed.

Sometimes having a small meal an hour before bed helps. As one knows after a heavy meal during the day, one often feels very drowsy. This is because hormones released after eating can also stimulate the sleep centres. These hormones are controlled by the hypothalamus which is, as we have seen, the main part of the brain disturbed in ME/CFS and FMS. Eating food can calm the hypothalamus and help induce sleep.

The best position for sleep is lying on one's side, which places minimal strain on to the spine. It has also been shown that neuro-lymphatic drainage occurs more when lying on one's side (no particular side, just the one you feel most comfortable on).

Some patients may develop sleep apnoea which is when one stops breathing during one's sleep for short periods. This obviously can be dangerous…we need to breathe; so contact your GP if you think you have this problem. You may need an aid to support breathing at night called a continuous positive airway pressure machine (CPAP), which is the most effective treatment if you have moderate to severe sleep apnoea.

Sleeping pills and low-dose tricyclic antidepressants, such as 10 mg amitriptyline, are prescribed by GPs to be taken an hour before bed. Some patients taking amitriptyline report feeling very drowsy the next morning, so if you have a problem inform your GP.

As mentioned in the beginning of this section, the hormone melatonin is important for sleep so sometimes this is prescribed by physicians around the world to help ME/CFS patients sleep, but the SAD light may be the best help.

How much exercise and activity can I do?

Post-*exertion* malaise (PEM) is the most common symptom in ME/CFS… not, as I have said on many occasions throughout this book, post-*exercise* malaise. Any activity that does not over-exert you will be okay and activity is actively encouraged if possible, as long as it does not exhaust you. PEM may not be immediate; the malaise may kick in up to three days following exertion, so beware of this problem.

It is best to avoid all exertive exercise and sport until you are virtually symptom-free and then you can revitalise your deconditioned body by gradually increasing your activity. The dreaded graded exercise therapy (GET) helps only ME/CFS and FMS patients who are fortunate enough to have recovered from most of their symptoms, but due to the forced reduction of activity over a protracted period are deconditioned. Even when their concentration returns and when feeling much more energetic, they still often remain basically unfit and one of the best ways of reconditioning the body is by gradually increasing physical activity.

Rehabilitation and reconditioning patients' weakened bodies has to be done safely. The best rehabilitative activity for the recovering ME/CFS and FMS patient is a swimming stroke known as adapted back sculling (see Figure 57), which is done lying on the back and gently wafting the arms along just beneath the water surface, slowly propelling you backwards; however, with this rehabilitative exercise you should slowly move your legs up and down as well.

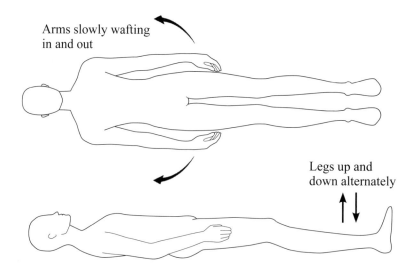

Arms slowly wafting in and out

Legs up and down alternately

Fig. 57 Adapted back sculling technique

Avoid breaststroke as this is just wrong on so many levels. When I was specialising in sports injuries the top-level swimmers that I saw most were the breast-stroke swimmers. This is the most common stroke among casual swimmers but places unnatural strain on the neck, shoulders, spine, pelvis, hips and knees ... besides that, it's okay.

As you are able to do more, then you can introduce backstroke and front crawl but try not to break any speed and distance records. One of my patients once threw caution to the wind and as soon as she felt able to swim a few lengths she decided to swim a couple of kilometres and spent the next few months in bed, recovering. Swimming in a saltwater pool, if one is available, or the sea if it is not too cold, is preferable to a chlorinated pool due to the toxic effects of the chlorine.

As the symptoms continue to improve, both the patient and the practitioner will be greatly encouraged. By steadily improving the mobility of the spine, and by relaxing all the irritated surrounding tissues, the function of the sympathetic nervous system should finally be restored to full working order. The patient once again enjoys health, vigour and a good quality of life and hopefully can go back to a more active lifestyle exercising in gyms and playing sports.

However, ... never forget my golden rule for any activity – what I call the 'half rule', i.e. only do 50% of what you feel capable of. This rule applies to every activity, including walking, talking, reading, writing and watching television. However, when it comes to aerobic exercise such as running and swimming, the patient has to be absolutely sure that they will not go over the half rule or risk a major relapse.

As I always say to my patients, and I said above: 'Half of more is still more'. In other words, when increasing exercise, doing a little at a time if you are well within your safe boundaries, will still increase your stamina and general fitness, with no risk.

The half rule is so difficult to adhere to, since once on the mend it is as though the patient's prison door has been unlocked for the first time in maybe years and then they are only allowed to walk around the courtyard and then go back into their cell. However, if one were to run out of the prison gates too quickly the guns and dogs of ME/CFS and FMS would be there ready to stop the fleeing prisoner in their tracks.

Much better to walk calmly out through the gates at a very gentle pace and then stop and return for a while and then go a bit further the next time, continually returning to the safety of the cell for a while, until one can slowly but surely leave the ME/CFS or FMS prison without alerting the sympathetic nervous system's 'prison guards' that one has escaped their clutches.

Patients who are eager to resume some form of aerobic exercise and can't swim, or live too far from a swimming pool or suitable beach, or remain sensitive to chlorine, should begin by gentle walks up and down the street and gradually build-up the distance. Walking should be on the flat at the beginning of rehabilitation and if possible wearing a pedometer, which is a device that counts each step a person takes by detecting movement of the arms or hips and is a very useful tool to monitor the gentle progress that you should be aiming for.

A pedometer can simply be downloaded as an app for your phone or you can buy a simple pedometer in most sports supply shops. Gradually increase the activity, keeping to walking and not jogging: shifting all one's weight onto first one side and then the other places too much strain on the spine whereas walking avoids this jarring effect.

Cycling should only be done on the flat. As with walking, avoid hills to begin with, as this may over-exert your back and leg muscles. A basic exercise bike with a little resistance is also a good form of rehabilitation.

REMEMBER: graded activity does not help ME/CFS and FMS patients recover but helps re-condition the recovered patient!

What hobbies can I do safely?

Hobbies and pastimes are very important for patients' sense of purpose and sanity, especially if housebound. They can also be a crucial part of rehabilitation, re-introducing physical and mental activity to a life that was just about existing from day to day. If the hobby involves arts and crafts, the patient may be suffering neurotoxicity from the paint, paint thinners and solvents they use. These and many other hobbies involving toxins should be kept to a minimum for obvious reasons. Patients should wear a mask if there is any danger of exposure to poisonous fumes.

Playing musical instruments is a favourite among some patients as they increase their abilities. This is highly recommended, but again try to space out the sessions whatever instrument you enjoy playing, and when playing the piano, to begin with, use a supportive chair rather than a standard piano stool as sitting with no back support will place extra strain on your spine.

If recovering patients take to the garden, they have to be careful not to expose themselves to organophosphates, such as pesticides and herbicides. Also, patients should invest in tools with long handles that reduce the need to stretch and bend. Be careful when carrying out repetitive actions to prevent overstraining weakened muscles.

Is technology safe to use?

People always think watching TV is a very passive activity and cannot overload the nervous system. They couldn't be more wrong. TV images create a hive of neuronal activity in the brain as one has to digest what is going on in each scene of a play, film or even a gameshow or the news. Screens also send out 'blue light', which has been shown to stimulate alpha waves, as mentioned in Chapter 3. During the morning the blue light is beneficial as it boosts mood, reaction times and concentration, but in the evening, and especially just before bed, it reduces good restorative sleep, so the advice to all patients is: do not watch TV for at least an hour before bed. A recent survey by a leading phone manufacturer found that almost nine out of 10 18–34-year-olds have trouble sleeping because they use their smartphones at bedtime. Technology firms have acknowledged the problem, with some major mobile tech providers introducing special settings that reduce blue light. Special yellow or orange tinted glasses can be used to filter out the harmful blue light.

Blue light filter glasses or blue light filter apps should definitely be used if using a computer for long periods. Many of my younger patients spend much of their day playing on computer games or looking at their phones. These screens should be set up with filters that shield the blue light as the day draws to a close. As with TV, all screens should be avoided for an hour before bed even when using the filter.

I recommend listening to relaxing music, reading or, if reading is difficult, listening to a talking book last thing at night is a good alternative.

Any screen-time should be restricted during the day as spending too long in one position can lead to postural strain on the spine and repetitive strain injuries when using game consoles or texting. Muscles are much more susceptible to damage from constant repetitive trauma, especially in fibromyalgia

As also explained in Chapter 7, hands-free options and non-metal cases on phones should be used to reduce radio frequency exposure.

When can I return to work?

If you have been off sick from work for a protracted amount of time, as you improve and are well enough to start work, you should never consider just returning to work full-time as soon as you feel better. You need to gradually increase hours in a phased return-to-work programme, such as that shown in Table 11.1. The phased return schedule depends on many factors and differs from patient to patient. This is an example of a recommended schedule I have used in clinic.

Table 11.1 Example of a phased return to work programme

Week	Monday	Tuesday	Wednesday	Thursday	Friday
1	1 hour		1 hour		1 hour
2	2 hours		2 hours		2 hours
3	3 hours		3 hours		3 hours
4	4 hours		4 hours		4 hours
5	4 hours		4 hours		4 hours
6	4 hours		4 hours		6 hours
7	6 hours		4 hours		6 hours
8	6 hours		6 hours		6 hours
9	6 hours		6 hours		8 hours
10	8 hours		6 hours		8 hours
11	8 hours		8 hours		8 hours
12	8 hours		8 hours	2 hours	8 hours
13	8 hours		8 hours	4 hours	8 hours
14	8 hours		8 hours	6 hours	8 hours
15	8 hours		8 hours	8 hours	8 hours
16	8 hours	2 hours	8 hours	8 hours	8 hours
17	8 hours	4 hours	8 hours	8 hours	8 hours
18	8 hours	6 hours	8 hours	8 hours	8 hours
19	8 hours	8 hours	8 hours	8 hours	8 hours

The rule of thumb is that you should listen to your body and symptoms. In other words, if you are struggling mid-way through the phased return programme and find four hours a day too much, you can go back a week or two in the schedule.

A similar situation occurs when a young patient is out of full-time or part-time education due to ME/CFS and FMS. Pressure to place the young person back into school is often compounded by social services becoming involved. Parents continue to be suspected of making their child worse than they actually are. As discussed in the previous chapters, conditions like 'Munchausen's disease by proxy' and 'fictitious illness syndrome' have been mentioned by the authorities, almost accusing patients' parents of making their children feel ill without any real physical cause of the disease.

Once the young person begins to improve, they can return to school, maybe just at break-time to begin with, so that there is some social interaction with their peer group. Little by little, add an extra class into the phased return schedule and as long as the young person feels that they are not getting too tired, they should continue to build-up their attendance.

University courses often present a problem as one cannot usually attend full-time degrees in a part-time capacity unless one joins a part-time course. This should sometimes be considered if the illness is too severe to continue. Another alternative is for severe patients to defer their university place for a time and hopefully they will be able to return to their studies once recovered. This has been the case with many of my student patients and most go on to receive a much better degree than if they had tried to struggle through. I am so proud of many of my patients who defer their university course and end up with excellent final exam results going on to flourishing careers.

Are there any dos and don'ts on commuting?

Travelling to and from work and school should always be factored into any phased return. Any travelling that places the patient under too much strain should be avoided. Going by train for long distances is usually better than driving as sitting for long periods can easily harm the spine. On the train the patient can get up and walk around a little as well as have a rest without the extra stress of traffic jams.

If I am improving can I go on holiday?

When you are well enough to take a vacation, it shouldn't first be a long-haul flight to a country that is very hot. Patients need to shelter from too much sun. ME/CFS and FMS symptoms are both exacerbated by jet lag, excessive temperatures and sunburn.

Often it's not the holiday that harms the patient, and a beach with fresh air and some sun and shelter, with the occasional dip into the sea, is often the best place to be. The problem lies in getting there and airports with their queues, and the long distances to the gate can be very damaging to the patient.

So, when flying I always advise patients who haven't yet recovered to order wheelchair support at airports. However much the patient may dislike the public display of their illness, they never regret following this advice since most airport staff look after wheelchair passengers and their families really well and take all the stress out of the airport experience.

If you have to go on a long-haul flight that may induce jet lag, ask your doctor or pharmacist about melatonin to take after the long flight, especially one that is travelling eastwards, such as from the USA to Europe. Melatonin helps to regulate the body's circadian rhythm and helps some patients' sleep problems. It is prescribed off-label for jet lag in many countries, but it is best to ask your doctor's advice before taking it.

When on holiday in a hot climate, make sure you keep in the shade as much as possible and use the highest rated sunblock. Sunburn will aggravate the pain in FMS and ME/CFS so you need to avoid the sun when possible. Try to avoid overheating and going to winter resorts that are too cold, as both will strain your hypothalamus, which is the body's thermostat, as discussed earlier. The best option is to go on vacation where the weather isn't too extreme.

Is it safe to get pregnant with ME/CFS or FMS?

There are two viewpoints concerning pregnancy and ME/CFS. Some experts believe that pregnancy is a time when a better balance is achieved within the woman's body and it can help reduce the symptoms of ME/CFS. However, this is unpredictable. Some healthy women blossom when pregnant; if the ME/CFS patient is lucky enough to be that type, her symptoms will probably reduce during pregnancy. However, if the mother-to be is one of those who generally have a difficult pregnancy, her ME/CFS symptoms may worsen for most of the nine months as her hormone levels fluctuate, producing more nausea and fatigue.

ME/CFS and especially FMS present a problem for the actual delivery of the baby as the natural pain in childbirth will be exacerbated and aggravate the widespread pain due to the illness. Gas and air or hypnosis should be considered before opting for any other forms of anaesthetic for the birth itself.

From a positional point of view, the best position for patients giving birth is the left lateral position, which is still commonly used and reduces strain on the spine compared with any other position.

If local or general anaesthetics are used in the labour, then one should check that they are safe and are non-adrenaline (epinephrine) based.

If there is a choice between having a spinal block or electing to have a Caesarean section, I would opt for the latter as injecting an anaesthetic directly into the spine is definitely not recommended for patients with ME/CFS and FMS.

A study published in 2004 showed that ME/CFS symptoms improve in about one third of pregnant ME/CFS patients, usually after the first trimester, and are unchanged in about one third and worsen in about one third, with worsening symptoms in their second and later pregnancies[8]. Any supplements taken for ME/CFS should be confirmed by your doctor as safe to take during pregnancy.

It's not just the pregnancy; it's the baby afterwards that obviously places more strain on the mother, and this is more of a problem. I would usually advise a patient to wait until they are well on the mend before they consider pregnancy. A survey found that 21% of a group of ME/CFS patients decided not to have a child because they thought that their debility would interfere with their ability to raise their child.

Breastfeeding carries the risk of toxins being transferred from mother to baby, as mentioned in Chapter 7. So, the best advice regarding this factor is for the mother to have as much detox treatment before she plans on getting pregnant.

There is also the genetic factor to consider. As mentioned earlier in Chapter 3, there is a 15% chance of ME/CFS being familial (running in families). However, I would never advise patients not to have children because they didn't want the risk of them also getting the disease. I do believe ME/CFS is preventable, with the physical signs appearing before the symptoms, so if a patient is worried about his/her child developing the illness, the child can be assessed for the five physical signs and if there is a problem they can be treated with the manual techniques listed in Chapter 10 before any symptoms arise. The physical signs will reduce quickly, and the child should remain healthy[9, 10].

If I require surgery, what precautions are needed?

You may have other problems that require an operation. If surgery is not essential, I would advise a delay as long as possible until you have improved with my treatment. However, occasionally surgery is crucial and needs to be done as soon as possible. In these cases, the advice I give to patients about general anaesthetics is that the anaesthetist should be aware of the illness and to follow the advice of one of the leading experts in this field, American physician and ME/CFS specialist Dr Charles Lapp.

Some patients have low magnesium and potassium levels so Dr Lapp recommends pre-operative tests for serum magnesium and potassium should be done as low levels can affect the heart under anaesthesia.

Many ME/CFS and FMS patients, especially the very severe, housebound patients, have a problem with their hypothalamic-pituitary-adrenal axis affecting their adrenal glands. Therefore, Dr Lapp also advises that cortisol levels should be tested before any operation, as low levels could place the patient at risk, so supplements may be required before surgery can commence.

All supplements should be discussed with the anaesthetist to check that they will be safe to take and that they will not interfere with the surgery or the anaesthetic. If possible, it is usually sensible to avoid most supplements for two weeks before surgery, especially garlic, ginseng and *Gingko biloba*, which increase bleeding.

Most of my patients have managed to recover quite quickly post-surgery, as long as they have taken things very easy and convalesced after their ordeal. The days of convalescent homes are long gone but when patients return home from hospital, they should be very careful to pace their activity to avoid a relapse of their symptoms.

How important are environmental factors?

All of us are exposed to a number of pollutants in our everyday lives. ME/CFS sufferers need to minimise as far as possible their exposure to these toxins (see Chapter 7, page 214, for a detailed list).

Sometimes it is not patients themselves who are directly exposed to a pollutant or environmental toxin. It can often be a family member who may be an engineer, a hairdresser or a car-paint sprayer. Many patients have had a possible neuro-lymphatic drainage problem since birth and have been harmed by living in a household where one or both parents have jobs that bring them into increased contact with toxins. The parents come home and may hug their baby and wash their clothes in the same machine as their child's clothes. This cross-contamination over the years can lead to the gradual build-up of neurotoxins in the brain and spinal cord, with the child eventually having sufficient exposure to trigger the onset of ME/CFS or FMS. Sometimes the onset of illness is many years later when the patient is an adult. Medicines for babies and children are given in minimal dosages since the young are much more susceptible to the effects of toxins, illustrating the fact that in the young toxic exposure does not have to be great to inflict harm.

When visiting the dentist, avoid having mercury amalgam dental fillings[11]. When going to have your hair done at the hair salon, the use of chemicals in your hair should be limited, especially since some have been shown to harm the actual hairdresser[12]. Remember that the scalp is very close to the brain and it is not advisable to massage poisons into the skin in this area. Take care to make sure that your neck is in a comfortable position, too, when your hair is being washed in a back basin.

Patients who are hairdressers themselves, or in other occupations that use large amounts of toxic materials, should take extra measures to avoid further exposure, such as wearing gloves, masks and having plenty of ventilation. This is advice that is all too familiar during the Covid-19 outbreak, but any patient working with toxins should continue to take these measures after the pandemic is over.

If you live in the countryside, take a trip away from home during crop spraying days[13]. If your work entails exposure to harmful toxins, you may need to consider a career change.

If both spouses or a few people in the same street develop ME/CFS or FMS, then try and see if there are any sources of pollution close by that may be a cause. One case that comes to mind is a couple who both were suffering from severe symptoms of ME/CFS. They were not blood related and yet both had been ill for a few years. They had been living in the same house for 20 years with their own little herb and vegetable garden, with no factories, farms or large roads nearby and their own market garden was 100% organic. They were not living under a flight path and they both had jobs that did not involve any contact with any toxins.

It seemed a very unusual case and, with the prevalence of ME/CFS on the increase, it could have been an unfortunate coincidence that the couple both had ME/CFS from other triggers rather than environmental. However, toxic screening at a local lab showed they both had high levels of nickel and cadmium in their blood samples. On questioning I found out that when they moved into their home it was a new build and further investigation revealed that it was built on a landfill site. I enquired about what the estate was built on and it was not so surprising they were being poisoned as the house was directly on top of a demolished car battery factory! Nickel and cadmium are used in the production of rechargeable batteries and obviously there was a seepage from the factory ruins into the soil. Sadly, this husband and wife both had different previous mechanical problems that had compromised their neuro-lymphatic pathways. However, the large amount of vegetables and herbs grown in this poisoned soil, and eaten for many years by this unfortunate couple, lay behind their illness.

As I said above, candles and scented products at home should be used sparingly as they are full of petrochemicals. If you move into a new home and you have new carpets, curtains and other soft furnishings then make sure you have plenty of ventilation. When decorating, use low-odour paint and again it is best to stay out of the house when the paint is being applied, especially the gloss. Make sure any home gas appliances are not emitting harmful carbon monoxide; ensure that you have detectors fitted in your home. Also, if you live in a damp, older property have an environmental check for mould.

When using mobile phones make sure you use a hands-free option as much as possible as holding it close to the head has been shown to damage the blood–brain barrier, making the brain more vulnerable to toxins.

Can the Perrin Technique help with other conditions?

This is a tricky question to answer. The simple answer is yes. Over the years, I have had the wonderful pleasure of working alongside some amazing doctors. One is leading neurologist Dr Margareta Griesz-Brisson in Harley Street, London. She always says: 'Ray, we are treating the physiology not the pathology'. In other words, the treatment is designed to aid the restoration of a healthy neuro-lymphatic system, which physiologically will encourage the central nervous system to work better. So, many problems affecting the nervous system should be helped by the Perrin Technique.

There are other diseases linked to problems affecting the lymphatic drainage of the brain. Scans in 2012 revealed visible proof of the drainage of beta amyloid proteins out of the brains of mice via the perivascular spaces into the lymphatic system. This showed how these large molecules could stagnate in diseases such as Alzheimer's, which has been linked to the accumulation of beta amyloid plaques, which destroy connections between the brain's neurones, affecting thinking, memory and behaviour.

I have treated a few patients with Alzheimer's disease and one elderly man in the early stages of the disorder received once a month treatment for four years with no deterioration in his symptoms throughout the four years. In fact, he sometimes came in for his monthly session saying he had had the best month yet, with increased energy and concentration and memory as good as ever. Sadly, he subsequently had a fall and injured his head which led to a speedy deterioration in his condition.

Another condition that I have helped many patients with over the years is Lyme disease; with this infection, the reverse flow of lymphatic drainage leads to a build-up of the bacterium *Borrelia burgdorferi* in the central nervous system. Research has also shown that problems with lymphatic drainage of the brain may also lead to some forms of clinical depression and rarer conditions such as Creutzfeldt-Jakob disease (CJD).

The neuro-lymphatic drainage pathway was shown to be affected in patients with the severe acute respiratory syndrome (SARS) caused by the corona virus infection of 2003, with some developing a ME/CFS-like illness. The coronavirus in Covid-19 seems to be causing the same post-viral fatigue states, leading to a post-Covid-19 syndrome (long Covid)[14], which has all the hallmarks of ME/CFS, and could very well affect the drainage in the olfactory pathway leading to loss of smell and taste, and an effect on the hypothalamus leading to high fever. In May 2020, I saw a 42-year-old man in clinic who responded very well to neuro-lymphatic treatment a month after having had severe post-Covid-19 symptoms and who was completely symptom-free two months later. We are seeing more and more post Covid-19 patients in clinic with all the physical signs and many symptoms of ME/CFS and most will respond very quickly to the Perrin Technique if caught in the first few months after coming down with the virus.

As the lymphatic drainage of the brain is being further investigated by neuroscientists around the world, more conditions will probably be connected to the dysfunction of this important process. This will probably indicate the validity in using the techniques shown in this book to treat many other neurological diseases that, at the time of writing, have no successful treatment and continue to baffle the medical world.

Once I have recovered, can the illness recur?

As patients recover, if they overdo things, suffer from infections or have to cope with too much stress, their symptoms may return or worsen. Some patients do suffer recurrences when they have significantly improved, but few experience relapses once they have been discharged, unless they push themselves too far day after day. ME/CFS and FMS patients, once recovered, need to reassess their lifestyle and take steps to reduce the continual stress that may have been part of what led to the illness in the first place. One should be able to exert oneself when better, but knowing when to stop is important.

Patients who have been discharged (10/10 on Table 10.3 in Chapter 10 – page 317) should continue the dorsal rotation exercises three times a day for life. Self-massage to the chest and neck should be done once a week in the shower. An annual check-up is advisable.

Should a relapse occur, it may take a long time to reverse, but remember that, if the treatment worked the first time, it should work again and perhaps more quickly the second time. Psychologists and counsellors are invaluable in these cases. The important rule in treatment, and even more so after relapse, is to remain as positive as possible. Negative thoughts create further neurotoxicity.

To secure a permanent remission and to remain in good health, one has to focus on the task ahead by means of sensible pacing (the '50% rule'), thus achieving a slow, sure return to good health.

Following a graded exercise programme, but only when better, is a good idea, not to treat the ME/CFS or FMS itself, but to help recondition the body and to remain fit and well in the future.

Can ME/CFS and FMS be prevented?

I am one of the few practitioners who maintain that ME/CFS and FMS can be prevented. The physical signs are very real and usually are seen long before the symptoms begin (see Chapter 8). This is why in the very early stages of the disorder only a physical and postural-based examination can detect the development of these disorders before the sympathetic nervous system breaks down.

If ME/CFS or FMS is found in more than one family member, there is probably a genetic predisposition that leads to a restricted flow of toxins from the brain and spine. I have discovered when examining children, siblings or even parents of the patient that they present some or all of the five physical signs of ME/CFS and FMS detailed in Chapter 8 (page 254).

When treating pre-ME, as I call it, the signs significantly reduce, usually with only a few weeks or months of treatment. For this reason, I believe that ME/CFS is preventable if treated and managed properly in the early stages.

The advice to physicians given by the International Association of CFS/ME states that establishing a diagnosis of ME/CFS as soon as possible will usually give the patient a much greater chance of relief[15].

The very severe cases of patients in bed all day and night in silent, darkened rooms should never happen, as early diagnosis should then be followed up quickly with advice on pacing and the appropriate treatment. The severe cases may be as a result of the wrong treatment or bad advice being given in the early stages of the illness, with patients being instructed and sometimes coerced to increase their activity, and sometimes medicated with drugs that have severe effects on the central nervous system.

If all practitioners around the world were taught to examine patients for the early physical signs, which are evidence-based, and to carefully review the patient's history and symptoms for indications and signs of neurotoxicity, there would be far fewer severe cases. If patients were given advice to pace at the outset, together with prompt treatment to restore a healthy neuro-lymphatic system, it could help prevent ME/CFS and FMS developing in the first place, and one day make these terribly cruel illnesses a thing of the past.

Case: Lorna's story

My first consultation with Dr Perrin six years ago, following a recommendation, was the turning point in my life, setting the path I was to follow to improve the quality of my life, which at that time, was nothing short of dire.

My life was overwhelmed by a myriad of 'confusing' symptoms, underpinned by fatigue and minimal stamina that I'd had probably since late teenager-hood. This situation culminated, in my early 50s, with long-term sickness absence from a 'professional' desk job in local government, following a seemingly innocuous virus on top of long-term sustained stress from the job itself and other various environmental and social sources. I was merely struggling into work and little else. It was purgatory. I could barely function and was sinking into a depression contrary to my normally bubbly and driven personality. My poor health was affecting my personal relationships to the detriment of my performance at work and socially and as a result, my self-esteem.

Dr Perrin's confirmation that I had ME/CFS through physical examination and careful regard to my medical and social history was sheer relief; his explanation was such a 'eureka' moment – it made utter sense that a structural defect was inhibiting my body's lymphatic drainage system from ridding itself of the ever-increasing toxic load of 21st century living and the overproduction of toxins being made by my own body due to the physical and emotional stress I was going through – the toxins had finally built up in my brain and spinal cord and were sufficiently concentrated so as to significantly debilitate me. I was in a vicious circle and downward spiral and had no chance of ever hoping to improve my chances without effective intervention, which was just not being, and is still not being, provided by the NHS. The unproven GET (graded exercise) regime offered at the time to me on the NHS had just stressed my body even further and no amount of CBT (cognitive behavioural talking therapy) I undertook (which is still being delivered) was going to address an organic, chronic medical crisis.

Reading Dr Perrin's first book (*The Perrin Technique*), a manageable read, further consolidated my understanding, based on his sound and unequivocal peer-reviewed research and proof of the root cause – the inadequate structural integrity of my spine and injury to my nose as a child led to an eventual build-up of toxins, irritating the 'all controlling' sympathetic nervous system and overloading the autonomic nervous system, which precipitated my relentless multifarious symptoms, characterised by utter fatigue of ALL my bodily functions. I was helpless but the Perrin Technique offered a plausible and scientifically proven remedy.

Following my moderate score given by Dr Perrin of around 4/10, I was then treated regularly for the next four years by Gail Sumner, a former patient of Dr Perrin and chartered physiotherapist, using the Perrin Technique as a method to break the cycle and assist my body to reduce and reverse the build-up of the toxic load that was ravaging me. Crucially, I appreciated that this was not about some miraculous 'cure'; rather, a measured, controlled restoration of my bodily functions to an acceptable level, sufficient to improve my quality of life.

My treatment over the last six years comprised of regular (at first weekly, then monthly) massages to the chest, neck and head using a special lymphatic drainage and manipulation technique devised by Dr Perrin, taking the complementary requisite supplements (milk thistle, EPA and EPO, vitamins C and B and others), the 'self-massage' and rotations of my torso routine, and pacing, whereby I should only do half or so of an activity I felt capable of doing. Adhering to all this advice rigorously within the confines of my job and running my home independently was difficult whilst coping with my symptoms, but I got great psychological comfort too from my visits to the Perrin Clinic in this regard.

I enjoyed my treatment (and still do every couple of months or so) and felt in very safe hands. At last, I was having proper treatment from practitioners with the knowledge and skills (and personal experience) to tackle this demon head on. It was the only real 'hands on' treatment and it gave me hope to keep going, miraculously.

Over the years, the Perrin Technique stabilised me enough to keep me in my job, however, life at work was getting harder in an ever-increasingly hostile working environment under austerity and I was also ageing, not being far off 60. In spite of our determination, it was evident that continuing to work under these circumstances was continually detrimental to my health and wellbeing and I ultimately succumbed to sick leave again. How could I pace sufficiently when the workload and other demands on me were increasing and where there was no intrinsic recognition of the severity of my situation in the workplace apart from mere lip service, that in itself being unduly stressful?

Dr Perrin provided the essential evidence I needed to convince my employer's medical advisors that I was unfit for any job in the workforce for the foreseeable future and as such, my employers for the Council were able, under Local Government regulations, to release my occupational pension early on grounds of ill health. My relief was nothing short of phenomenal after initial resistance from the

Council's medics. Sadly, there was no marking or 'celebration' of my leaving after 40 years of 'graft', not even a leaving card, yet again a reflection of the lack of recognition or appreciation of this debilitating and devastating condition.

Since I ceased paid employment last year, my stress levels have plummeted and I am able to pace and rest when I need to without ramifications or guilt. Coupled with continuous Perrin treatment once every three months or so and implementing my self-help measures, I'd say that the most troubling symptoms of malaise and feeling constantly 'poorly' have tailed off and I feel markedly better in myself and am able to accept and cope with my other troubling symptoms more readily. As one poignant example, just before Xmas, I was able to actually shop with enthusiasm for an outfit for my daughter's wedding and fully participate in (well almost) and actually enjoy the wedding itself, a far cry from having missed her graduation previously and barely enjoying and appreciating other notable milestones and events.

I'll be forever indebted to Dr Perrin and his ground-breaking research and tireless, compassionate team, especially Gail, who gave me my life back, not my old life, but a different, more circumspect life, and one which I intend to savour every moment. I'm currently planning my joint 60th birthday bash with two friends, but never far from my thoughts are those poor, abandoned and neglected souls, fellow sufferers in less fortunate positions than my own, having been unable to access the Perrin Technique and of course also the families of those who have met their untimely demise due to the neglect by the 'authorities' and society in general of this cruel condition.

Lorna Goulding, Manchester, UK
Patient of Dr Perrin and Gail Sumner, Chartered Physiotherapist and Licensed Perrin Technique Practitioner

Case: Noel's story

From a young age I had always been really sporty, running my first 10k race at 11 and making the school basketball team, right up to studying sports science at university, where I participated in boxing, swimming, running, basketball and coaching the wheelchair basketball team. Even after starting a career in medical sales, I still maintained my passion to keep fit and compete. Especially in running; I always loved to run, and I loved to win.

It's hard to say when my health started to suffer. I'd always seemed to pick up a virus here and there. But as I worked in the health industry it wasn't too surprising. However, my busy work schedule seemed to be taking its toll and I was getting more and more tired and no amount of rest would improve things. I would still run. But recovery was taking longer and longer.

I'd been to the GP several times and they always steered the diagnosis towards either a nasty virus or depression. Unconvinced, I started to research possible illnesses and realised that ME appeared to describe the symptoms I'd been suffering. When I presented this to the GP I was told that it could well be ME, but that the waiting list for the ME or CFS clinic was nine months. In the meantime, I underwent a series of blood tests to rule out anything else.

I remembered that a friend of mine had suffered from ME many years before and had been treated effectively by an osteopath in Manchester.

At the first consultation Dr Perrin was absolutely convinced that I had ME. He rated me as quite severe, a 3 or 4 I think, on the scale of 1 to 10, despite my best efforts to appear perfectly well.

Dr Perrin spelled out the course of treatment that would be required to get me back to a 10. He explained that it would get worse before it got better and that it would take 2 years. I admitted to my wife Laura, later at home, that I planned to be better in 18 months. Always competing!

Treatment began and the restrictions that I had to adhere to were difficult. There was very limited exercise and a new diet and supplements had to be adopted. Plus, a daily regime of hot and cold therapy and twice daily lymphatic massages; lovingly provided by Laura. She became quite the expert and had my routine down to a fine art. I really couldn't have done it without her. She was my rock.

The first few treatments from Raymond were the worst as we would travel to Manchester for the therapy and then head back to Yorkshire. Laura would drive as on the return journey I would be almost comatose. The following day would be no better and I'd often be unable to get out of bed.

Slowly but surely over the coming months we progressed. Our daily routine was carried out with military precision. Our diets and lifestyles drastically changed – all in a bid to get me healthy again.

Despite the recovery being gradual, there was a tipping point, around 12 months I think, when I started to feel much better. It was at this stage that I would quiz Dr Perrin about when I could start to run again. Raymond was very measured with his responses and encouraged me to be very careful. Walking at first and only doing half of what I thought I was able. As ever I was totally compliant, never pushing things too far, never wanting to risk a relapse.

After 18 months of treatment, Raymond signed me off. I can't explain the elation we felt at this point. We knew the treatment was working. However, to see the end result and feeling fully fit, back to myself again, was very special and we can't thank Raymond enough.

It has been seven years since I was signed off. In that time, I have completed several 10k runs, triathlons and ultra-marathons. My new passion is CrossFit, which is a strength and conditioning workout incorporating functional movement, Olympic lifting and gymnastics at high intensity. It's the most extreme sport I could find to push myself further than ever before. There's really no stopping me now!

Noel Brennan, York, UK

APPENDICES

- The ABC of symptoms
- Common pathological and radiological tests
- Glossary
- The Perrin Questionnaire (PQ-CFS)

ME/CFS and FMS:
The ABC of symptoms

I have included this section on the symptoms of ME/CFS and FMS as a useful guide to patients and physicians. It lists the complaints that occur in these conditions with a short explanation as to the cause of each one. Once you have read this book, ME/CFS and FMS should no longer be a mystery. By understanding the mechanisms that cause these disorders one can logically explain all the varied symptoms that patients suffer from. Over the years many patients have enquired whether a particular symptom is due to their illness 'I started with this itching in my leg last week…could it be due to my fibromyalgia?' or 'I have been diagnosed with sleep apnoea and my GP doesn't know if this has anything to do with my ME'.

To make this section as user-friendly as possible, I have compiled the list in alphabetical order to simply answer all those questions that patients or practitioners may raise regarding the symptoms that could be related to ME/CFS and FMS. I say 'could', because of course there is always a possibility of a comorbidity being present. In other words, the patient could be suffering from more than one condition and the symptom may be due to a completely different disease as well as the ME/CFS or FMS.

Any new complaint should always be thoroughly investigated to rule out any serious pathology, and there are plenty of comorbidities that require their own specific treatment approach which is discussed in detail in Chapter 6. As a general rule I would suspect the onset of a different disease if new symptoms seem to begin out of the blue and gradually worsen, when the major symptoms of the ME/CFS or FMS are responding well to treatment.

A

Acne: This skin condition is very common in ME/CFS and FMS, particularly in teenagers, primarily due to overstimulation of the sympathetic nerve supply to sebaceous glands leading to excess oil production. The backflow of the lymphatic system in ME/CFS and FMS can lead to hair follicles being congested with the excess oil plus, toxins including bacteria from prior infections which also can cause acne. Due to a backflow of the neuro-lymphatic (glymphatic) system in ME/CFS and FMS, there is a dysfunction of the hypothalamus which can lead to the over-production of hormones such as testosterone, leading to further acne in both male and female patients.

Allergies: Many patients with ME/CFS and FMS have sensitivities that may become allergies over time due to over-activation of the immune system, often seen in the early stages of the disease. The increased production of histamine in the mast cells can lead to one or sometimes many allergic responses with some extreme cases leading to mast cell activation syndrome (MCAS). For further information see Chapter 6.

Alopecia (see **Hair loss**)

Amenorrhoea (loss of periods): The absence of menstrual periods is rare in ME/CFS and FMS but I have seen the occasional case in clinic over the years. More common is painful menstruation (see **Dysmenorrhoea**). The reason why some women with ME/CFS and FMS suffer from amenorrhoea is mostly due to the dysfunction of the hormonal control in the hypothalamus due to increased neurotoxicity. Deficiency of the hormone leptin that regulates appetite can also be a major factor leading to an absence of periods, and research has pointed to high or low levels of leptin being found in ME/CFS and FMS (see Chapter 4).

Anosmia (loss of smell): This has been a common symptom in the Covid-19 outbreak and is caused by the same pathophysiological process as in ME/CFS and FMS. The pro-inflammatory cytokines produced by the immune system become congested within the perivascular lymphatic drainage through the olfactory pathway in the perforations of the cribriform plate, part of the ethmoid bone lying above the nasal cavity. This is one of the main neuro-lymphatic drainage points in the cranium. The increased toxicity and inflammation will result in damaging the olfactory nerves, leading to a disturbed sense of smell and, in some extreme cases, total loss of smell (see stages leading to ME/CFS and FMS in Chapter 8).

Anxiety (not primary, but secondary to the disease): This is a very common symptom in ME/CFS and FMS. The limbic system in the brain controls the emotions and is the main region targeted by neurotoxins when there is a backflow and congestion of the neuro-lymphatic system. This is compounded by the stress caused by the condition and the worry that the symptoms will worsen if the patient exerts him/herself. The resultant inactivity in severe cases aggravates the anxiety state.

Aphasia (problems with the production and/or comprehension of speech). Most patients with ME/CFS and FMS have cognitive impairment from neurotoxic overload due to backflow of neuro-lymphatic drainage. In some patients it can cause a dysfunction in Broca's area which is situated in the front part of the left hemisphere which is associated with speech. The patient's ability to turn thoughts into spoken language is affected, leading to difficulty or inability in finding the correct word or saying the wrong word during conversation. This is known as Broca's aphasia.

Arrhythmia (irregular heart beat): This condition is due to disturbance in the autonomic nervous system control of the cardiac rhythm, leading to an increase (tachycardia) or decrease (bradycardia) in the normal heart rate. In ME/CFS and FMS, there is a dysfunction of the central control of the autonomic nervous system leading to bodily disturbances including of the heart rate.

Arthralgia (joint pain): Arthralgia is usually present in many areas of the body in patients with ME/CFS and FMS. The pain is due to two factors: (i) the areas controlling pain in the thalamus and basal ganglia of the brain have become dysfunctional due to neurotoxins, exacerbating pain throughout the body; and (ii) disturbed sympathetic nerves affecting sensory nerves and local nociceptors (pain receptors) in the joints. The joints become painful but not swollen unlike in arthritis. ME/CFS and FMS are not arthritic diseases, so if the joints of the patient are swollen then it is due to another condition, possibly SLE (lupus). Sometimes the patient will complain of swollen hands or feet, but this is usually due to oedematous changes due to problems with their lymphatic drainage and not arthritis.

B

Back pain: Widespread pain is the cardinal symptom of FMS and nearly always present in ME/CFS. The back is the most common region for pain in these conditions, with symptoms usually in the mid and upper thoracic region, but many people have pain all along their back. This is often aggravated by postural problems, always found in the patient's thoracic spine and further exacerbated by toxins affecting the pain control centres in the brain, such as the thalamus and the basal ganglia (see Chapter 3 for more details).

Bad breath (halitosis): This is due to central autonomic disturbance in ME/CFS and FMS leading to a reduction in salivation and resultant dry mouth. A lack of salivary enzymes reduces the antibacterial function of the saliva, leading to a build-up of odour-causing bacteria.

Bloating of the abdomen: In ME/CFS and FMS there is a backflow of the lymphatics in the gut due to disturbed sympathetic nervous system control of the lymph vessels. Larger molecules such as yeast, gluten and casein (the protein in milk) need to drain away in the lymphatics. However, due to the retrograde flow of lymph this does not happen, leading to a build-up of these macromolecules; this in turn leads to fermentation and the production of gas and resultant bloating of the abdomen. There is also a problem with the blood–gut barrier, with leaky gut being a common finding in ME/CFS and FMS and is often due to an overgrowth of microbiota or gut flora.

Blurred vision: One of the main drainage pathways of the neuro-lymphatic system is the perivascular space alongside the blood vessels supplying the optic nerve. Due to the neuro-lymphatic backflow, inflammatory toxins can build-up around the optic nerve leading to blurred vision.

Body odour (BO): This is the result of bacteria breaking down protein on the skin into carboxylic acids, such as amino acids and fatty acids. With the retrograde lymph flow due to disturbed sympathetic control of the lymphatic system in ME/CFS and FMS, there will be a build-up of bacteria and large molecules such as cytokines and other proteins. This toxic soup in the sweat glands creates a large amount of carboxylic acids, leading to severe BO in some patients.

Bradycardia: This is a condition where the heart rate is slower than the accepted normal lowest rate, i.e. less than 60 beats a minute. Although many ME/CFS and FMS patients have an abnormal increase in the heart rate (tachycardia) some do suffer from bradycardia due to hormonal problems caused by a dysfunctional hypothalamus and possibly an over-stimulation of the dorsal vagus nerve in the suboccipital region of the neck (see the polyvagal theory, Chapter 3, page 73).

Brain fog: One of the most common symptoms of ME/CFS and FMS is described by many patients as 'brain fog', or as I like to call it 'muzziness'. Their ability to think properly about anything is usually disturbed. Scientists have examined the cognitive symptoms of ME/CFS for many years and have come to the conclusion that it is partly due to altered blood flow to parts of the brain, due to sympathetic dysfunction coupled with disturbed neurotransmission within the brain[1]. The main parts of the brain affected by neuro-lymphatic drainage problems are the frontal and prefrontal lobes concerned with thought, plus the basal ganglia and thalamus, which are concerned with emotion and relay messages from the frontal region to all over the brain. This leads to the brain fog that some patients find the worst of all the symptoms, especially if prior to their illness they had a job that required major cognitive skills, and owing to the connection with the limbic system it makes them even more depressed.

Breathlessness (also known as dyspnoea or dyspnea): Breathlessness is a common symptom in ME/CFS[2] due to the autonomic dysfunction leading to disturbance in the control of the cardiovascular system and ventilation. In FMS the fatigue and pain in the muscles of respiration can bio-mechanically lead to shortness of breath[3].

Bruising: Bruising spontaneously is often a sign of connective tissue disorders such as Ehlers-Danlos syndrome, which is a common comorbidity in cases of ME/CFS[4]. Sometimes spontaneous bruising is a sign of vitamin C and/or K deficiency. Bruising for no apparent reason does also occur in hormonal problems such as thyroid deficiency, diabetes and overactive adrenal function, which can be due to the dysfunction in the hypothalamus that takes place in ME/CFS and FMS.

Bruit: A 'bruit' is the name for an audible sound associated with turbulent blood flow and is sometimes present in the head in ME/CFS and FMS patients due to autonomic disturbance which can cause an increase in blood flow around the ears of the patient giving the characteristic 'wooshing' or beating noise.

Bulging eyes (exophthalmos, also known as proptosis): This is due to hyperthyroidism, which in ME/CFS and FMS would be due to the overstimulation of the hypothalamus in the brain which controls the thyroid via the pituitary gland.

Burning sensation: Some patients with ME/CFS and FMS will complain of many unusual sensory symptoms, including a burning feeling as if their skin is on fire. This is due to over-activity of the sympathetic nervous system caused by neurotoxicity in the brain. Superficial sympathetic nerves lie adjacent to somatic sensory nerves which can lead to a crossover of neurological activity just below the skin passing between the two nerve fibres in what are known as ephapses leading to these sensory disturbances (for more details see Chapter 3).

C

Candidiasis (thrush or other yeast and fungal infections): Excess yeast and fungi need to be removed by the lymphatic system and in ME/CFS and FMS there is a reversal of sympathetic nervous system control of the lymphatic drainage. This leads to a build-up of excess yeast and fungi in the body.

Chemical sensitivity: Many ME/CFS and FMS patients find they become sensitive to more and more chemicals as their illness deteriorates. They eventually may receive a diagnosis of 'multiple chemical sensitivity' (MCS). Some scientists believe ME/CFS, FMS and MCS are all different presentations of a group of environmental illnesses which are now termed 'central sensitivity syndromes'. MCS is probably caused by excess toxicity in the brain and an overloaded immune system which both occur in ME/CFS and FMS (see Chapter 6 for further details).

Clumsiness: Patients with ME/CFS and FMS often suffer from a lack of coordination with similar symptoms of developmental co-ordination disorder (DSD), the neurological condition known as dyspraxia, which affects the ability to plan and process motor tasks. In ME/CFS and FMS when there is a backflow of the neuro-lymphatic system, toxins accumulate in the thalamus of the brain which affects its function of relaying sensory and motor signals to the cerebral cortex. This causes a major disturbance in the patient's control over all activity and makes many everyday simple tasks such as walking, talking, and reading become difficult chores.

Coated/furry tongue: This is a feature in some patients with ME/CFS and FMS due to the build-up of bacterial infection due to a compromised immune system and reduced lymphatic drainage from the mouth.

Cognitive dysfunction: The prefrontal cortex in the front of the brain modulates cognitive processes, and is directly above the neurological pathways controlling smell that contain the main neuro-lymphatic drainage routes through the cribriform plate in the ethmoid bone of the cranium, via perivascular spaces alongside blood vessels supplying the olfactory nerves. In ME/CFS and FMS there is a backflow of toxins affecting this drainage which will eventually have a profound effect on the prefrontal cortex, leading to the cognitive problems which can be the most troubling of the many symptoms affecting patients, especially if they had a job that required major concentration and cognitive skills (see also **Brain fog**).

Cold hands and feet: Cold extremities are extremely common symptoms in both ME/CFS and FMS due to disturbance of the sympathetic nervous system which controls blood flow throughout the body. When the sympathetic nervous system is overloaded it leads to constriction of the blood vessels supplying the arms and legs. This problem is exacerbated by the dysfunction of the arteriole-venule shunts, which are tiny muscular valves controlled by sympathetic nerves which form a direct connection between arterioles (the smallest arterial vessels) and venules (the smallest veins), bypassing the capillary bed for the major purpose of regulating body temperature. These shunts open in times of hot weather, causing blood to flow through the hands and feet, leading to red clammy extremities which allow the blood to lose more heat and reducing the overall body temperature. The opposite happens in very cold weather when the shunts close, leading to whitened cold hands and feet whilst maintaining the blood flow to the major organs of the body. It has been proven that the cold extremities in FMS are also associated with more severe pain in the hands and feet due to disturbed sympathetic nerves at these AV shunts[5].

Cold sores: Seen frequently in ME/CFS and FMS, a cold sore is caused by the human herpes simplex virus type HSV-1 and HSV-2. After the initial infection has receded the virus lies dormant in the trigeminal nerve in the face and can lead to the complication of trigeminal neuralgia (nerve pain). With ME/CFS and FMS, the neuro-lymphatic system is dysfunctional and so viruses lying dormant in the nervous system can lead to increased pro-inflammatory cytokine activity which require a healthy lymphatic system to drain away, preventing further neuro-inflammation. Unfortunately, with ME/CFS and FMS this drainage is moving in the wrong direction, leading to the worsening of any viral presentation.

Constipation: This can be due to irritable bowel syndrome, which is a very common complaint in many of my patients. The autonomic disturbance in ME/CFS and FMS can lead to sluggish bowel movements and resultant constipation.

Cough: A persistent cough that may or may not be dry is a symptom of ME/CFS and FMS and is usually a result of sensitivities or allergies that are more common in these conditions. Sometimes patients experience post-nasal drip when excess mucus drains down the throat, causing coughing, especially if it contains neurotoxins. Occasionally, in some patients I have seen irritation of the nerves supplying the diaphragm and intercostal muscles, leading to a chronic cough.

Craving for certain foods: In ME/CFS, the severity of fatigue has been shown to be associated with daily cytokine fluctuation, driven by leptin. High levels of leptin have also been shown in FMS. Leptin is a hormone released from fat cells that regulate energy balance by inhibiting hunger via signals to the brain, especially the hypothalamus, and if disturbed leads to neurotoxic damage of the fatty glial cells in the brain. This leads to increase or decrease in feelings of satiety, thereby affecting the appetite of the patient and can lead to major cravings (see Chapter 4).

D

Dark patches around the eyes (periorbital dark circles): Many patients with ME/CFS and FMS present with dark patches, usually below their eyes, and often with puffy eyelids which are due to a combination of factors. In ME/CFS and FMS there is central autonomic nerve disturbance resulting in blood vessel dilation and lung dysfunction leading to disturbed blood flow and oxygen levels in the blood, which are both causes of the dark patches. The sympathetic control of lymphatic vessels leads to retrograde (backwards) flow and oedematous changes (swelling) in the orbit, which is one of the main drainage points of the neuro-lymphatic system, thus leading to the puffiness. The backflow can lead to a build-up of many different types of toxins clogging up this region and occasionally leading to a multi-coloured toxic soup that creates a collage of greens and greys on the skin in this region.

Dehydration: Patients with ME/CFS and FMS need to drink plenty of fluids every day (around 2 litres for an adult). In these disorders there is a toxic overload affecting the hypothalamus which controls the overall metabolic processes in the body via autonomic nerves and hormonal activity. This can badly affect the balance in body fluids, leading to possible dehydration.

Depression: The limbic system in the brain has been shown to be the most affected part of the brain when there is a restriction or backflow of the neuro-lymphatic system. This leads to most patients suffering from symptoms of depression. However, there is another major secondary cause of depression in ME/CFS and FMS. My name for this is TPOS ('thoroughly p****d off syndrome'!) and it is usually brought about by frustration – not being able to do any activity without suffering and not having any real proof of the illness, with many getting worse and becoming less active, which only aggravates their depression. It is a sad fact that most ME/CFS and FMS patients never receive 'get well' cards, as even their closest friends and family do not really understand why they are so ill, which leads to further frustration and depression.

Diarrhoea: As with constipation, diarrhoea can be due to irritable bowel syndrome, which is a very common complaint among my patients. The autonomic nerve disturbance in ME/CFS and FMS can lead to overstimulation of bowel movements and resultant diarrhoea.

Dizziness (also termed vertigo): Dizziness can be due to problems in the brain, blood flow to the head and /or a disturbance in the vestibular apparatus, the balance mechanism within the ear. In ME/CFS and FMS there is a toxic overload in the central nervous system affecting the brain, plus there is a disturbance of the autonomic control of the cerebral circulation and, to make matters even worse, one of the main pathways of the neuro-lymphatic drainage is the perivascular space of the blood vessels supplying the 8th cranial nerve, the vestibulocochlear, which controls balance. A build-up of toxins when there is a backflow of the drainage lead to dizziness.

Drowsiness: ME/CFS and FMS patients do not have much delta wave sleep at night, which reduces the neuro-lymphatic drainage and therefore they do not feel refreshed when they wake up. Rather they experience delta waves during the day leading to more toxic drainage, causing drowsiness. Even though people think FMS patients don't get tired… they do, and as well as ME/CFS patients, FMS patients may suffer unrelenting drowsiness from morning to night.

Dry eyes: Dry eyes are a common feature, especially in ME/CFS. Some types of antihistamine and antidepressant and contraceptive can cause the condition. Dry eyes can also be a symptom of both eye disease and medical conditions that affect the production of tears by the lacrimal glands in the eyes, such as the autoimmune disease Sjogren's syndrome. There is a separate condition known as 'dry eye syndrome' (DES), with symptoms of burning sensation, itchy eyes, aching, heavy, fatigued, sore red eyes with photophobia and blurred vision which has been shown to possibly be a risk factor for developing ME/CFS. This is due to the fact that some neurotoxic drainage is via perivascular spaces down the optic nerve pathways. Increased inflammation in this area could overload the neurotoxic backflow in vulnerable patients leading to ME/CFS and FMS. Increased computer use, contact lenses, ageing, menopause, smoking and frequent flying could all be aggravating or causal factors in dry eye syndrome (see Chapter 6 for further details).

Dry mouth: A dry mouth is a common symptom due to a disturbance in autonomic nerves supplying the salivary glands. It can also be aggravated by medications that have anticholinergic properties, such as some tricyclic antidepressants, muscle relaxants and antihistamines. Dry mouth and dry eyes can also be due to the autoimmune disorder Sjogren's syndrome, which can sometimes occur together with ME/CFS and FMS, so some symptoms may overlap and cause confusion in the diagnosis.

Dry skin: This has been reported in both ME/CFS and FMS and is due to either levels of toxins affecting the integrity of the skin or an increase in mast cell activation in the skin that leads to it becoming dry.

Dysmenorrhoea (irregular periods): Painful, heavy and irregular periods are all too common in ME/CFS and FMS. This is caused by disturbance to the autonomic nervous system and hormonal disturbance, both causes of primary dysmenorrhoea due to a build-up of neurotoxins in the hypothalamus following a backflow of the neuro-lymphatic system. Endometriosis and polycystic ovary syndrome (PCOS) are common comorbidities of ME/CFS and FMS that can both cause secondary dysmenorrhoea.

Dysphasia: see **Aphasia**

Dyspnoea: see **Breathlessness**

E

Earache: As discussed in detail in the book (see page 31), one of the main pathways of the neuro-lymphatic drainage system is the perivascular space around the blood vessels supplying the 8th cranial nerve, the vestibulocochlear, which controls hearing and balance. In both ME/CFS and FMS there is a build-up of inflammatory neurotoxins in this region due to backflow of the drainage which can cause occasionally severe earache.

Electro-sensitivity also known as **electromagnetic hypersensitivity (EHS)**: Growing numbers of ME/CFS and FMS patients find their symptoms worsen when exposed to low-dose electromagnetic radiation. The cause of EHS is unknown but researchers have shown that it may be due to impaired detoxification[6]. With ME/CFS and FMS there is an increase in neurotoxicity due to impaired neuro-lymphatic drainage, which can lead to the patient having to avoid exposure to mobile phones, WiFi and sometimes all electrical devices, making their lives intolerable (see Chapter 6 for further details).

Erectile dysfunction: ME/CFS and FMS both often affect libido in both sexes due to hormonal disturbances. However, a research study showed that erectile dysfunction was around twice as likely to occur in ME/CFS[7]. The reason for this is neurotoxicity causing central autonomic disturbance affecting blood flow to the penis. Problems with sexual intercourse are common in both ME/CFS and FMS, but they are more often due to lack of libido, pain or just plain exhaustion.

F

Fainting (syncope): When you stand up from sitting or lying down, your blood pressure should automatically increase to maintain a healthy blood flow in your head. This alteration in blood pressure is controlled by the autonomic nervous system. Most ME/CFS and FMS patient suffer different levels of neurally-mediated hypotension – that is, a drop in blood pressure due to autonomic nerve dysfunction. Neurally-mediated syncope (also known as vaso-vagal syncope) occurs when the drop in blood pressure results in fainting. The overall symptoms in patients with neurally-mediated hypotension usually worsen when standing and are relieved by lying down, which is known as orthostatic intolerance. Some patients with ME/CFS and FMS also suffer from a severe form of neurally-mediated hypotension know as POTS (postural orthostatic tachycardia syndrome). This causes the heart to race when standing up as well as a severe drop in blood pressure that leads to frequent fainting (see Chapter 6 for more details on POTS).

Fatigue: Obviously, as the name suggests, fatigue is one of the main symptoms of chronic fatigue syndrome. Even though widespread pain is the main feature of FMS, patients with fibromyalgia nearly always complain of fatigue. The fatigue in ME/CFS and FMS is typically both physical and mental and is aggravated by exertion and not relieved by rest (see **Post-exertional malaise**). The lymphatic system should drain away excess lactic acid created by exertion; however, in ME/CFS and FMS, neurotoxins affect the central autonomic control in the brain which disturbs the sympathetic nerve control of lymphatic vessels. This leads to a retrograde flow of lymph, resulting in a raised level of lactic acid following low-level exercise, plus a reduced clearance after exercise in ME/CFS[8] and FMS[9]. The mental fatigue is due partly to altered blood flow to parts of the brain resulting from sympathetic nerve dysfunction and partly to disturbed neurotransmission within the brain due to neurotoxic overload caused by backflow of the neuro-lymphatic system (see **Brain fog**). For more details, see Chapter 6: Defining fatigue.

Fever: ME/CFS is often triggered by a virus and it is the build-up of toxins, i.e. the pathogen and pro-inflammatory cytokines, passing through the blood–brain barrier in circumventricular organs such as the hypothalamus which leads to autonomic nervous system breakdown and can cause a high fever due to the infection and cytokines overstimulating the median preoptic nucleus of the hypothalamus.

Floaters: Floaters are spots in your vision which appear as black or grey specks, strings or cobwebs. They are usually age-related but can be caused by inflammation at the back of the eye which can occur in ME/CFS and FMS due to neurotoxic drainage problems in the perivascular spaces down the optic nerve pathways.

Forgetfulness: Many patients with ME/CFS and FMS enter a room to get something but forget what it was when they enter, or halfway through a conversation forget what they were talking about. A major area in the brain shown to be affected directly when neuro-lymphatic drainage is disturbed is the part called the basal ganglia, which has several interrelationships with the memory centres of the hippocampus. Another major region affected is the frontal lobe. This area via its connections with the hippocampus also become dysfunctional leading to short-term memory loss and other neurocognitive problems[10].

G
Gastroparesis: Delayed gastric emptying is due to autonomic disturbance in ME/CFS and FMS causing a premature full feeling while eating, nausea, gastric reflux and occasional vomiting.

Gum sores/ulcers: A major neuro-lymphatic pathway out from the cranium is via the perivascular space along blood vessels supplying the trigeminal nerve. In ME/CFS and FMS this pathway may become congested with a backflow of toxins draining into the mouth, specifically in the upper jaw region, which can cause gum sores and ulcers more frequently in the upper gums but may show up anywhere in the mouth.

H
Hair loss, Alopecia or general thinning: This may be due to lack of absorption of certain nutrients. Some of my patients who have low levels of iron have suffered hair thinning. The condition telogen effluvium, when the normal cycle of hair follicle production and hair shedding is disturbed due to autonomic dysfunction, occurs in ME/CFS and FMS when the body is under emotional and physical stress, but thankfully it is usually reversible.

Hallucinations: The thalamus is one of the main areas of the brain to be affected by a build-up of toxicity due to a dysfunctional neuro-lymphatic system, which occurs in ME/CFS and FMS. The thalamus controls dream states and if there is a problem in this region of the brain one can have very vivid dreams which in severe cases can present as hallucinations when awake.

Headache: This is one of the most frequent symptoms of ME/CFS and FMS. It can be similar to migraine headache and is often due to the increase or decrease of blood flow in the head due to autonomic nervous system dysfunction. Congested toxins in the cranium outside of the brain can stimulate nociceptors (pain receptors) that can lead to severe piercing headaches, especially in the region of the forehead. Due to metabolic changes patients may often be dehydrated or hypoglycaemic (low sugar), both common causes of headaches in ME/CFS and FMS. With a backflow of cerebrospinal fluid drainage in ME/CFS and FMS some symptoms such as headaches and nausea may be due to a very slight increase in intracranial pressure as hypothesised by other studies[11].

Hearing problems: One of the main pathways of neuro-lymphatic drainage is the perivascular space of the blood vessels supplying the 8th cranial nerve, the vestibulocochlear which controls hearing as well as balance. A build-up of toxins due to a backflow of the drainage in ME/CFS and FMS can lead to loss of hearing, tinnitus and also, more commonly, hyperacusis when the patient experiences a heightened sensitivity to sounds and finds loud noise unbearable.

Heartburn: This can be a problem in ME/CFS and FMS due to a disturbance in the autonomic nervous system's control of gastrointestinal processes. This can cause an overstimulation of goblet cells in the stomach, producing more acid than required, and a dysfunction of the control of the lower oesophageal sphincter, the muscular ring which joins the food pipe to the stomach. The resultant acid reflux – that is, backflow of the excess hydrochloric acid from the stomach into the oesophagus – causes the heartburn.

High blood pressure: see hypertension

Hives: Hives, also known as urticaria or nettle rash, are where welts or weals appear as a raised, itchy rash on the skin. In ME/CFS and FMS they can appear anywhere, but usually on the back and front of the thorax, and are caused by allergic reactions due to the release of histamine from mast cells which, due to overactivation of the immune system, are often seen in ME/CFS and FMS.

Hyperacusis (sensitivity to loud noise): One of the main pathways of neuro-lymphatic drainage is the perivascular space around the blood vessels supplying the 8th cranial nerve, the vestibulocochlear nerve, which controls hearing as well as balance. A build-up of toxins due to a backflow of this drainage in ME/CFS and FMS can lead to hyperacusis when the patient experiences a heightened sensitivity to sounds and finds loud noise unbearable.

Hyperosmia (sensitivity to smell): This is a common symptom of ME/CFS and FMS. The olfactory pathway is one of the main neuro-lymphatic drainage points in the cranium. The increased neurotoxicity and/or inflammation in this region will result in irritation of olfactory nerves leading to a heightened sensitivity to smell in some patients, with others finding a lessening of their senses and in some a total loss of smell and taste (see **anosmia**).

Hypertension: High blood pressure in ME/CFS and FMS sometimes occurs but is much less common than low blood pressure and is due to central dysfunction of the autonomic nervous system which leads to disturbed blood pressure.

Hyperventilation: This is shallow, rapid breathing and leads to low blood levels of CO_2. ME/CFS and FMS patients are often under terrible stress due to their illness that can precipitate a long-term state of hyperventilation; this in turn will exacerbate many of their symptoms, including fatigue and pain (see Chapters 4 and 6).

Hypotension: Low blood pressure is much more common in ME/CFS and FMS than high blood pressure and is due to central dysfunction of the autonomic nervous system which leads to a disturbance in blood pressure. Patients often present with postural hypotension which occurs when they stand up from sitting or lying, causing light-headedness and in, some cases, fainting.

I

Irritable bladder: Irritable bladder, also known as overactive bladder, is due to the smooth muscle walls of the bladder contracting even when the bladder isn't full, with the patient feeling that they have to urinate frequently. In ME/CFS and FMS a dysfunction of the hypothalamus due to increased neurotoxicity often leads to overstimulation of the sympathetic nerves and disturbance of hormonal control that can lead to an overactive bladder.

Irritable bowel: Irritable bowel is one of the most common symptoms of ME/CFS and FMS. Many patients are actually diagnosed with irritable bowel syndrome (IBS), discussed in detail in Chapter 5, causing loose bowels and/or constipation, bloating and pain in any part of the abdomen. This is due to the dysfunction of the autonomic nerves controlling the smooth muscles of the bowel wall. The irritable bowel in ME/CFS and FMS usually occurs together with gut dysbiosis where there is an imbalance of the flora (microbes) in the gut, with normally dominating healthy bacteria in the gastrointestinal tract overtaken by harmful bacteria, viruses and fungi (see Chapter 5).

Itchiness (also known as pruritus): Some patients with ME/CFS and FMS will complain of many unusual sensory symptoms, including itchy skin, often in different parts of their body. This is due to overactivity of the sympathetic nervous system due to neurotoxicity in the brain. Superficial sympathetic nerves lie adjacent to somatic sensory nerves and so near the skin surface there can be a crossover of neurological activity passing between the two nerves in what are known as ephapses leading to these sensory disturbances (see Chapter 3).

J
Joint pain: see **Arthralgia**

L
Light-headedness: This is a very common complaint in ME/CFS and FMS that usually occurs when the patient tries to get up too quickly from sitting or lying. This is due to the disturbed sympathetic nerve control of the blood pressure and leads to a momentary reduction in blood flow to the head when standing, causing the patient to feel very faint (see **Fainting** for more information).

Low blood pressure: see **Hypotension**

M
Mastalgia: Breast pain in ME/CFS and FMS is more common in female patients due to hormonal changes putting stress on the areas of the brain controlling the hormones, especially the hypothalamus which becomes dysfunctional due to an overload of neurotoxicity. Mastalgia in ME/CFS and FMS in both male and female patients is also due to a backflow of the breast lymphatics caused by disturbed sympathetic control

of the lymphatic drainage that leads to a build-up of inflammatory toxins causing mastitis and more pain in the breasts as a whole. One of the reasons why many more women develop ME/CFS and FMS than men is the presence of many more lymph vessels in this region. Sympathetic nerve irritation is a third reason for mastalgia in all patients with ME/CFS and FMS, affecting adjacent sensory nerves near to the surface of the breasts, especially lateral and superior to the left nipple. This is known as Perrin's Point and is one of the physical signs of ME/CFS reviewed in an NHS-sponsored clinical trial published in the *BMJ open*[12].

Mastitis: Inflammation in the breast can occur in both male and female patients with ME/CFS and FMS and is due to a backflow of the breast lymphatics. This in turn is due to disturbed sympathetic nerve control of the smooth muscle walls that control the flow in the lymphatic vessels, especially the main lymphatic ducts into the subclavian veins. The retrograde flow causes a build-up of pro-inflammatory toxins, such as cytokines, in the lymphatics and the first port of call in the body with many lymphatic vessels are the breasts, causing mastitis.

Memory problems…usually short term: see **Forgetfulness**

Migraine: Migrainous headaches are prevalent in ME/CFS and FMS[13]. This is partly due to the fact that trigger factors for migraines include hormonal, physical and psychological problems, all seen in ME/CFS and FMS, but also to central sensitisation which triggers some of the very severe migraines with or without visual auras (see **Headaches**).

Mood swings: Patients with ME/CFS and FMS often suffer from mood swings and this is due to the fact that when the neuro-lymphatic system is disturbed, neurotoxins affect the limbic system, the emotional centres in the brain (see **Anxiety** and **Depression** for further details).

Muscular pain (myalgia): As detailed in Chapter 2, FMS is diagnosed if there is muscular pain present in all four quadrants of the body, plus many other symptoms. Myalgia is nearly always present in patients with ME/CFS, thus the term myalgic encephalomyelitis (ME), but not usually as widespread as with FMS. Clinically I find most of the pain is in the upper trunk and the limbs, aggravated by exertion. The pain is due to two factors: (i) the control areas of pain in the thalamus and basal ganglia of the brain have become dysfunctional due to neurotoxins exacerbating pain throughout the body and (ii) disturbed sympathetic nerves affecting sensory nerves and local nociceptors (pain receptors) in the muscles and tendons. This disturbance of sympathetic nerve activity can reduce blood flow in the muscles. The resultant ischaemia further irritates the nociceptors, leading to worsening pain.

Muzziness in the head: see **Brain fog**

N

Nausea: In ME/CFS and FMS the toxic overload of the brain due to disturbed neuro-lymphatic drainage can lead to symptoms such as nausea when the patient is upright – in other words, this is an aspect of orthostatic intolerance (see later).The vestibular pathway in the ear may also be affected leading to dizziness and nausea. Any toxic overload and disturbed autonomic control of the liver and gastrointestinal system can also lead to nausea.

Neuralgia (nerve pain): This can be in the form of burning, shooting and sometimes a 'toothache-type pain. This is due to the central pain areas in the brain being affected by neurotoxins when the drainage of the brain becomes disturbed, which also leads to over-activity of the sympathetic nervous system. Superficial sympathetic nerves lie adjacent to somatic sensory nerves and in ME/CFS and FMS there is a crossover of neurological activity passing just beneath the skin surface between the two nerves in what are known as ephapses. This leads to pain that does not seem to follow the dermatomes – that is, the normal distribution of areas of skin supplied by the specific sensory nerves (see Chapter 3).

Nipple discharge (galactorrhoea): Some female patients with either ME/CFS or FMS complain of a milky nipple discharge not related to pregnancy. This is due to a disturbed hypothalamus caused by neurotoxic overload leading to the abnormal production of the hormone prolactin. Sometimes the discharge is smelly and discoloured which is most probably caused by the milky fluid mixing with all manner of toxins in the congested breast.

Numbness: Some patients with ME/CFS and/or FMS will complain of many unusual sensory symptoms, including numbness, often in different parts of their body. This is due to over-activity of the sympathetic nervous system due to neurotoxicity in the brain. Superficial sympathetic nerves lie adjacent to somatic sensory nerves and so near the skin surface there can be a crossover of neurological activity passing between the two nerves in what are known as ephapses. This leads to these sensory disturbances which don't seem to follow the dermatomes – the normal distribution of areas of skin supplied by the specific sensory nerves (see Chapter 3).

Nosebleeds: In both ME/CFS and FMS, nosebleeds can occur because of inflamed mucous membranes of the nasal cavity (rhinitis) due to a backflow of pro-inflammatory toxins along the olfactory pathway of the neuro-lymphatic system.

O
Obesity: see **Weight gain/loss**

Orthostatic intolerance: This occurs due to disturbed autonomic control of blood pressure, which occurs in many patients with ME/CFS and/or FMS. The body's inability to correctly calculate blood pressure leads to worsening symptoms when standing or sometimes when sitting and is relieved by lying down. (see **Dizziness** and **Fainting**).

Overstimulation: see **Sensory overload**

P
Pain: Patients with CFS /ME, and especially those with FMS suffer, with 'allodynia', which is the name given to pain due to no obvious stimulus, and also from general exacerbation of any pain stimulus (hyperalgesia); both are due to central sensitisation. It has been shown that when there is a cessation of normal drainage within the neuro-lymphatic system, the two main areas first affected in the brain are the thalamus and the basal ganglia in the brain which are both areas involved in the central control of pain (as detailed in Chapter 2).

Palpitations: Many patients with ME/CFS and/or FMS have noticeable rapid, strong, or irregular heartbeats that are aggravated by exertion, or stress. The palpitations are caused by the build-up of neurotoxicity in the brain leading to disturbance in the sympathetic and parasympathetic nervous control of the heart via the cardiac plexus situated at the base of the heart. In fact, the link made between ME/CFS and the autonomic control of the heart goes back to the American Civil War, when the condition was known as 'irritable heart disease' or 'soldier's heart' (see page 38).

Panic attacks: This is different to an anxiety attack as it is unprovoked and not a reaction to any particular stressor. Patients complain of physical problems, including palpitations, trembling, sweating, shortness of breath and other symptoms of sympathetic nerve overdrive that occur in ME/CFS and FMS. These are due to the neurotoxic overload in the brain affecting autonomic nerve control and the emotional centres of the brain.

Perspiration problems: Increased sweating, known as 'hyperhidrosis', is common in ME/CFS and FMS due to overstimulation of the sympathetic nerves supplying the sweat glands around the body. Increased perspiration also occurs due to a disturbed hypothalamus, which is the body's thermostat; the neurotoxic overload in ME/CFS and FMS leads to disturbed thermoregulation, with many patients feeling too hot constantly. On the other hand, in some cases, the dysfunctional hypothalamus causes the patient to feel cold most of the time, together with the sympathetic nerves supplying the sweat glands becoming underactive. This can lead to reduced perspiration (hypohidrosis) and, in extreme cases, anhidrosis when the patient is unable to sweat at all.

Photophobia (over-sensitivity to light): Many ME/CFS and FMS patients have dilated pupils due to neurotoxicity leading to an overload of the sympathetic nerves supplying the eye. The neurotoxins will also increase the pain and pressure behind the eye, worsening the overall symptom.

Some patients, however, have reduced sympathetic nerve activity leading to pupil constriction but dilated pupils are much more frequent with the patient needing to avoid bright lights and sunshine. Some ME/CFS and FMS patients need to wear sunglasses all the time, with the worst cases so photophobic that they need to wear blackout eye masks.

Pins-and-needles/tingling in the skin (paraesthesia): Some patients with either ME/CFS or FMS will complain of many unusual sensory symptoms, including pins-and-needles, often in different parts of their body. This is due to over-activity of the sympathetic nervous system due to neurotoxicity in the brain. Superficial sympathetic nerves lie adjacent to somatic sensory nerves and so near the skin surface there can be a crossover of neurological activity passing between the two nerves in what are known as ephapses. This leads to these sensory disturbances which don't seem to follow the dermatomes – the normal distribution of areas of skin supplied by the specific sensory nerves.

Post-exertional malaise (PEM): This is the main symptom of ME/CFS and also a major feature of FMS. It is both physical exertion and mental exertion that aggravate the symptoms, but not always immediately afterwards. It could be up to three days after a patient exerts him/herself that their condition suddenly worsens. Also, it is important to realise that it is 'exertion' and not simply exercise that triggers the PEM. Many patients with ME/CFS and FMS can cope with gentle exercise, such as a stroll in the park or swimming a few lengths in the local pool. Some patients can manage to do seemingly strenuous exercise, but for them it isn't exertion. Exertion involves doing any activity that means the individual patient pushes him/herself over the limit of what they consider normal healthy exercise. The reason why PEM occurs is that, when patients exert themselves, they overstrain the sympathetic nervous system, which in both ME/CFS and FMS is already overloaded. This is due to the build-up of neurotoxins in the brain affecting the central control of the autonomic nervous system of which the sympathetic nervous system is a part.

Post-nasal drip: The constant accumulation at the back of the throat of mucus from the sinuses is caused by the inflamed mucous membranes of the nasal cavity (rhinitis). This is extremely common in both ME/CFS and FMS due to a backflow of the main pathway of the neurolymphatic system. Lymph drains from the brain through the cribriform plate in the ethmoid bone (see Figure 4 on page 19) into the lymphatic vessels in the nasal cavity's mucous membrane. Other associated symptoms are a stuffy nose and/or sneezing. In ME/CFS and FMS, sensitivities and allergies are commonplace, leading to many patients having the condition allergic rhinitis which leads in turn to post-nasal drip.

Pre-menstrual syndrome (PMS): This is a collection of symptoms such as mood swings bloating, skin rashes and headaches, that affect many women but particularly female ME/CFS and FMS patients about a week or two before their period due to the obvious hormonal changes that take place during this time. This will disturb an already dysfunctional hypothalamus due to neurotoxic overload.

Pressure behind the eyes and nose: This feeling of pressure occurs in ME/CFS and FMS due to the reversal of normal lymph flow and subsequent build-up of neuro-lymphatic drainage via spaces lying around blood vessels supplying the optic nerves behind the eyes and the olfactory nerves above the nose. Increased toxicity in this region will cause further pain and possible inflammation in the sinuses and eyes.

R
Rosacea: This is an inflammatory chronic skin condition seen in ME/CFS and FMS leading to redness and raised spots. It is similar to acne and usually found on the face but can appear in all other parts of the body. It can be triggered by stress but has been linked mainly to types of pro-inflammatory and environmental toxins[14].

S
Sensory overload: Patients with either ME/CFS or FMS often feel much worse in crowded or loud places, such as parties, or when watching TV, and sometimes even when just going for a drive in a car. This is because of using too many of the senses at once, which with ME/CFS and FMS are overstimulated due to the build-up of neurotoxins

Sleep disturbance: Sleep disturbance in both ME/CFS and FMS usually takes the form of insomnia that includes difficulty getting to sleep or waking throughout the night; however, sometimes it involves too much sleep (hypersomnia). Sleep is controlled in the brain at areas specifically targeted by toxins, such as the hypothalamus, pineal gland, thalamus and locus coeruleus; consequently sleep/awake patterns and the quality of the sleep are affected.

Skin rashes and spots: Many patients with either ME/CFS or FMS develop rashes and spots on the skin, mostly on the face, upper back and/or chest, but they can be anywhere on the body. These can be atopic skin reactions such as eczema and can also be caused by reactions to or side effects of some medicines commonly prescribed, but in ME/CFS and FMS they are more commonly due to toxic overload affecting the control of the superficial lymphatic system which can cause many types of skin eruptions (see also **Acne** and **Rosacea**).

Sore throat: Listed in the NHS online information on ME/CFS as one of the main symptoms, sore throats can also occur in FMS. The post-nasal drip often complained of can lead to toxins draining from the inflamed nasal mucous membranes down to the throat. The neuro-immune system is compromised in ME/CFS and FMS, leading to lymphatic congestion in the neck; this in turn leads to the build-up of post infectious toxins that can cause sore throats. Some patients with ME/CFS and FMS suffer from sore throats as part of **chronic co-infections** such as coxsackie-B and human herpes viruses, or chronic bacterial illnesses, such as borreliosis (Lyme disease) (see Chapter 6).

Swollen glands/lymph nodes: Patients with either ME/CFS or FMS may have enlarged lymph nodes, usually in the neck or armpit. These are not the same as the enlarged varicose lymphatic vessels that are explained in detail earlier in the book that are easily palpated in the superficial breast tissue and the neck (see Chapter 8: The physical signs of ME/CFS). The swollen lymph nodes could be a result of an infection that possibly triggered the illness in the first place but also as a direct result of the backflow of lymphatic drainage that occurs in ME/CFS and FMS.

T

Tachycardia: Many patients with either ME/CFS or FMS have a rapid heartbeat of over 100 beats per minute; this is due to the build-up of neurotoxicity in the brain leading to disturbance in the sympathetic and parasympathetic nerve control of the heart via the cardiac plexus situated at the base of the heart. While an overly rapid heartbeat is most common in ME/CFS and FMS, as explained earlier, there are some patients who have the opposite problem of too low a heart rate (see **Bradycardia**).

Temperature dysregulation: Thermoregulatory disorders are extremely common in ME/CFS and FMS. with some patients feeling too hot and some too cold for most of the time, regardless of the external temperature. This is due to the neurotoxic overload in ME/CFS and FMS and the resultant disturbed hypothalamus, which is the body's thermostat, leading to dysfunctional thermoregulation.

Tinnitus: One of the main pathways of neuro-lymphatic drainage is the perivascular space of the blood vessels supplying the 8th cranial nerve, the vestibulocochlear nerve, which controls hearing. A build-up of toxins due to a backflow of the drainage in ME/CFS and FMS can lead to continuous buzzing or ringing in the ears as well as other associated symptoms (see **Hearing problems**).

Toothache: Patients with ME/CFS and FMS may have more sensitive teeth, especially heightened hot and cold sensitivity due to referred pain from hypertonic, fatigued facial muscles. Also, many patients have pain in their temporomandibular joint (TMJ), which can cause occlusion (closing) problems in the bite and lead to toothache as well as severe headaches.

Trembling/twitching (fasciculation): Muscle spasms are most commonly due to raised lactic acid levels. Extremely high levels of lactic acid have been shown in research studies on ME/CFS and FMS patients. The reason for this accumulation is that excess would normally be drained off via the lymphatics, but in ME/CFS and FMS lactic acid builds up in the muscles due to to the reversal of healthy lymph flow (see Chapter 6, page 161)[15, 16].

U

Unrefreshed sleep: ME/CFS and FMS patients often wake up after a night in bed feeling that they haven't slept at all. We now know that in health, neuro-lymphatic drainage occurs mostly during deep restorative delta wave sleep, which allows us to get rid of the poisons in our brain when we are asleep and wake up feeling refreshed. Unfortunately, ME/CFS and FMS patients have little delta-wave sleep at night, with delta-waves occurring during the day, making them feel more tired and more toxic during their waking hours (page 64).

V

Vertigo: see **Dizziness**

Vivid dreams: Many patients with either ME/CFS or FMS have much more vivid dreams than they did before they were ill. Sometimes these dreams are very weird ones or nightmares. The reason for this is the build-up of toxins in the thalamus, which controls dream states, and is one of the main areas of the brain to be affected by a dysfunctional neuro-lymphatic system.

Voice loss (dysphonia): The voice of ME/CFS and FMS patients may become very weak, with some severe cases only able to muster up a whisper and with the worst cases completely losing their ability to speak[17]. There are several reasons for this. The disturbed neuro-lymphatic drainage in ME/CFS and FMS affects the central autonomic control as well as the local autonomic control of the laryngeal muscles, which has been shown to be a major reason for dysphonia[18]. Loss of speech may also be due to fatigue of the muscles of respiration, especially the internal intercostal muscles (the muscles between the ribs) that are needed to propel the correct amount of air out through the mouth in order to speak.

Vomiting: In ME/CFS and FMS the toxic overload of the brain due to disturbed neuro-lymphatic drainage can lead to symptoms such as nausea and in severe cases this can lead to vomiting which may also be due the neuro-lymphatic drainage around the ear being affected. Any toxic overload and disturbed autonomic control of the gastrointestinal system can cause vomiting. The liver in ME/CFS and FMS will be struggling to cope with an increase in toxicity which may also lead to nausea and vomiting.

W

Weight gain/loss: Many patients with ME/CFS and FMS seem to put on weight when their illness strikes. Obviously, the patient is less active and so may increase their weight due to the inactivity. However, many patients have hormonal imbalances due to hormonal control by the hypothalamus in the brain being affected in neuro-lymphatic disorders. This can lead to thyroid and adrenal imbalances that can cause weight gain. In some patients, however, there is a substantive weight loss due to opposite hormonal changes occurring. Also it has been shown in ME/CFS and FMS that there is an abnormal amount of the hormone leptin found in the brain which affects satiety and hunger and is associated with both weight gain and weight loss (see Chapter 4).

Common pathological and radiological tests

Around the world, most ME/CFS and FMS patients are diagnosed by exclusion, since there is no definitive diagnostic pathological test from blood or other body fluid samples that can accurately diagnose these disorders. Hopefully, by using the methods detailed in this book, clinicians will be able to reach a definite positive diagnosis, but since there are many comorbidities that can cause similar symptoms to ME/CFS and FMS one has to initially carry out many pathological tests to see the complete picture. Clinically, due to the overall disturbance in the general metabolic processes in ME/CFS and FMS patients, many of the blood tests carried out are usually in the high or low range, but the values tend to remain just within the normal boundaries.

Many of my patients when we first meet hand me the results of dozens of lab tests ordered by their doctor without really understanding what they were for. Over and above what I include here, there are many more blood, urine, stool and salivary tests plus an incredible array of scans that can now be carried out to test for all sorts of conditions that may be the cause of some of the patient's symptoms. However, this section deals with the most frequent tests that doctors usually request when they are looking for an explanation of some or many of the symptoms which present in ME/CFS.

Since there is a difference from lab to lab across the world regarding what is considered a normal healthy range I have purposely left out a reference range. Most labs include reference ranges for normal on individual test results so make sure you have the results explained to you by the lab or your own GP.

Antibody tests

- **Rheumatoid factor (RF):** rheumatoid factor is an antibody that is measurable in the blood that can bind to other antibodies. Up to 70–90% of patients with rheumatoid arthritis (RA) have a positive RF test. The RF test is not diagnostic. It must be interpreted in conjunction with the patient's symptoms and history, and with tests of inflammation such as ESR or CRP. RF is also present in patients with other conditions, including other connective tissue diseases (such as systemic lupus erythematosus), some infectious diseases, liver disease and sarcoidosis. RF can also sometimes be present in healthy people who have RA in the family.
- **ANF (anti-nuclear factor) or ANA (anti-nuclear antibody):** the ANF or ANA test is carried out to check for systemic lupus erythematosus (SLE) or other connective tissue disorders. However, a positive ANF test by itself is not proof of SLE. Another test – antibody to double stranded DNA measurement – is used to determine if the symptoms may be due to SLE.
- **Complement component 3 and 4:** Complement component is a blood test that measures the activity of a certain protein that is part of the innate immune complement system that plays a part in the development of inflammation. C3 and C4 are the most commonly measured complement components. Complement activity may be measured to determine how severe a disease is or if treatment is working.
- **Endomysial antibody:** This is a test for the autoimmune response to gluten seen in coeliac disease.

Full blood count

In a full blood count, the blood sample is well mixed and placed on a rack of an analyser which is an instrument that measures different elements in the blood. The detailed analysis will examine the blood cells for the following values.

Red blood cells (the oxygen-carrying cells in blood)

- **Total red blood cells:** The numbers of red blood cells (RBCs) are given as an absolute number per litre.

- **Haemoglobin:** The amount of haemoglobin in the blood, expressed in grams per decilitre (low haemoglobin = anaemia).
- **Haematocrit or packed cell volume (PCV):** This is the fraction of whole blood volume that consists of red blood cells.
- **Red blood cell indices or mean corpuscular volume (MCV):** The average volume of the red cells, measured in femtolitres (10^{-15} litres). Anaemia is classified as microcytic or macrocytic based on whether this value is above or below the expected normal range.
- **Mean corpuscular haemoglobin (MCH):** The average amount of haemoglobin per red blood cell, measured in picograms (10-15 of a kilogram).
- **Mean corpuscular haemoglobin concentration (MCHC):** The average concentration of haemoglobin in the cells.
- **Red blood cell distribution width (RDW):** This is a measure of the variation across the RBC population.

Other blood cell counts

- **White blood cells** (the cells in the blood needed for the immune system): The total white blood cells are given as a percentage and as an absolute number per litre.
- **Platelets** (the cells in the blood needed for clotting).
- **Immune cells:** a complete blood count will include the numbers of specific immune cells, such as neutrophils, lymphocytes, monocytes, eosinophils and basophils.

Other common blood tests

- **Calcium (Ca):** A calcium blood test is important as calcium is one of the main minerals needed for bone and muscle integrity and is also essential for proper functioning of your nerves and heart.
- **C-reactive protein (CRP):** CRP is produced in the liver and its level in the blood will rise in response to inflammation, so it is a very accurate marker for any inflammatory state. Typically, patients with ME/CFS and FMS have a low to normal CRP; however, a higher than normal level can occur but usually indicates a comorbidity or another diagnosis.
- **Creatine kinase (CK):** CK is the most widely used enzyme to diagnose and

monitor neuromuscular diseases. The other muscle enzyme tests are for the levels of aldolase and LDH, which are all important when diagnosing ME/ CFS and especially FMS in ruling out other muscle pathologies. Aldolase is involved in the breakdown of glucose, fructose and galactose. LDH helps convert lactic acid to pyruvic acid.

- **Cholesterol:** Lipoproteins are combinations of lipids (fats) and proteins that transport cholesterol in the blood. High-density lipoproteins (HDL) transport cholesterol from the tissues of the body to the liver. HDL cholesterol is therefore considered the 'good' cholesterol. The higher the HDL cholesterol level, the lower the risk of coronary artery disease. Low-density lipoprotein (LDL) transports cholesterol from the liver to the tissues of the body. LDL cholesterol is therefore considered the 'bad' cholesterol.

- **ESR:** The erythrocyte sedimentation rate (also known as SED rate) also measures inflammation in the body but is much cruder than the CRP. The SED rate actually measures how fast red blood cells fall to the bottom of a test tube. An ESR is usually high during flare ups of inflammatory diseases such as rheumatoid arthritis. As with CRP, it is normally low or normal in ME/CFS and FMS patients.

- **Polymerase chain reaction (PCR)**: This is a universally used technique to rapidly multiply millions of copies from a small DNA sample, allowing scientists to amplify it so it can be analysed much more accurately. It is an extremely versatile test and can use other body fluids as well as blood to screen for bacteria, fungi and parasitic infection as well as viruses (as plenty of people who have had PCR testing for Covid-19 will testify).

- **Triglycerides:** The major form of fat. A triglyceride consists of three molecules of fatty acid combined with a molecule of the alcohol glycerol. The levels if high may indicate an imbalance of free radicals and antioxidants in the body. In 2012 a study showed that ME/CFS patients have higher levels of triglycerides than a control group[19]. The research team concluded this was due to oxidative stress induced damage to lipids and proteins.

- **U&Es (urea and electrolyte balance):** Urea is the major organic component of human urine comprised of broken-down amino acids. A U&E test is commonly used to detect abnormalities in blood chemistry, primarily kidney (renal) function and dehydration.

Hormone tests

In both ME/CFS and FMS the hypothalamus and the pituitary gland are both affected by toxic overload which can lead to many hormonal problems affecting any endocrine (hormone-producing) gland. Tests for the main hormones can identify a problem which may be due to a problem in the central control rather than a disease in the individual endocrine organ. I therefore advise patients who start the Perrin Technique to have a retest periodically to see if the hormonal disturbance has rectified after a course of treatment.

- **Thyroid tests:** There are two main thyroid tests, for triiodothyronine (T3) and for thyroxine (T4). There are three different types of T3 test: total T3, free T3 and T3 uptake. The two most common blood tests for hypothyroidism in men and women are a T4 blood test and a serum TSH (thyroid stimulating hormone) blood test. A T4 blood test will measure the level of T4 hormones in the blood.

- **Adrenal tests:** By measuring levels of the adrenal hormones cortisol and dehydroepiandrosterone (DHEA) in the saliva one can assess how the body responds to stress. Cortisol levels can be tested at home by taking a saliva sample immediately on waking, and then four further samples throughout the day. The **short synacthen test** screens for adrenal insufficiency by measuring serum cortisol before and after an injection of synthetic adrenocorticotrophic hormone (ACTH), normally secreted from the anterior pituitary gland.

- **Prolactin** is a single-chain protein hormone closely related to growth hormone. It is secreted by the anterior pituitary gland. It is also synthesised and secreted by a broad range of other cells in the body, most prominently various immune cells, the brain and the decidua (remains) of the pregnant uterus after birth.

- **Folicle stimulating hormone (FSH)** is released by the pituitary gland into the bloodstream and stimulates the growth of ovarian follicles before the release of an egg at ovulation. In men it stimulates sperm production.

- **Luteinising hormone (LH)** is a protein hormone that causes ovulation; it is released by the anterior pituitary gland in women. In men, LH stimulates production of testosterone.

- **Insulin:** This hormone is produced in the pancreas and causes glucose to leave the blood and enter the cells for use as energy or for storage, glucose being the body's main source of energy. Testing for glucose levels is important for establishing whether or not the patient is diabetic. Diabetes is the most common cause of abnormal glucose levels. Too little insulin, or too much, may be a sign of diabetes of which there are two types:

o Type 1 diabetes is an autoimmune disease that causes the insulin producing beta cells in the pancreas to be destroyed leading to little or no insulin at all. It is commonly diagnosed in children; however, the condition can develop at any age.

o With type 2 diabetes, the body still makes insulin but the person develops 'insulin resistance'. This is when cells in your body don't respond well to insulin and can't use glucose for energy leading to more insulin being produced in a vicious circle. Eventually, sugar levels in the blood go up leading to type 2 diabetes.

Liver function tests (LFTs)

Liver enzymes are proteins that help trigger chemical reactions that your body needs to function. Too much or too little of the following enzymes found in the blood may signal a problem with the liver that needs further investigation.

- **Albumin (Alb)** is the main protein produced by the liver found in the blood. It keeps fluid from leaking out of blood vessels; nourishes tissues; and transports hormones and other chemicals through the blood.
- **Alanine transaminase (ALT)** converts alanine, an amino acid found in proteins, into pyruvate, important for several metabolic pathways including energy production. In healthy people ALT levels in the blood are low.
- **Aspartate transaminase (AST)** is found mostly in the liver and muscles and is released into the blood when the liver is damaged. There is a small amount of AST found in healthy blood but higher-than-normal amounts may be a sign of a health problem.
- **Alkaline phosphatase (ALP)** is also found at high levels in bones and varies with age and gender. High levels of ALP are seen in pregnant women and children undergoing growth spurts.
- **Gamma glutamyl transpeptidase (GGT)** helps transport other molecules around the body. It plays a significant part in helping the liver metabolise drugs and other toxins and is affected by alcohol intake. GGT is often

measured relative to another enzyme, such as ALP. That is, both GGT and ALP are raised in liver problems whereas if GGT levels are normal and ALP high, it indicates possible bone disease.

- **Total bilirubin (TBIL):** Bilirubin is an orange-yellow pigment that occurs when part of your red blood cells are broken down by the liver. It travels through your liver, gallbladder, and digestive tract before being excreted. It is used to detect jaundice, anaemia and liver disease but can be naturally high due to a genetic condition, Gilbert's syndrome (see page 198).

Parasitic infection tests

Some patients with ME/CFS and FMS have been found to suffer from parasitic disorders which need to be tested for as stringently as viral, bacterial or fungal infections. As discussed in detail in Chapter 6, parasites that could occur alongside or actually lead to ME/CFS or FMS, can be nematodes (round worms) or other invading microscopic parasites causing infections that may require further investigation, such as specialised blood tests for *Toxoplasma protozoa, Giardia lamblia* or *Babesia* or for nematode infection (see page 187).

Virology tests

As a viral infection is a common trigger for both ME/CFS and FMS, tests for viral infections are most important in helping understand some of the symptoms of the condition. If one suspects a virus is still active and in the acute phase this will be revealed by an antibody test known as IgM (immunoglobulin M).

It may be that a new virus has recently infected the patient who already has ME/CFS or FMS, aggravating the pre-existing condition and exacerbating symptoms already present. However, if the test shows a positive IgG (immunoglobin G) this detects antibodies from a past infection and is important in identifying the possible viral infection that led to the start or worsening of the symptoms. The IgG test is the antibody test that has become so familiar during the Covid-19 pandemic.

- **Coronavirus-B (Covid-19):** Coronaviruses (CoV), which thanks to the pandemic of 2020 need no introduction, are a large family of viruses that cause illness ranging from the common cold to more severe diseases. A novel coronavirus (nCoV) is a new strain that has not been previously identified in humans. The novel coronavirus causing severe acute respiratory coronavirus 2 (SARS-CoV-2) was first discovered in China in 2019 and is better known as COVID-19.

- **Cytomegalovirus (CMV) antibody tests:** CMV is a herpes virus that can sometimes cause similar symptoms to EBV. The test detects current active CMV infection IgM, or past CMV infection IgG.

- **Epstein-Barr virus (EBV) test:** Glandular fever, also known as infectious mononucleosis or just 'mono', can be diagnosed with an antibody blood test called a Paul Bunnel test which reacts to blood cells of the sheep, or monospot tests which uses horse's blood to cause the positive test reaction for the Epstein-Barr virus (EBV).

- **Hepatitis:** Most cases of acute hepatitis are due to viral infections: hepatitis B is caused by a hepadna virus; hepatitis C is caused by a flaviviridae virus. Both hepatitis B and C may lead to a chronic form of hepatitis, culminating in liver cirrhosis.

- **Rubella:** The presence of IgM antibodies means a current or recent rubella (German measles) infection. The presence of IgG antibodies confirms immunity against the infection. If the patient has little or no immunity to rubella, the antibody titre will be 1:8 or less.

Bacteriology tests

One of the main chronic bacterial infections that is being detected in patients with severe ME/CFS and FMS is Lyme disease, also known as borreliosis, as detailed in Chapter 6 (page 183). To make a diagnosis of Lyme disease the doctor may take a blood sample. The most common screening tools in clinics worldwide are the ELISA and Western Blot tests which miss many positive cases. However, there are a few private specialised labs that carry out much more accurate tests, such as the Elispot (see page 184).

Many other bacterial infections can trigger ME/CFS and FMS and a simple blood culture can be done via your family doctor to screen your blood for bacteria or yeast that might be causing the infection. Gut bacteria play an important part and many studies on ME/CFS and FMS have shown a major disturbance with the microbiome (see Chapter 4).

Fungal infection tests

Most patients and health practitioners don't even think of testing for mycotoxins yet it was crucial for one of my younger patients who was brought up in a very old house which was full of mould. This teenage boy had a simple urine test at a specialist private lab which detected mycotoxins which were then treated by antifungal and detox regimes. A thorough investigation into fungal infections examines mycotoxins associated with *Aspergillus* (aflatoxin, ochratoxin and gliotoxin); *Penicillum* (sterigmatocystin and mycophenolic acid); *Tachybotrys* (roridin), *Fusarium* (enniatin and zealalenone), *Chaeomium globosum* (chaetoglobosin) and multiple other mould species (ciritin).

Other medical tests – scans and X-rays

Note: both CT and MRI imaging techniques may sometimes deploy the use of chemicals that are injected into the patient before the procedure that enhances the image. This may not be tolerated well in some ME/CFS and FMS patients and so should be discussed with the doctor before any such procedure is carried out.

- **CT scan:** A computerised tomography scan, also known as a CAT scan, uses computers and rotating X-ray machines to create cross-sectional images of all parts of the body. These images provide more detailed information than normal X-ray images and are better at examining bones and joints three-dimensionally than are MRI scans.
- **Echocardiogram**, also known as an 'echo', is a type of ultrasound scan used to examine the heart and nearby blood vessels. A small probe is used to send out high-frequency sound waves that create echoes when they bounce off different parts of the body. These echoes are picked up by the probe and turned into a moving image on a monitor while the scan is carried out. An echocardiogram may be requested by a heart specialist (cardiologist) or any doctor, including a GP, who thinks there might be a problem with the heart. The test is usually carried out at a hospital or clinic by a cardiologist or a trained specialist called a cardiac physiologist.
- **EEG** or electroencephalogram is a painless test used to find problems related to electrical activity of the brain. Small electrodes are placed on the scalp

which then send signals to a computer to record the wave patterns of the
brain.

- **ECG** or electrocardiogram checks the heart's rhythm and electrical activity.
It is used to investigate symptoms of a possible heart problem, such as chest
pain, palpitations, dizziness and shortness of breath, and arrhythmias which
all can occur in ME/CFS and FMS.

- **fMRI:** A functional magnetic resonance imaging scan is a type of MR scan
(see below) that is used to measure and map the brain's activity.

- **HRV** or heart rate variability is the the variation in the time interval between
consecutive heartbeats measured in milliseconds. HRV changes with exercise,
hormonal reactions, cognitive processes, plus other metabolic processes and,
of course, stress. It can be measured by sophisticated equipment in a hospital
setting but can be also monitored with certain strap-on portable devices one
can buy online. There are plenty of practitioners world-wide that use HRV
for many different disease processes to monitor autonomic disturbance and
therefore this may be very useful in monitoring patients with either ME/CFS
or FMS.

- **MRI** or magnetic resonance imaging scan uses strong magnetic fields
and radio waves to produce detailed images of the inside of the body.
It takes longer than the CT scans and makes a much louder noise so is
more challenging for many ME/CFS and FMS patients who suffer from
hyperacusis (see page 383). However, it can be more accurate in detecting
problems within the brain and nervous system that are hard to see on CT
images.

- **PET** or positron emission tomography scan is an imaging technique that uses
a radioactive tracer that can detect the functioning of different internal organs,
mainly used to show if the brain is functioning correctly

- **SPECT**, or single photon emission computed tomography scan, is another
type of nuclear imaging test looking at the functioning of the brain. It uses
a radioactive substance and a special camera to create 3-D pictures. It is
excellent in showing blood flow to tissues and organs. Since 2012 dual
photon emission computerised tomography has been used in research to
image the neuro-lymphatic drainage of cerebrospinal fluid in perivascular
and paravascular spaces but the clinical use of these advanced scanning
techniques remains rare at the present time (2020).

- **Ultrasound** scans use a small probe to send out high-frequency sound waves that create echoes when they bounce off different parts of the body which are turned into an image on a monitor while the scan is carried out. They are most often used to examine the foetus in pregnancy but can be used to examine the health of most organs in the body.
- **X-rays** are a type of invisible radiation that can pass through the body, being absorbed at different rates by different parts of the body usually for the examination of bones and joints.

Glossary

A

ACT   Acceptance and commitment therapy

ACTH   Adrenocorticotrophic hormone

AfME   Action for ME (see Useful names and addresses, page 427)

ANS   (see Autonomic nervous system)

AOA   American Osteopathic Association (see Useful names and addresses, page 435)

AP   Anterior posterior

ARA   Arachidonic acid

ATP   Adenosine triphosphate

ABDOMEN: The lower part of the trunk that lies between the thorax and the pelvis. The abdominal cavity contains the stomach and intestines, plus other internal organs and glands, including the liver and pancreas.

ACUPUNCTURE: The puncture of the body by one or more needles to relieve pain, induce anaesthesia and improve the health of a person. It is based on the Chinese philosophy of chi (the energy of life) that is a balance of the positive yin and the negative yang. The acupuncture takes place along meridians, which are pathways of energy under the skin. The flow of energy is obstructed in disease states. By inserting a gold, copper or silver needle into a blocked meridian, the flow of energy is improved.

ACETYLCHOLINE: One of the substances that aids the transmission of impulses from one nerve to another, and from a nerve to its target organ.

ACID: A substance that forms hydrogen ions in solution and combines with an alkaline material to form a salt. Acids have a pH value of less than 7.

ACYCLOVIR: A drug used against viruses. It is known to be helpful in the treatment of herpes infections.

ADRENALINE (called epinephrine in the USA): a hormone secreted by the adrenal gland that acts as a neurotransmitter, stimulating the sympathetic nervous system along with noradrenaline. It is also manufactured synthetically and used for its stimulating properties.

ADRENERGIC RECEPTORS: Areas in the body which are targeted by adrenaline (also known as epinephrine) and noradrenaline (norepinephrine), mainly in the nervous system but also found in the various organs of the body aside from the brain.

ADRENO-MEDULLARY: Pertaining to or arising from the medulla of the adrenal gland.

AETIOLOGY: The cause of a disorder.

AGRANULAR: Not consisting of granules or grains.

ALBICANS: White.

ALKALI: A compound that forms a salt when mixed with an acid. Alkalis possess a pH value of more than 7.

ALLOSTASIS: The process of maintaining physiological equilibrium in response to stressors.

ALLOSTATIC LOAD: The wear and tear on the bodily systems after repeated stress.

AMPHETAMINE: A powerful and addictive drug which has a similar effect to adrenaline and stimulates the sympathetic nervous system.

ANAEMIA (US – ANEMIA): The condition that arises when the red blood cell and/or haemoglobin count falls below the normal level.

ANATOMICAL: Pertaining to the body's structure.

ANATOMY: The science dealing with the structure of the human and animal body.

ANTAGONIST: A substance that neutralises the action of another; A muscle that counteracts the action of another muscle (its agonist).

ANTERIOR: In front of; at the front.

ANTERIOR HORN CELL: A horn-shaped region found in the front part of the spinal cord.

ANTERO-LATERAL: positioned towards the front and outside of a structure.

ANTIBODIES: Substances in the blood that fight against different toxins or foreign bodies (known as antigens).

ANTIDEPRESSANTS: The collective name given to those drugs that prevent or relieve depression.

ANTIVIRAL: Working against viruses.

AROMATHERAPY: The treatment of certain disorders by the use of aromatic essential oils during massage.

ARTERY: A tube or vessel that conveys blood from the heart to the rest of the body.

ARTHRITIS: Inflammation of a joint, due to either a disease or the process of wear and tear.

AUSCULTATION: Listening for certain sounds within the body by using either the ear or a stethoscope.

AUTONOMIC: Not under voluntary control.

AUTONOMIC NERVOUS SYSTEM (ANS): A section of the nervous system that regulates the systems of the body that are not under voluntary control, such as the heart, gut, blood and lymphatic vessels.

B

BIT   Bojungikki-tang: An Asian herbal medicine used to aid the digestive system

BPM   Beats per minute

BETA BLOCKER: A type of drug that prevents the stimulation of receptors in certain autonomic nerves responsible for increased cardiac activity. They are usually prescribed to reduce blood pressure, and control heart rhythm.

BORRELIA BURGDORFERI: This is a bacterium of the spirochete class that is most commonly transmitted to humans by the deer tick and leads to Lyme disease.

BORRELIOSIS: Lyme disease due to infection with the bacterium *Borrelia burgdorferi*.

BRONCHUS: One of the larger tubes, in which air passes through from the windpipe (trachea) to the smaller bronchioles within the lungs.

BUFFER: A chemical system that prevents change in the concentration of other chemical substances. Usually to keep acid/alkali levels in equilibrium.

C

CAB   Carotid basilar

CBT   Cognitive behavioural therapy

CCFP Chronic ciguatera fish poisoning

CCHS Chronic candidiasis hypersensitivity syndrome

CDC   Centers for Disease Control and Prevention (see Useful names and addresses, page 431)

CFC   Chlorofluorocarbon

CFIDS Chronic fatigue immune dysfunction syndrome

CFS   Chronic fatigue syndrome

CNS   Central nervous system

CP   Control patient

CRH   Corticotropin releasing hormone

CRI   Cranial rhythmic impulse

CSF   Cerebrospinal fluid

CT   Computerised tomography

CV4   Compression of fourth ventricle

CANDIDA: Yeast-like fungi that naturally occur in a healthy body but are capable of causing disease.

CANDIDIASIS: Infection caused by candida.

CANTHUS: Part of the facial bone to the side of the eye.

CARBONIC ACID: A solution of carbon dioxide and water.

CARDIAC: Pertaining to the heart.

CARDIOLOGIST: A heart specialist.

CARDIOVASCULAR SYSTEM: The system composed of the heart and the blood vessels.

CEREBROSPINAL FLUID (CSF): The fluid surrounding and bathing the brain and spinal cord.

CERVICAL: Pertaining to the neck (note: also a medical term referring to the 'neck' of the uterus).

CHOLINERGIC: The nerves that release the transmitter substance acetylcholine; an agent that stimulates the release of acetylcholine.

CHRONIC: Long-lasting.

COCCYX: The triangular bone at the tail-end of the spine formed by the fusion of 3–5 vertebrae.

COMORBIDITY: More than one disease process affecting the body at the same time.

CONTRACTILE: Possessing the ability to contract, e.g. muscle.

CONTRACTION: A shortening (pulling together) of tissue.

CORTEX: The outer layer of a structure.

CRANIAL: Pertaining to the skeleton of the head (the cranium).

CRANIO-SACRAL: Pertaining to the cranium and the sacrum. Used mostly in relation to the rhythm of the CSF which travels from the head to the sacrum at the base of the spine.

CRIBRIFORM PLATE: A perforated bony plate in the centre of the ethmoid bone of the skull through which blood vessels and the olfactory nerve pass.

CYTOKINE: Cytokines are a category of proteins that act as signalling molecules, coordinating the body's response against infection and triggering inflammation.

CYTOTOXIC: Having a poisonous effect on cells.

D

DHA   Docosahexaenoic acid

DHEA Dehydroepiandrosterone

DWMH Deep white matter hyperintensity

DECEREBRATE: Stopping the function of the cerebrum (the main portion of the brain) by severing the brain stem, or by cutting off the blood supply to the brain.

DIETETIC: Pertaining to the diet for health purposes.

DILATION: The act of expanding.

DISC (DISK): A flat, thin, circular structure. Intervertebral discs contain fibrous outer layers surrounding soft, jelly-like centres. They lie between the bodies of adjacent vertebrae in the spinal column and act as shock absorbers.

DISTAL: At the further end.

DORSAL: Pertaining to the back; positioned on the back surface. Another name for thoracic, e.g. the dorsal spine.

DYSFUNCTION: An impairment or abnormality in the functioning of an organ or system in the body.

E

EBV   (see Epstein-Barr virus)

EFA   Essential fatty acid

EMG   Electromyography

ELECTRON MICROSCOPY: Examination with a microscope that emits a beam of electrons (negatively charged particles of an atom). This beam forms an image for viewing on a fluorescent screen and can be used for ultra-small structures that are too small to be seen under a light microscope.

EPSTEIN-BARR VIRUS (EBV): A herpes virus that is believed to cause infectious mononucleosis (glandular fever).

ENDOCRINE: Pertaining to specific organs, or the complete system, that secretes hormones into the circulation.

ERECTOR-SPINAE: The name applied to a group of muscles that extend along the length of the spine. As the name suggests, their main function is to keep the spine erect.

F

FES   Functional electrical stimulation

FORME Fund for Osteopathic Research into Myalgic Encephalomyelitis (see Useful names and addresses, page 428)

FOV   Field of view

FIBROUS: Composed of or containing fibres. Fibrous tissue is present in many different structures throughout the body. It is also formed in scar tissue during the natural healing process.

FIBROSITIS: An inflammatory condition affecting white fibrous tissue within chronically damaged muscle. The inflammation is combined with an increase in the volume of the tissue to cause a very tight, enlarged and tender area. The shoulders are the most common site for fibrositis to occur.

FORAMEN: An opening or hole, usually found in bone, that forms a natural passageway.

FATTY ACID: An acid that contains only carbon, hydrogen and oxygen which combines with glycerine to form fat.

FUNCTIONAL ANATOMY: Anatomy as applied to the interaction between different structures of the body during any activity.

G

GABA   Gamma aminobutyric acid

GWVs   Gulf War veterans

GALL-BLADDER: A small pear-shaped sac which lies beneath the liver. Its function is to store bile that is produced by the liver.

GANGLION: A bundle of nerve cell bodies that lie outside the brain and spinal cord (plural = ganglia).

GANGLIONATED: Structures that contain ganglia.

GANGLION IMPAR: The ganglion which unites the two chains of the sympathetic nervous system. It is found in front of the coccyx.

GASTROINTESTINAL: Pertaining to the gut.

GENITALIA: The organs of reproduction.

H

HPA   Hypothalamic-pituitary-adrenal

HVLA   High velocity low amplitude

HVT   High velocity thrust

HAEMOTOXIC: Poisonous to the blood.

HEPATITIS: Inflammation of the liver.

HERPES VIRUS: A large group of DNA viruses, which includes herpes simplex (causes cold sores) and herpes zoster (causes chicken pox and shingles).

HIGHER CENTRES: The controlling mechanisms of the central nervous system within the brain.

HOMEOPATHY: A system of medicine whereby a minute dose of the drug stimulates the body to fight the disorder from within. It is based on the philosophy of treating like with like.

HOMEOSTASIS: The ability of the body to keep all functions working in a state of dynamic equilibrium.

HORMONE: An internal secretion which produces a specific physiological action on a target organ.

HIGH VELOCITY THRUST (HVT): The manipulative technique that produces a speedy gapping of a joint, usually accompanied by a loud 'crack'.

HYPERMOBILE: Abnormal increase of movement/flexibility in a joint.

HYSTERECTOMY: The surgical removal of the uterus (the womb).

I

IBS   Irritable bowel syndrome

ICD   International Classification of Disease

ICP   Intracranial pressure

IGC   Item group checklist

IGF   Insulin-like growth factor

IF   Interferon

IL   Interleukin

IMMUNE SYSTEM: The system in the body responsible for fighting infection and disease.

IMMUNOGLOBULIN: A type of animal protein which produces antibodies. It is used in combating disease processes.

IMPAR: Not paired.

IMPULSES: The electrochemical process that travels along nerve fibres.

INFARCTION: An obstruction of blood supply leading to local death of the tissue.

INFLUENZA: The 'flu'is an acute viral infection primarily of the respiratory tract but it can affect other systems in the body too.

INHIBITORY DRUGS: Chemicals that interfere with the normal physiological mechanism.

INTERSPINAL NERVES: Nerves that pass between two segments of the spine.

INTERVERTEBRAL: Between two adjacent vertebrae.

INTRADERMAL: Within the layers of the skin.

INTRAMUSCULAR: Within a muscle.

INTRAVENOUS: Within a vein.

INVOLUNTARY MECHANISM: The mechanism of the flow of cerebrospinal fluid from the cranium to the sacrum, and its influence on other tissues.

K

KYPHOSIS: The convex curvature of the spine when viewed from the side. The dorsal spine is said to be KYPHOTIC if its naturally convex curvature is abnormally exaggerated.

L

LC   Locus coeruleus

LACRIMAL: Pertaining to tears.

LATERAL: To the side; in a position further away from the midline of the body.

LESION: A damaged area of tissue.

LEVATOR SCAPULAE: A muscle that attaches to the shoulder-blade and the upper neck. Its function is to raise the shoulder-blade.

LIGAMENT: A strong band of fibrous tissue that holds bones together.

LOBE: A divided portion of an organ, as in the brain or the liver.

LORDOSIS: The concave curvature of part of the spine when viewed from the side.

LUMBAR: Pertaining to the lower part of the back, i.e. the area of the spine between the thorax and the pelvis.

M

MAP   Muscle action potential

ME   Myalgic encephalomyelitis/encephalomyelopathy (see below)

MIA   Membrane immunobead assay

MMR   Measles-mumps-rubella

MPTP   1-methyl-4-phenyl-1,2,3,6-tetrahydropyridinium

MR   Magnetic resonance

MRI   Magnetic resonance imaging

MANIPULATION: The expert treatment of the body by the hands.

MAOIs: Mono amino oxidase inhibitors – a group of antidepressant drugs.

MEDULLA: The innermost portion of a structure.

METABOLISM: The chemical and physical process by which the living body is maintained.

MITOCHONDRIA: Organelles within cells that produce about 90% of the chemical energy that cells need to survive.

MONONUCLEAR: Containing only one nucleus.

MOTOR NEURONE: A nerve that supplies a skeletal muscle to stimulate motion.

MUSCULOSKELETAL: Pertaining to the muscles and skeleton.

MUZZINESS: The state of being confused and unable to think clearly often referred to as 'brain fog'.

MYALGIC ENCEPHALOMYELOPATHY (ME): An alternative term for ME indicating that inflammation of the spine need not always be present.

MYELIN: The fatty substances surrounding part of particular nerve fibres (known as MYELINATED fibres).

MYELOPATHY: A disease process affecting the spinal cord.

N

NADH   Nicotinamide adenine dinucleotide H

NIAC   Neuro imaging analysis centre

NK   Natural killer

NMDA N-methyl-D-aspartate

NEUROCHEMICAL: Pertaining to the chemistry of the nervous system.

NEUROCOGNITIVE: Pertaining to thought processes of the nervous system.

NEUROENDOCRINE: Pertaining to hormonal control by the nervous system.

NEUROLOGIST: A specialist in disorders of the nervous system.

NEUROMUSCULAR-SKELETAL SYSTEM: The system in the body comprising of nerves, muscles and the skeleton.

NEURON: A nerve cell.

NEURORADIOLOGY: A division of radiology that specialises in investigating and diagnosing abnormalities in the nervous system.

NEUROTRANSMITTER: A chemical which stimulates activity when released at nerve endings, either transmitting between two nerves or between nerves and target tissues.

NORADRENALINE: (Norepinephrine in the US) is the main neurotransmitter for the sympathetic nervous system, and some central nerve endings. In the brain it is produced by small nuclei, the most significant one being the locus coeruleus in the brain stem. It is also a hormone produced in the central part of the adrenal glands (the adrenal medulla). Its main role is to increase heart rate. It also increases blood pressure, helps break down fat and increases blood sugar levels.

O

OIS   Osteopathic Information Service (see Useful names and addresses)

OLFACTORY: Pertaining to the sense of smell.

ORGANOPHOSPHATES: Chemicals formed of phosphoric acid and alcohol that are major components of some pesticides and herbicides.

P

PC   Phased contrast

PCB   Polychlorinated biphenyl

PET   Positron emission tomography

PFRS   Profile of fatigue related states

PVH   Periventricular hyperintensity

PVN   Paraventricular nucleus

PTSD   Post traumatic stress disorder

PALPITATION: An increased awareness of the heartbeat.

PANACEA: A global remedy; a cure-all.

PARALYSIS: Total or partial loss of movement in the body.

PARASYMPATHETIC NERVES: Autonomic nerves that stem from the cranium and the sacral regions and have different functions to sympathetic nerves.

PARAVASCULAR PATHWAY: Part of the pathway of the neuro-lymphatic system. Also known as the 'glymphatic' pathway containing cerebrospinal fluid (CSF) surrounding penetrating arteries of the brain and draining toxins via paravenous spaces out of the brain.

PATHOGENIC: Pertaining to any organism that causes a disease.

PAUL-BUNNELL TEST: A blood test which confirms the diagnosis of glandular fever (infectious mononucleosis), in which antibody reaction to red blood cells of sheep are examined.

PECTORALS: The collective name for the muscles of the chest, i.e. the pectoralis major and minor.

PEPTIC: Pertaining to the juices of the stomach and digestion.

PERIVASCULAR: Situated or occurring around a blood vessel.

PERIVASCULAR SPACE: also known as a Virchow-Robin space, is an interstitial fluid-filled space within the wall of blood vessels in the brain and spinal cord and is involved in the drainage of toxins from the central nervous system.

PHYSIOLOGIST: A specialist in physiology, the functioning of the body.

PHYSIOLOGY: The science of the function of living organisms, and how the body works.

PLACEBO: The beneficial response to treatment due to the patient's belief in its value. Placebo drugs are inactive substances that are given to gratify the patient.

PLASMA: The fluid part of the blood.

PLEXUS: A network of nerves.

POSTERIOR: At, or towards the back.

POSTGANGLIONIC: Positioned after (distal to) a ganglion.

PREGANGLIONIC: Positioned before (proximal to) a ganglion.

PROLAPSE: The downward fall of part, or all, of an organ.

PROXIMAL: Nearer to a particular point. (The opposite of 'distal'.)

Q

QUADRICEPS: The large four-headed muscle in the front of the thigh. Its main function is to extend and straighten the knee joint. Its tendon contains the patella (the kneecap).

R

REM   Rapid eye movement

RNase L Ribonuclease L

RSD   Reflex sympathetic dystrophy

RSI   Repetitive strain injury

RAMI COMMUNICANTES: A branch that connects two nerves.

RAMUS: A branch.

RECEPTORS: Receivers of certain nervous or chemical stimuli. They are situated at the ends of particular sensory nerves and on cells.

REFLEX: The automatic reaction that occurs in response to nervous stimulation.

REFLEXOLOGY: An alternative system of diagnosis and therapy. It is based on reflex points in the foot that correspond to different parts of the body.

REMISSION: The lull or cessation of the symptoms of a disease.

S

sEMG   Surface electromyography

SNS   Sympathetic nervous system

SPECT   Single photon emission computerised tomography

SPET   Single positron emission tomography

SACRUM: The wedge-shaped bone situated directly beneath the lumbar spine. It comprises of five sacral bones fused together and is the back part of the pelvis.

SCAPULA: The shoulder blade (plural: Scapulae).

SHIATSU: A form of oriental massage which concentrates on acupuncture points in the body.

SOFT TISSUE: The term used to describe the structural and connective tissue that is not bone, e.g. muscles and ligaments.

SOLAR PLEXUS: Also known as the coeliac plexus; it is the sympathetic nerve plexus situated in the upper central region of the abdomen. It supplies and receives messages to and from the internal organs of the abdomen.

SOMATIC: Pertaining to the body; pertaining to the body wall as opposed to the internal organs.

SYNAPSE: A junction between two nerve cells.

SYNDROME: A collection of different symptoms that occur together.

T

Tc   Cytotoxic T lymphocytes

TD   Thoracic duct

TE   Time to echo

Th   T-helper cells

TR   Time of repetition

TENDON: A fibrous continuation of the muscle body. It attaches muscle to bone.

TENNIS ELBOW: Lateral epicondylitis; an inflammation of the common tendon of the extensor muscles of the forearm due to an overuse injury.

THORACIC: Pertaining to the thorax.

THORAX: The chest; the section of the body between the neck and the abdomen. It is enclosed by the rib cage.

TRAPEZIUS (plural TRAPEZII): A muscle that attaches the neck to the shoulder blade and the collar bone. Its main function is to raise the shoulder.

U

URTICARIA: A breakout of hives – raised and red swellings on the skin. The cause may be unknown but can be due to an allergic response.

V

VAGUS: The vagus nerve, the 10th cranial nerve which has sensory, motor and parasympathetic fibres. It travels down from the head to supply structures in the neck, thorax and abdomen.

VASOCONSTRICTION: A decrease in the diameter of the blood vessels.

VASODILATION: An increase in the diameter of the blood vessels.

VENTRAL: Towards the front (opposite of dorsal).

VENTRICLE: The term applied to a cavity or chamber in the brain or the heart.

VERTEBA: The individual bones of the spinal column.

VIRCHOW-ROBIN SPACE: See perivascular space.

VISCERA: The internal organs of the chest and abdomen such as the heart, lungs, liver and intestines.

VISCERAL: Pertaining to viscera.

VITAMIN: A group of organic substances that occur mainly in small amounts in food, and which are vital for the healthy functioning of the body.

Y

YANG: Chinese philosophical concept as half of the complete whole, being the male half associated with heaven, heat and light.

YIN: Chinese philosophical term which is the opposite but complementary to the Yang. It is the female half associated with earth, cold and dark.

Z

ZEOLITE: A mineral with many different crystalline structures composed of mainly aluminium, oxygen and silicon. Zeolites help detox heavy metals and radiation.

The Perrin Questionnaire for chronic fatigue syndrome/ ME (PQ-CFS)

The following is the Questionnaire I use as part of the assessment of new ME/CFS and FMS patients. (Note that joint swelling (Question 16) is not a symptom of ME/CFS or FMS. There may be joint pain or swelling in a limb due to oedema but arthritic-type joint swelling means that there is a comorbidity of arthritis, especially if the swelling is in more than one joint, or other conditions causing joint inflammation such as SLE.) The maximum score is therefore 49 for women, 47 for men. Also note that the scores are part of the assessment and do not always reflect the actual severity of the patient's condition but generally <15 = a mild case; 15-25 = average; 25-35 = severe and 35+ = very severe. To make a more accurate prognostic score one should follow the system detailed in Chapter10 and, better still, see a licensed Perrin Technique practitioner if possible.

> Please take your time and make sure you answer all the questions. You do not have to complete the questionnaire all at once, as long as all questions are answered (male patients do not answer questions 49 and 50).
>
> Please tick the box only if the answer to each of the following is yes. Leave blank if the answer is no.

1. I suffer from physical fatigue ☐

2. My concentration is reduced ☐

3. I have difficulty getting to sleep ☐

4. I often have vivid/weird dreams ☐

5. My sleep is usually disturbed ☐

6. I have problems with short-term memory ☐

7. I find it difficult to read ☐

8. I get 'muzziness' in the head/brain fog ☐

9. I suffer from sinusitis ☐

10. I suffer from head pain ☐

11. I suffer from neck pain ☐

12. I suffer from shoulder pain ☐

13. I suffer from upper back pain ☐

14. I suffer from lower back pain ☐

15. I suffer from other joint pain ☐

16. I suffer from joint swelling ☐

17. I suffer from general muscle pain ☐

18. I often suffer from numbness ☐

19. I often suffer from pins and needles ☐

20. I suffer from redness in the face ☐

21. I suffer from frequent rashes ☐

22. I suffer from dry skin ☐

23. I suffer from frequent spots on my forehead ☐

24. I suffer from frequent spots on my back ☐

25. I suffer from frequent spots on my chest ☐

26. I feel depressed ☐

27. I feel anxious ☐

28. I suffer from panic attacks ☐

29. I am sensitive to bright light ☐

30. I am sensitive to loud noise/suffer tinnitus ☐

31. My temperature fluctuates ☐

32. I suffer from bad breath ☐

33. I suffer from thrush ☐

34. I have problems with my bowels ☐

35. I have problems with my bladder ☐

36. I am sensitive to smells ☐

37. I have food intolerances/allergies ☐

38. I have lumpy breasts ☐

39. I have tenderness/pain in the chest ☐

40. I am frequently breathless ☐

41. I suffer from palpitations ☐

42. I suffer from sore throats ☐

43. I suffer from nausea ☐

44. I suffer from dry eyes ☐

45. I suffer from dry mouth ☐

46. I sweat a lot ☐

47. I suffer from cold hands/feet ☐

48. I suffer from mood swings ☐

(The final 2 questions are for female patients only)

49. I suffer from PMS ☐

50. My symptoms are worse during periods ☐

The following supplementary question should always be used together with the PQ-CFS as it screens patients for possible disorders such as clinical depression, anxiety or bipolar who will answer (a) or (b) positively; ME/CFS and FMS patients will answer (c), (d) or (e) positively. If they tick (b) and (d) they may have both depression and ME/CFS. Also remember, this question is investigating if the patient suffers from post-exertional malaise (PEM) – not post-exercise fatigue! Make sure that the patient understands that they must think how they feel after pushing themselves physically or mentally. Also, the reaction may take up to three days to surface as reflected in the response to (e). See Chapter 10 for further details.

Supplementary question

Please tick the box that you feel best describes your symptom picture.
Following exertion do your symptoms:

a. always improve ☐

b. sometimes improve ☐

c. always worsen ☐

d. sometimes worsen ☐

e. sometimes initially improve but worsen within three days ☐ .

Useful names and addresses

ME/CFS and FMS organisations

UK

Action for ME
Action for ME is a UK charity working to improve the lives of adults and children with ME. They campaign for more research, better services and treatments.
42 Temple Street
Keynsham
BS31 1EH
Tel: +44(0)117 927 9551
questions@actionforme.org.uk
www.afme.org.uk

Association of Young People with ME
The Association of Young People with ME (AYME) is a UK charity that provides support for children and young people aged up to 26 who have ME. AYME also offers help and support to parents, carers and professionals in health, education and social care.
PO Box 5766
Milton Keynes
MK10 1AQ
Tel: +44(0)8451 23 23 89
info@ayme.org.uk
www.ayme.org.uk

Fibromyalgia Association UK

FMA UK provides information and support to patients and their families. It also provides medical information for professionals and operates a national helpline. They aim to encourage NHS and other funding sources to fund new research projects; helplines are manned mostly by volunteers most of whom are FMS sufferers themselves.

Studio 3007

MileEnd Mill

12 Seedhill Road

Paisley

PA1 1JS

Tel: +44(0)844 826 9022 (not for support calls)

www.fmauk.org

FORME (Fund for Osteopathic Research into ME)

FORME is a UK charity dedicated to helping osteopathic research into chronic fatigue syndrome (ME/CFS). It has funded research that has led to the scientific support of the Perrin Technique and aims to support further projects looking into the physical nature of ME/CFS. One of its main aims now is to disseminate the findings of Dr Perrin's ongoing research.

www.forme-cfs.co.uk

ME Association

The ME Association (MEA), founded in 1976, funds and supports research and provides information and support, education and training in the field of ME/CFS. It aims to avoid duplicating the work undertaken by other voluntary and statutory agencies. It has a very useful website with listings of local societies throughout the world.

7 Apollo Office Court

Radclive Road

Gawcott

Bucks

MK18 4DF

Tel: +44(0)1280 818963

www.meassociation.org.uk

ME Research UK (MERGE)
MERGE holds the database on all research into ME since 1956, in archive form.
meruk@pkavs.org.uk, www.meresearch.org.uk

The Young ME Sufferers Trust (Tymes Trust)
A charity dedicated to children and young people with ME and their families. Their entire team work pro bono and in 2010 they received the Queen's Golden Jubilee Award for Voluntary Service, for pursuing the educational rights and advancing the care of children with ME. They played a major role in producing the children's section of the Dept of Health Report on CFS/ME (2002).
PO Box 4347, Stock, Ingatestone, CM4 9TE
www.tymestrust.org

AUSTRALIA

Emerge Australia
A national organisation providing information, support and advocacy.
www.emerge.org.au/

CANADA

FM-CFS Canada
Provides information about research, connects fellow sufferers and raises awareness about ME/CFS and FMS.
310-1500 Bank Street,
Ottawa, Ontario K1H 1B8
office@fm-cfs.ca
Tel (toll-free): 1-877-437-HOPE (4673)

EUROPE

European ME Alliance
A grouping of European national charities and organisations that actively supports patients and campaigns for funding for biomedical research to provide better treatment.
www.euro-me.org/

IRELAND

FibroIreland

FibroIreland has been created for people affected by fibromyalgia. It provides general information to help sufferers understand how fibromyalgia affects them and what they can do to manage it. It also explains where to find further information.
https://fibroireland.com/

Irish ME/CFS Association

The Irish ME/CFS Association, through its various activities and awareness campaigns, strives to improve the situation for people with ME/CFS and to give them information to empower themselves. The group, which has been run entirely by volunteers for the last seven years, has approximately 400 members from the estimated 10,000 sufferers in the Republic of Ireland.
PO Box 3075
Dublin 2
Ireland.
Tel: +353 (0)1 235 0965
info@irishmecfs.org
www.irishmecfs.org

Irish ME Trust

The Irish ME Trust was established in 1989 to provide information and a counselling service to those affected with ME as well as targeting individual problems on behalf of sufferers. It aims to create awareness in the general public and the medical profession as to the plight of ME sufferers in Ireland and contribute to quality biomedical research studies.
Carmichael House
North Brunswick Street
Dublin 7
Ireland
Tel: +353 (0)1 890 200 912
info@imet.ie
www.imet.ie/index.html

NEW ZEALAND

The Associated New Zealand ME Society (ANZMES)

ANZMES was established to provide support for and publish and distribute information to groups and individuals suffering from or interested in ME/CFS including their families and carers. Also to provide a national focus for and to represent individual sufferers and support groups for ME/CFS in New Zealand. It promotes research into the study of ME/CFS , and into its causes and treatments and liaises internationally, keeps abreast of current research and helps educate health professionals about ME/CFS.

PO Box 36 307
Northcote
Auckland 1309
New Zealand
www.anzmes.org.nz

SOUTH AFRICA

ME CFS Foundation South Africa

Supports people with ME/CFS, FMS and other comorbidities such as POTS (postural orthostatic tachycardia syndrome).

info@mecfssa.org
mecfssafoundation@gmail.com

USA

Centers for Disease Control and Prevention

As the USA's health protection agency, the CDC is a federal agency that conducts health promotion, prevention and preparedness activities in the USA with the goal of improving overall public health.

1600 Clifton Road
Atlanta
GA 30329
USA
Tel: +1-800-CDC-INFO (800-232-4636); TTY: (888) 232-6348

The National CFIDS Foundation
CFIDS is a national non-profit organisation that funds research and provides information, education and support to people who have ME/CFS (NB: CFIDS is a former name for ME in the USA). The Foundation publishes a quarterly newsletter, *The National Forum.*
103 Aletha Road
Needham
MA 02492
Tel: +1-(781) 449-3535
info@ncf-net.org
www.ncf-net.org/

PANDORA
(Patient Alliance for Neuroendocrine-immune Disorders Organization for Research & Advocacy)
PANDORA is a grassroots advocacy organisation that promotes awareness of and research into/ME/CFS, fibromyalgia, Gulf War illnesses (GWI), multiple chemical sensitivities (MCS) and chronic Lyme disease.
PANDORA Org, Inc
3209 Charlesgate Ave SW
Wyoming
MI 49509
Tel: +1-(231) 360-6830
www.pandoraorg.net/

Solve ME/CFS Initiative (formerly The CFIDS Association of America)
This organisation has a great monthly e-newsletter *Research 1st*, as well as a print publication, the *Chronicle*, which comes out three times a year. Both publications contain articles on research developments, public policy and media reports, personal stories and a wealth of information vital to people living with CFS. Archived issues are available on the website in an easy-to-read digital publishing format. The organisation also offers a free webinar series and has a vibrant social media community, where patients can stay connected and share information with one another.

350 N Glendale Avenue
Suite B #368
Glendale, CA 91206
+1-704-364-0016
SolveCFS@SolveCFS.org
http://solvecfs.org/

The International Association for CFS/ME (IACFS/ME)
The IACFS/ME is a non-profit international organisation geared towards the professional community which promotes and coordinates the exchange of ideas related to CFS, ME and fibromyalgia (FM) research, patient care and treatment. The IACFS/ME publishes a peer review online journal, the *Bulletin of the IACFS/ME*. The IACFS/ME holds major international conferences which are attended by Dr Perrin, and many of the leading scientists and doctors in the field of ME/CFS, FMS and related illnesses.
27 N Wacker Drive Suite 416
Chicago
IL 60606
Tel:+1-(847) 258-7248
Admin@iacfsme.org
www.iacfsme.org/

OTHER COUNTRIES

ME/CFS is universal and there are dozens of countries which also have ME/CFS national support groups for patients. They can usually be found by searching on the internet. Alas, there are many more countries where the sufferer does not have any official organisation that recognises the existence of the disease. Hopefully, this book can be used to help lobby the relevant authorities in showing that ME/CFS is a real physical entity and should be taken more seriously.

PROFESSIONAL ORGANISATIONS

OSTEOPATHY

UK

General Osteopathic Council
176 Tower Bridge Road
London, SE1 3LU
Tel: +44 (0) 207 357 6655
info@osteopathy.org.uk

Australia

Osteopathy Australia
Postal Address:
PO Box 5044
Chatswood West NSW 1515
Tel: (Toll Free) 1800 467 836 Tel: 02 9410 0099
info@osteopathy.org.au

Ireland

Osteopathic Council of Ireland
Gray Office Park
Galway Retail Park,
Headford Road,
Galway
H91 WC1P
info@osteopathy.ie*
Tel: +353(0)1 6768819

Canada

Canadian Osteopathic Association
McKenzie Professional Centre
209 - 1595 McKenzie Avenue
Victoria, British Columbia

V8N 1A4
Tel: +1-250-595-7772
www.osteopathic.ca
osteopathic.ca@gmail.com

USA

American Osteopathic Association
The AOA also provides health information to patients and media interested in osteopathic medicine.
142 E Ontario St
Chicago
IL 60611-2864
Tel: +1-888-626-9262
www.osteopathic.org

Chiropractic

UK

General Chiropractic Council
Park House
186 Kennington Park Rd
London
SE11 4BT
UK
Tel: +44 (0) 20 7713 5155
enquiries@gcc-uk.org

Australia

Australian Chiropractors Association
Level 1 / 75 George Street
Parramatta
NSW 2150
PO Box 255, Parramatta NSW 2124
Tel: Toll free - 1800 075 003; Tel: +612 8844 0400

Canada

Canadian Chiropractic Association
186 Spadina Ave. Suite 6
Toronto
ON M5T 3B2
Tel: +1 (416) 585-7902; Toll-free: 1-877-222-9303
info@chiropractic.ca; membership@chiropractic.ca

Ireland

Chiropractic Association of Ireland
39 Clonard StreetBalbriggan
Co Dublin
K32 W729
Tel: +353 87 392 4275
caiadmin@chiropractic.ie

USA

The American Chiropractic Association
1701 Clarendon Blvd., Suite 200
Arlington
VA 22209
Tel: +1-703-276-8800
memberinfo@acatoday.org

Physiotherapy

UK

The Chartered Society of Physiotherapy
14 Bedford Row
London
WC1R 4ED
Tel: +44 (0)20 7306 6666
enquiries@csp.org.uk

Australia

Australian Physiotherapy Association
Level 1, 1175 Toorak Road
Camberwell
VIC 3124
PO Box 437 Hawthorn BC VIC 3122
Tel: 1300 306 622 (within Australia); (+61 3) 9092 0888 (international calls)

Canada

Canadian Physiotherapy Association
955 Green Valley Crescent, Suite 270
Ottawa, Ontario
K2C 3V4
Tel: +1 (613) 564-5454; (800) 387-8679
information@physiotherapy.ca

Ireland

Irish Society of Chartered Physiotherapists
Royal College of Surgeons in Ireland
St Stephen's Green
Dublin 2
D02 H903
Tel: +353 1 402 21 48
info@iscp.ie

USA

The American Physical Therapy Association
111North Fairfax Street
Alexandria
Virginia
22314-1488
Tel: +1-800-999-2782
memberservices@apta.org

Further reading

Bannister Sir R, Mathias C (eds). 2001. *Autonomic Failure* 4th Edition. Oxford Medical (OUP), Oxford, UK.

Bonica J. 1990. *The Management of Pain* 2nd Edition. Lea Febiger, Philadelphia, US.

Chikly B. 2011. *Silent Waves Theory and Practice of Lymph Drainage Therapy*. 2nd Edition . International Health and Healing Publishing.

Drake RL, Vogl AW, Mitchell AWM (Eds). 2019. *Grays Anatomy for Students*. Elsevier, Edinburgh, UK.

Gershon MD. 2020. *The Second Brain: The Scientific Basis of Gut Instinct.,* Harper Perennial, New York, US.

Goldstein JA. 1996. *Betrayal by the Brain: Neurological Basis of Chronic Fatigue Syndrome, Fibromyalgia Syndrome and Related Neural Network Disorders*. Routledge Publishers (Sage).

Greenhalgh S, Selfe J. 2019. *Red Flags and Blue Lights: Managing Serious Spinal Pathology* 2nd edition. Elsevier.

Hall JE, Hall ME. 2020. *Guyton and Hall's Textbook of Medical Physiology* 14th Edition. Elsevier.

Harris R. 2012 *The Reality Slap: How to find fulfilment when it hurts*. Robinson. US

Harry GJ, Tilson HA. 2016. *Neurotoxicology*. CRC Press, London, UK.

Hartman L. 1997. *Handbook of Osteopathic Technique*. 3rd edition. Springer, UK.

Kinmonth JB. 1982. *The Lymphatics*, 2nd Edition. Edward Arnold, London, UK.

Liem T. 2009 (Eng Lang ed) *Cranial Osteopathy: A practical textbook*. Eastland Press, Seattle Washington.

Lewis T. 1920. *The Soldier's Heart and the Effort Syndrome.* Paul B. Hober, New York, US.

Miller JB. 2002. Intradermal provocative-neutralizing food testing and subcutaneous food extract injection therapy. In: *Food Allergy and Intolerance.* 2nd edition. Brostoff J and Challacombe SJ (eds.). WB Saunders, London, UK.

Myhill S. 2018. *Diagnosis and Treatment of Chronic Fatigue Syndrome and Myalgic Encephalitis.* 2nd edition. Hammersmith Health Books Limited: London, UK. (US edition: Chelsea Green)

Pemberton S, Berry C (Eds). 2009 *Fighting Fatigue: a practical guide to managing the symptoms of ME/CFS.* Hammersmith Health Books, London, UK.

Richards J. 2008. *Biomechanics in Clinic and Research: An interactive teaching and learning course.* Churchil Livingstone, London, UK.

Rogers S. 1990. *Tired or Toxic?*: Syracuse, New York, US.

Seffinger MA (Executive Ed). 2018. *Foundations of Osteopathic Medicine* 4th edition, Wolters Kluwer.

Still AT. 1899. *Philosophy of Osteopathy,* Published by the Author, Kirksville, Mo, USA.

Still AT. 1902. *The Philosophy and Mechanical Principles of Osteopathy,* Hudson-Kimberly, Kansas City, Mo, USA.

Sutherland WG. 1990. *Teachings in the Science of Osteopathy,* Wales AL. (ed). Sutherland Cranial Teaching Foundation, Ft Worth, Texas, USA.

Upledger JE, Vredevoogd JD. 1983. *Cranio-Sacral Therapy.* Eastland Press, Chicago, USA.

Webster GV. 1928. *Sage Sayings of Still.* Wetzel Publishing Co, London, UK.

References

Chapter 1: The basics – how the Perrin Technique works

1. Schwalbe G. Die Arachnoidairaum ein Lymphraum und sein Zusammenhang mit den Perichorioidairaum. *Zbl med Wiss Zentralblatt fur die medizinschen Wissenschaften* 1869; 7: 465–467.

2. Kida S, Pantazis A, Weller RO. CSF drains directly from the subarachnoid space into nasal lymphatics in the rat: anatomy, histology and immunological significance. *Neuropathology and Applied Neurobiology* 1993; 19: 480–488.

3. Johnston M, Zakharov A, Papaiconomou C, Salmasi G, Armstrong D. Evidence of connections between cerebrospinal fluid and nasal lymphatic vessels in humans, non-human primates and other mammalian species. *Cerebrospinal Fluid Res* 2004; 1: 2.

4. Miura M, Kato S, Von Ludinghausen M. Lymphatic drainage of the cerebrospinal fluid from monkey spinal meninges with special reference to the distribution of epidural lymphatics. *Arch Histol Cytol* 1998; 61: 277–286.

5. Bozanovic SR, Mollanji R, Johnston MG. Spinal and cranial contributions to total cerebrospinal fluid transport. *American Journal of Physiology* 2001; 281(3–2): R909–R916.

6. Boulton M, Flessner M, Armstrong D, Hay J, Johnston M. Determination of volumetric cerebrospinal fluid absorption into extracranial lymphatics in sheep. *American Journal of Physiology* 1998; 274: 1(2): R88–R96.

7. Bradbury MWB, Cole DF. The role of the lymphatic system in drainage of

cerebrospinal fluid and aqueous humour. *Journal of Physiology* 1980; 299: 353–365.

8. Mokri B, Aksamit AJ, Atkinson JL. Paradoxical postural headaches in cerebrospinal fluid leaks. *Cephalalgia* 2004; 24(10): 883.

9. Czerniaswska A. Experimental investigations on the penetration of 198Au from nasal mucous membrane into cerebrospinal fluids. *ACTA Otolaryngologica* 1970; 70: 58–61.

10. Silver I, Li B, Szalai J, Johnston M. Relationship between intracranial pressure and cervical lymphatic pressure and flow rates in sheep, *American Journal. of Physiology* 1999; 277(6–2): R1712–R1717.

11. Jones HC, Lopman BA. The relation between CSF pressure and ventricular dilatation in hydrocephalic HTx rats. *European Journal of Pediatric Surgery* 1998; 8(S1): 55–58.

12. Cserr HF, Knopf PM. Cervical lymphatics, the blood-brain barrier and immunoreactivity of the brain: a new view. *Immunology Today* 1992; 13: 507–512.

13. McComb JG, Davson H, Hyman S, Weiss MH. Cerebrospinal fluid drainage as influenced by ventricular pressure in the rabbit. *Journal of Neurosurgery* 1982; 56: 790–797.

14. Knopf PM, Cserr HF. Physiology and immunology of lymphatic drainage of interstitial and cerebrospinal fluid from the brain. *Neuropathology and applied Neurobiology* 1995; 21: 175–180.

15. Koh L, Zakharov A, Johnston M. Integration of the subarachnoid space and lymphatics: Is it time to embrace a new concept of cerebrospinal fluid absorption? *Cerebrospinal Fluid Research* 2005; 2: 6.

16. Mascagni P, Bellini GB. *Istoria Completa Dei Vasi Linfatici.* Vol. II. Florence: Presso Eusebio Pacini e Figlio; 1816.

17. Iliff J, Wang M, Liao Y, Plogg B, Peng W, Gunderson GA, Benveniste H, Vates E, Deane R, Goldman SA, Nagelhus EA, Nedergaard M. A paravascular pathway facilitates CSF flow through the brain parenchyma and the clearance of interstitial solutes, including amyloid beta. *Sci Transl Med* 2012; 4 (147): 147ra111.

18. Xie L, Kang H, Xu Q, Chen MJ, Liao Y, Thiyagarajan M, O'Donnell J, Christensen DJ, Nicholson C, Iliff JJ, Takano T, Deane R, Nedergaard M. Sleep drives metabolite clearance from the adult brain. *Science* 2013; 342: 373–377.

19. Louveau A, Smirnov I, Keyes TJ, Eccles JD, Rouhani SJ, Peske JD, Derecki NC, Castle D, Mandell JW, Lee KS, Harris TH, Kipnis J. Structural and functional features of central nervous system lymphatic vessels. *Nature* 2015. doi: 10.1038/nature14432

20. Aspenlund A, Antila A, Proulx ST, Karlson TV, Karaman S, Detmar M, Wiig H, Alitalo K. A dural lymphatic vascular system that drains brain interstitial fluid and macromolecules. *Journal of Experimental Medicine* 2015; 212 (7): 991–999. doi:10.1084/jem.20142290

21. Absinta M, Ha S-K, Nair G, Sati P, Luciano NJ, Palisoc M, Louveau A, Zaghloul KA, Pittaluga S. Human and nonhuman primate meninges harbor lymphatic vessels that can be visualized noninvasively by MRI. *eLife* 2017; 6: e29738.

22. Bell GH, Emslie-Smith D, Paterson CR. *Textbook of Physiology.* 10th edn. Edinburgh: Churchill Livingstone; 1980: 343.

23. Chikly B. *Silent Waves: Theory and Practice of Lymph drainage Therapy.* 2nd edn (revised). Scotsdale, Arizona: IHH Publishing; 2011.

24. Kinmonth JB. *The Lymphatics.* 2nd edn. London: Edward Arnold, London; 1982: 80.

25. Kinmonth JB. Some aspects of cardiovascular surgery. *J. Royal College of Surgery. Edinb* 1960; 5: 287–297.

26. Kinmonth JB, Sharpey-Schafer EP. Manometry of human thoracic duct. *J Physiol* 1959; 177: 41.

27. Browse NL. Response of lymphatics to sympathetic nerve stimulation. *J Physiol* 1968; 19: 25.

28. Davson H, Segal MB. *Physiology of the CSF and Blood-Brain Barriers.* New York: CRC Press; 1996.

29. Bingham EM, Hopkins D, Smith D, Pernet A, Hallett W, Reed L, Marsden PK, Amiel SA. The role of insulin in human brain glucose metabolism: an 18 fleurodeoxyglucose positron emission tomography study. *Diabetes* 2002; 51(12): 3384–90.

30. Obici S, Feng Z, Karkanias G, Baskin DG, Rossetti L. Decreasing hypothalamic insulin receptors causes hyperphagia and insulin resistance in rats. *Nature Neuroscience* 2002; 5: 566–572.

31. Rogers SA. *Tired or Toxic: A Blueprint for Health.* Syracuse, New York: Prestige Publishing; 1990.

32. Lopachin RM, Aschner M. Glial-neuronal interactions: relevance to neurotoxic mechanisms. *Toxicology and Applied Pharmacology* 1993; 118: 141–158.

33. Iacono RF, Berria MI, Lascono EF. A triple staining procedure to evaluate phagocitic role of differentiated astrocytes. *Journal of Neuroscience Methods* 1991; 139: 225–230.

34. Morganti-Kossman MC, Kossman T, Wahl SM. Cytokines and neuropathology. *Trends in Pharmaceutical Sciences* 1992; 13: 286–291.

35. Lindholm D, Castren E, Kiefer R, Zafra F, Thoenen H. Transforming growth factor-B1 in the rat brain; increase after injury and inhibition of astrocyte proliferation. *Journal of Cell Biology* 1992; 117: 395–400.

36. Sawada M, Suzumura A, Ohno K, Marunouchi T. Regulation of astrocyte proliferation by prostaglandin E2 and the a-subtype of protein kinase C. *Brain Research* 1993; 613: 67–73.

37. Wei Z. Neurotoxicology of the brain barrier system: new implications. *J. Toxicol Clin Toxicol*. 2001; 39(7): 711–719.

38. Montaya JG, Holmes TH, Anderson JN, Maecker HT, Rosenberg-Hasson Y, Valencia IJ, Chu L, Younger JW, Tato CM, Davis MM. Cytokine signature associated with disease severity in chronic fatigue syndrome patients. *Proc Natl Acad Sci*. 2017; 114(34): E7150–E7158. doi: 10.1073/pnas.1710519114

39. Bakker EN, Arbel-Ornath M, Aldea R, Bedussi B, Morris AW, Weller RO, Carare RO. Lymphatic clearance of the brain: perivascular, paravascular and significance for neurodegenerative diseases. *Cell Mol Neurobiol*. 2016; 36(2): 181–194.

40. Barkhof F. Enlarged Virchow-Robin spaces: do they matter? *Journal of Neurology, Neurosurgery & Psychiatry* 2004; 75: 1516–1517.

41. Perrin RN. Chronic fatigue syndrome: a review from the biomechanical perspective. *British Osteopathic Journal* 1993; 11: 15–23.

42. Perrin RN, Edwards J, Hartley P. An evaluation of the effectiveness of osteopathic treatment on symptoms associated with myalgic encephalomyelitis: a preliminary report. *Journal of Medical Engineering and Technology* 1998; 22(1): 1–13.

43. Perrin RN. *The Involvement of Cerebrospinal Fluid and Lymphatic Drainage in Chronic Fatigue Syndrome/ME* (PhD Thesis). University of Salford, UK. 2005.

44. Perrin RN. Lymphatic drainage of the neuraxis and the CRI: a hypothetical model. *Journal of the American Osteopathic Association* 2007; 107(06): 218–224.

Chapter 2: ME/CFS – what it is

1. Craig AD, Bushnell MC, Zhang ET, Blomqvist A. A thalamic nucleus specific for pain and temperature sensation. *Nature* 1994; 372(6508): 770–773.
2. Pall M. Elevated nitric oxide/peroxynitrite theory of multiple chemical sensitivity: central role of N-methyl-D-aspartate receptors in the sensitivity mechanisms. *Environmental Health Perspectives* 2003. doi: org/10.1289/ehp.5935
3. Littlejohn G, Guymer E. Modulation of NMDA receptor activity in fibromyalgia. *Biomedicines* 2017; 5(2): 15. doi: 10.3390/biomedicines5020015
4. Lui H, Mantyh PW, Basbaum AI. NMDA-receptor regulation of substance P release from primary afferent nociceptors. *Nature* 1997; 386(6626): 721–724.
5. Chaudhuri A, Condon BR, Gow JW, Brennan D, Hadley DM. Proton magnetic resonance spectroscopy of basal ganglia in chronic fatigue syndrome. *Neuroreport* 2003; 14(2): 225–228.
6. Ocon AJ. Caught in the thickness of brain fog: exploring the cognitive symptoms of chronic fatigue syndrome. *Frontiers in Physiology* 2013; 4: 63.
7. Eidelman D. Chronic fatigue syndrome – medical fact or artefact. *Medical Hypotheses* 2003; 60: 840–842.
8. Bell DS. *The disease of a thousand names: CFIDS – chronic fatigue/immune dysfunction syndrome.* Lyndonville, NY: Pollard Publications; 1991.
9. Ramsay AM, O'Sullivan E. Encephalomyelitis simulating poliomyelitis. *Lancet* 1956; 270(6926): 761–764.
10. Hutchinson A, Pinching L, Chambers T, Waterman J, Wayne N (eds). *A Report of the CFS/ME Working Group to the Chief Medical Officer.* 2002.
11. Fukuda K, Straus SE, Hickie I, Sharpe MC, Dobbins JG, Komaroff A. The chronic fatigue syndrome: a comprehensive approach to its definition and study. *Annals of Internal Medicine* 1994; 121(12): 953–959.
12. Sharpe M, Archard L, Banatvala J. A report: chronic fatigue syndrome: guidelines for research. *J R Soc Med* 1991; 84: 118–121.

13. Carruthers BM. Definitions and aetiology of myalgic encephalomyelitis (ME): how the Canadian consensus clinical definition of ME works. *J Clin Pathol* 2007; 60(2): 117–119.

14. Da Costa JM. A clinical study of a form of functional cardiac disorder and its consequences. *American Journal of Medical Science* 1871; 61: 17–52.

15. Lewis T. *The Soldiers Heart and the Effort Syndrome.* New York: Paul B Hober; 1920.

16. Wesseley S, Chalder T, Hiersch S, Wallace P, Wright D. The prevalence and morbidity of chronic fatigue and chronic fatigue syndrome: a prospective primary care study. *Am J Public Health* 1997; 87: 1449–1455.

17. Van Houdenhove B, Onghena P, Neerinckx E, Hellin J. Does high 'action-proneness' make people more vulnerable to CFS? A controlled psychometric study. *J Psychosom Res* 1995; 39(5): 633–640.

18. Silver A, Haeney M, Vijayadurai P, Wilks D, Pattrick M, Main CJ. The role of fear of physical movement and activity in chronic fatigue syndrome. *J Psychosom Res* 2002; 52(6): 485–493.

19. Metzger FA, Denney DR. Perception of cognitive performance in patients with chronic fatigue syndrome. *Ann Behav Med* 2002; 24(2): 106–112.

20. Fisher L, Chalder T. Childhood experiences of illness and parenting in adults with chronic fatigue syndrome. *Journal of Psychosomatic Research* 2003; 54(5): 439–443.

21. Carruthers BM, van de Sande MI, De Meirleir KL et al. Myalgic encephalomyelitis: international consensus criteria. *J Intern Med* 2011; 270(4): 327–338. doi: 10.1111/j.1365-2796.2011.02428.x

22. Clayton EW (Chair) et al. Beyond myalgic encephalomyelitis/chronic fatigue syndrome: redefining an illness. Committee on the Diagnostic Criteria for Myalgic Encephalomyelitis/Chronic Fatigue Syndrome; Board on the Health of Select Populations; *Institute of Medicine.* Washington DC: National Academies Press; 2014.

23. Stevens S, Snell C, Stevens J, Keller B, VanNess JM. Cardiopulmonary exercise test methodology for assessing exertion intolerance in myalgic encephalomyelitis/chronic fatigue syndrome. *Front Pediatr* 2018; 6: 242.

24. Van Ness JM, Snell CR, Stevens SR. Diminished cardiopulmonary capacity during post-exertional malaise. *J Chronic Fatigue Syndr* 2007; 14: 77–85.

25. Van Oosterwijck J, Nijs J, Meeus M, Lefever I, Huybrechts L, et al. Pain

inhibition and postexertional malaise in myalgic encephalomyelitis/chronic fatigue syndrome; an experimental study. *J Intern Med* 2010; 268: 265–278.

26. McCrone P, Darbishire L, Ridsdale L, Seed P. The economic cost of chronic fatigue and chronic fatigue syndrome in UK primary care. *Psychol Med* 2003; 33(2): 197–201.

27. Bierl C, Nisenbaum R, Hoaglin DC, Randall B, Jones AB, Unger ER, Reeves WC. Regional distribution of fatiguing illnesses in the United States: a pilot study. *Popul Health Metr* 2004; 2: 1.

28. Pinching AJ. AIDS and CFS/ME: a tale of two syndromes. *Clin Med* 2003; 3(2): 188.

29. Naschitz JE, Sabo E, Dreyfuss D, Yeshurun D, Rosner I. The head-up tilt test in the diagnosis and management of chronic fatigue syndrome. *Isr Med Assoc J* 2003; 5(11): 807–811.

30. Lloyd AR, Broughton C, Dwyer J, Wakefield D. What is myalgic encephalomyelitis? *Lancet* 1988; 1(8597): 1286–1287.

31. Gershon S, Shaw FH. Psychiatric sequelae of chronic exposure to organophosphorus insecticides. *Lancet* 1961; 1: 1371–1374.

32. Dunstan RH Donohoe M, Taylor W, Roberts TK, Murdoch RN, Watkins JA, McGregor NR. A preliminary investigation of chlorinated hydrocarbons and chronic fatigue syndrome. *Medical Journal of Australia* 1995; 163(6): 294–297.

33. Tahmaz N, Soutar A, Cherrie JW. Chronic fatigue and organophosphate pesticides in sheep farming: a retrospective study amongst people reporting to a UK pharmacovigilance scheme. *Ann Occup Hyg* 2003; 47(4): 261–267.

34. Rogers S. *Tired or Toxic*. Syracuse, New York: Prestige Publishing; 1990.

35. Fiedler N, Kipen M, DeLuca J, Kelly-McNeil K, Natelson B. A controlled comparison of multiple chemical sensitivities and chronic fatigue syndrome. *Psychosomatic Medicine* 1996; 58: 38–49.

36. Buchwald D, Garrity D. Comparison of patients with chronic fatigue syndrome, fibromyalgia and multiple chemical sensitivities. *Archive of Internal Medicine* 1994; 154: 2049–2053.

37. Nawab SS, Miller CS, Dale JK, Greenberg BD, Friedman TC, Chrousos GP, Straus SE, Rosenthal NE. Self-reported sensitivity to chemical exposures in five clinical populations and healthy controls. *Psychiatry Research* 2000; 95(1): 67–74.

38. Hickie I, Lloyd A, Wakefield D. Immunological and psychological dysfunction in patients receiving immunotherapy for chronic fatigue syndrome. *Australia & New Zealand Journal of Psychiatry* 1992; 26(2): 249–256.

39. Kerr JR, Christian P, Hodgetts A et al. Current research priorities in chronic fatigue syndrome / myalgic encephalomyelitis (CFS/ME): disease mechanisms, a diagnostic test and specific treatments. *J Clin Pathol* 2007; 60(2): 113–116.

40. Harvey WT. A flight surgeon's personal view of an emerging illness. *Aviat Space Environ Med* 1989; 60(12): 1119–1201.

41. Simpson LO. Non-discocytic erythrocytes in myalgic encephalomyelitis. *NZ Med J* 1989; 102: 126–127.

42. Spurgin M. The role of blood cell morphology in the pathogenesis of ME/CFIDS. *The CFIDS Chronicle* 1995; 55–58.

43. Puri BK, Holmes J, Hamilton G. Eicosapentaenoic acid-rich essential fatty acid supplementation in chronic fatigue syndrome associated with symptom remission and structural brain changes. *Int J Clin Pract* 2004; 58(3): 297–299.

44. Harris WS. The omega-3 index: clinical utility for therapeutic intervention. *Cur Cardiol Rep* 2010; 12(6): 503–508.

45. Hokama Y, Uto GA, Palafox NA, Enlander D, Jordan E, Cocchetto A. Chronic phase lipids in sera of chronic fatigue syndrome, chronic ciguatera fish poisoning (CCFP), hepatitis B, and cancer with antigenic epitope resembling ciguatoxin, as assessed with Mab-CTX. *J Clin Lab Anal* 2003; 17(4): 132–139.

46. Smith S, Sullivan K. Examining the influence of biological and psychological factors on cognitive performance in chronic fatigue syndrome: a randomized, double-blind, placebo-controlled, crossover study. *International Journal of Behavioral Medicine* 2003; 10 (2): 162–173.

47. Hotopf A, David A, Hull L, Ismail K, Unwin C, Wessley S. Role of vaccinations as risk factors for ill health in veterans of the Gulf War: cross sectional study. *Br Med J* 2000; 320: 1363–1367.

48. Shaheen S. Shots in the desert and Gulf War Syndrome. *Br Med J* 2000; 320: 1351–1352.

49. Gowers W. Lumbago: its lessons and analogues. *Br Med J* 1904; 1: 117–121.

50. Wolfe F et al. The American College of Rheumatology preliminary diagnostic criteria for fibromyalgia and measurement of symptom severity. *Arthritis Care Res* 2010; 62(5): 600–610.
51. Di Franco M, Iannuccelli C, Valesini G. Neuroendocrine immunology of fibromyalgia. *Ann N Y Acad Sci* 2010; 1193: 84–90.
52. Clauw DJ, Arnold LM, McCarberg BH. The science of fibromyalgia. *Mayo Clin Proc* 2011; 86: 907–911.
53. Arnold LM. The pathophysiology, diagnosis, and treatment of fibromyalgia. *Psychiatr Clin North Am* 2010; 33: 375–408.

Chapter 3: The role of the sympathetic nervous system

1. Da Costa JM. A clinical study of a form of functional cardiac disorder and its consequences. *American Journal of Medical Science* 1871; 61: 17–52.
2. Häuser W et al. Post-traumatic stress disorder in fibromyalgia syndrome: prevalence, temporal relationship between posttraumatic stress and fibromyalgia symptoms, and impact on clinical outcome. *Pain* 2013; 154(8): 1216–1223.
3. Pellegrino MJ. *Understanding post-traumatic fibromyalgia.* Columbus, OH: Anadem Inc; 1996.
4. Dale HH, Gaddum JH. Reactions of denervated voluntary muscle, and their bearing on the mode of action of parasympathetic and related nerves. *J Physiol* 1930; 70(2): 109–144.
5. Feldberg W, Gaddum JH. 1934. The chemical transmitter at synapses in a sympathetic ganglion. *J Physiol* 1934; 81(3): 305–319.
6. Xie L et al. Sleep drives metabolite clearance from the adult brain. *Science* 2013; 342: 373–377.
7. Fultz NE et al. Coupled electrophysiological, hemodynamic, and cerebrospinal fluid oscillations in human sleep. *Science* 2019; 366: 628–631.
8. Van Hoof E et al. Defining the occurrence and influence of alpha-delta sleep in chronic fatigue syndrome. *Am J Med Sci* 2007; 333(2): 78–84.
9. Jason LA, Zinn ML and Zinn MA. Myalgic encephalomyelitis: symptoms and biomarkers. *Curr Neuropharmacol* 2015; 13(5): 701–734.
10. T Lee H et al. The effect of body posture on brain glymphatic transport. *J Neurosci* 2015; 35(31): 11034–11044.

11. Person E et al. A novel sleep positioning device reduces gastroesophageal reflux: a randomized controlled trial. *J Clin Gastroenterol* 2015; 49(8): 655–659.

12. Light KC et al. Adrenergic dysregulation and pain with and without acute beta-blockade in women with fibromyalgia and temporomandibular disorder. *J Pain* 2009; 10(5): 542–52. doi: 10.1016/j.jpain.2008.12.006

13. Korr IM. The spinal cord as organizer of disease processes: the peripheral autonomic nervous system. *Journal of American Osteopathic Association* 1979; 79: 82–90.

14. Korr IM (ed.). *Sustained Sympatheticonia as a Factor in Disease: The Neurobiological Mechanism in Manipulative Therapy.* New York: Plenum; 1978; 229–268.

15. Korr IM. The sympathetic nervous system as mediator between the somatic and supportive process. *The Physiological Basis of Osteopathic Medicine* 1970; 21–38.

16. Korr IM, Denslow JS, Krems AD. Quantitative studies of chronic facilitation in human motoneuron pools. *American Journal of Physiology* 1947; 150: 229–238.

17. Korr IM, Wright HM, Chase JA. Cutaneous patterns of sympathetic activity in clinical abnormalities of the musculoskeletal system. *Journal of Neural Transmission* 1964; 25: 589–606.

18. Gasser. Properties of dorsal root undmedullated fibres on the two sides of the ganglion. *Journal of General Physiology* 1955; 38: 709–728.

19. Chao CH, Chen HJ, Wang HY, Li TC, Kao CH. Increased risk of organic erectile dysfunction in patients with chronic fatigue syndrome: a nationwide population-based cohort study. *Andrology* 2015; 3(4): 666–671.

20. Bannister R, Mathias C (eds). *Autonomic Failure.* 3rd edn. Oxford: Oxford Medical; 1993.

21. Vizi ES, Orso E, Osipenko ON, Hasko G, Elenkov IJ. Neurochemical, electrophysiological and immunocytochemical evidence for a noradrenergic link between the sympathetic nervous system and thymocytes. *Neuroscience* 1995; 68(4): 1263–1276.

22. Lewis T. *The Soldiers Heart and the Effort Syndrome.* New York: Paul B Hober; 1920.

23. Vladutiu GD, Natelson BH. Association of medically unexplained fatigue

with ACE insertion/deletion polymorphism in Gulf War veterans. *Muscle Nerve* 2004; 30(1): 38–43.

24. Albright F, Light K, Light A, Bateman L, Cannon-Albright LA. Evidence for a heritable predisposition to chronic fatigue syndrome. *BMC Neurol.* 2011; 11: 62.

25. Park DJ, Lee SS. New insights into the genetics of fibromyalgia. *Korean J Intern Med* 2017; 32(6): 984–995.

26. Noguchi H, Kaname T, Sekimoto T, Senba K, Nagata Y, Araki M, Abe M, Nakagata N, Ono T, Yamamura K, Araki K. Naso-maxillary deformity due to frontonasal expression of human transthyretin gene in transgenic mice. *Genes Cells* 2002; 7(10): 1087–1098.

27. Chatel M, Menault F, Pecker J. Arguments in favor of the genetic origin of malformed syringohydromyelic pictures. *Neurochirurgie* 1979; 25(3): 160–165.

28. Goldstein. *Chronic Fatigue Syndromes: The Limbic Hypothesis.* New York: The Haworth Medical Press; 1993.

29. McKeown-Eyssen G, Baines C, Cole DE, Riley N, Tyndale RF, Marshall L, Jazmaji V. Case-control study of genotypes in multiple chemical sensitivity: CYP2D6, NAT1, NAT2, PON1, PON2 and MTHFR. *Int J Epidemiol* 2004; 33(5): 971–8. doi: 10.1093/ije/dyh251.

30. Morris G, Maes M, Berk M, Puri BK. Myalgic encephalomyelitis or chronic fatigue syndrome: how could the illness develop? *Metabolic Brain Disease* 2019; 34(2): 385–415. doi.org/10.1007/s11011-019-0388-6

31. Ramsay AM, O'Sullivan E. Encephalomyelitis simulating poliomyelitis. *Lancet* 1956; 270(6926): 761–764.

32. Moldofsky H, Patcai J. Chronic widespread musculoskeletal pain, fatigue, depression and disordered sleep in chronic post-SARS syndrome; a case-controlled study. *BMC Neurol* 2011; 11(1): 37. doi: 10.1186/1471–2377-11-37

32a. Meinhardt J, Radke J, Dittmayer C, et al. Olfactory transmucosal SARS-CoV-2 invasion as a port of central nervous system entry in individuals with COVID-19. *Nat Neurosci* 30 November 2020. https://doi.org/10.1038/s41593-020-00758-5

33. Hotchin NA, Read R, Smith DG, Crawford DH. Active Epstein-Barr virus infection in post-viral fatigue syndrome. *J Infect* 1989; 18(2): 143–150.

34. Richards AJ. Epstein-Barr virus and chronic fatigue syndrome. *J Rheumatol* 1988; 15(10): 1595.

35. Jones JF. Epstein-Barr virus and the chronic fatigue syndrome: a short review. *Microbiol Sci* 1988; 5(12): 366–369.

36. Nairn C, Galbraith DN, Clements GB. Comparison of Coxsackie B neutralisation and enteroviral PCR in chronic fatigue patients. *J Med Virol* 1995; 46(4): 310–313.

37. Soto NE, Straus SE. Chronic fatigue syndrome and herpes viruses: the fading evidence. *Journal of the IHMF* 2000; 7(2): 46–50.

Chapter 4: The causes of ME/CFS

1. Georgiades E, Behan WM, Kilduff LP, Hadjicharalambous M, Mackie EE, Wilson J, Ward SA, Pitsiladis YP. Chronic fatigue syndrome: new evidence for a central fatigue disorder. *Clin Sci* 2003; 105(2): 213–218.

2. Lerner AM, Beqaj SH, Deeter RG, Dworkin HJ, Zervos M, Chang CH, Fitzgerald JT, Goldstein J, O'Neill W. A six-month trial of valacyclovir in the Epstein-Barr virus subset of chronic fatigue syndrome: improvement in left ventricular function. *Drugs Today* 2002; 38(8): 549–561.

3. Agut H, Aubin JT. A new virus: the human herpesvirus 6. *Rev Prat* 1994; 44(7): 871–874.

4. Blondel-Hill E, Shafran SD. Treatment of the chronic fatigue syndrome: a review and practical guide. *Drugs* 1993; 46(4): 639–651.

5. Demettre E, Bastide L, D'Haese A, De Smet K, De Meirleir K, Tiev KP, Englebienne P, Lebleu B. Ribonuclease L proteolysis in peripheral blood mononuclear cells of chronic fatigue syndrome patients. *J Biol Chem* 2002; 277(38): 35746–35751.

6. Snell CR, Vanness JM, Strayer DR, Stevens SR. Physical performance and prediction of 2-5A synthetase/Rnase L antiviral pathway activity in patients with chronic fatigue syndrome. *In Vivo* 2002; 16(2): 107–109.

7. Suhadolnik RJ, Peterson DL, O'Brien K, Cheney PR, Herst CV, Reichenbach NL. Biochemical evidence for a novel low molecular weight 2-5 A-dependent Rnase L in chronic fatigue syndrome. *J Interferon Cytokine Res* 1997; 17(7): 377–385.

8. Peterson D, Brenu EW, Gottschalk G, Ramos S, Nguyen T, Staines D, et al. Cytokines in the cerebrospinal fluids of patients with chronic fatigue syndrome/myalgic encephalomyelitis. *Mediat Inflamm* 2015; 2015: 929720. doi: 10.1155/2015/929720

9. Hornig M, Gottschalk CG, Eddy ML, Che X, Ukaigwe JE, Peterson DL, et al. Immune network analysis of cerebrospinal fluid in myalgic encephalomyelitis/chronic fatigue syndrome with atypical and classical presentations. *Transl Psychiatry* 2017; 7: e1080. doi: 10.1038/tp.2017.44

10. Pall ML, Satterlee JD. Elevated nitric oxide/peroxynitrite mechanism for the common etiology of multiple chemical sensitivity, chronic fatigue syndrome and posttraumatic stress disorder. *Ann NY Acad Sci* 2001; 933: 323–329.

11. Pall ML. Elevated, sustained peroxynitrite levels as the cause of chronic fatigue syndrome. *Med Hypotheses* 2000; 54(1): 115–125.

12. Stringer EA et al. Daily cytokine fluctuations, driven by leptin, are associated with fatigue severity in chronic fatigue syndrome: evidence of inflammatory pathology. *J Transl Med* 2013; 11: 93.

13. Montaya JG, Holmes TH et al. Cytokine signature associated with disease severity in chronic fatigue syndrome patients. *Proc Natl Acad Sci* 2017; 114(34): E7150–E7158. doi: 10.1073/pnas.1710519114.

14. Lazarus M et al. EP3 prostaglandin receptors in the median preoptic nucleus are critical for fever responses. *Nat Neurosci* 2007; 10(9): 1131–1133.

15. Wakefield AJ, Puleston JM, Montgomery SM, Anthony A, O'Leary JJ, Murch SH. Review article: the concept of entero-colonic encephalopathy, autism and opioid receptor ligands. *Alimentary Pharmacology & Therapeutics* 2002; 16(4): 663–674.

16. Brierley SM, Hibberd TJ, Spencer NJ. Spinal afferent innervation of the colon and rectum. *Front Cell Neurosci* 2018; 12: 467.

17. Breit S et al., Vagus nerve as modulator of the brain–gut axis in psychiatric and inflammatory disorders. *Front Psychiatry* 2018; 9: 44. doi.org/10.3389/fpsyt.2018.00044

18. Holzer P. Neuropeptides, microbiota and behavior. *Int Rev Neurobiol* 2016; 131: 67–89.

19. Fung TC et al. Intestinal serotonin and fluoxetine exposure modulate bacterial colonization in the gut. *Nature Microbiology* 2019; 4(12): 1–10. doi: 10.1038/s41564-019-0540-4

20. Voigt RM et al. Circadian rhythm and the gut microbiome. *Int Rev Neurobiol* 2016; 131: 193–205.

21. Levine PH, Peterson D, McNamee FL, O'Brien K, Gridley G, Hagerty M, Brady J, Fears T, Atherton M, Hoover R. Does chronic fatigue syndrome

predispose to non-Hodgkin's lymphoma? *Cancer Res* 1992; 52(19): 5516s–5518s.

22. Eby NL, Grufferman S, Flannelly CM, Schold SC Jr, Vogel FS, Burger PC. Increasing incidence of primary brain lymphoma in the US. *Cancer* 1988; 62(11): 2461–2465.

23. Goldstein J. *Chronic Fatigue Syndromes: The Limbic Hypothesis.* New York: The Haworth Medical Press; 1993.

24. Schmaling KB, Lewis DH, Fiedelak JI, Mahurin R, Buchwald DS. Single-photon emission computerized tomography and neurocognitive function in patients with chronic fatigue syndrome. *Psychosom Med* 2003; 65(1): 129–136.

25. Iliff J, Wang M, Liao Y, Plogg B, Peng W, Gunderson GA, Benveniste H, Vates E, Deane R, Goldman SA, Nagelhus EA, Nedergaard M. A paravascular pathway facilitates CSF flow through the brain parenchyma and the clearance of interstitial solutes, including amyloid beta. *Sci Transl Med* 2012; 4(147): 147ra111.

26. Nairn C, Galbraith DN, Clements GB. Comparison of Coxsackie B neutralisation and enteroviral PCR in chronic fatigue patients. *J Med Virol* 1995; 46(4): 310–313.

27. Lerner AM, Beqaj SH, Deeter RG, Dworkin HJ, Zervos M, Chang CH, Fitzgerald JT, Goldstein J, O'Neill W. A six-month trial of valacyclovir in the Epstein-Barr virus subset of chronic fatigue syndrome: improvement in left ventricular function. *Drugs Today* 2002; 38(8): 549–561.

28. Straus SE, Dale JK, Tobi M, Lawley T, Preble O, Blaese RM, Hallahan C, Henle W. Acyclovir treatment of the CF: lack of efficacy in a placebo-controlled trial. *N Engl J Med* 1988; 319(26): 1692–1698.

29. Scott LV, Dinan TG. The neuroendocrinology of chronic fatigue syndrome: focus on the hypothalamic-pituitary-adrenal axis. *Funct Neurol* 1999; 14(1): 3–11.

30. Kuratsune H, Yamaguti K, Sawada M, Kodate S, Machii T, Kanakura Y, Kitani T. Dehydroepiandrosterone sulfate deficiency in chronic fatigue syndrome. *Int J Mol Med* 1998; 1(1): 143–146.

31. Knook L, Kavelaars A, Sinnema G, Kuis W, Heijnen CJ. High nocturnal melatonin in adolescents with chronic fatigue syndrome. *J Clin Endocrinol Metab* 2000; 85(10): 3690–3692.

,;,,,,,,,,

32. Shepherd C. *Living with ME, the Chronic Post-viral Syndrome.* London: Vermillion Press; 1998.
33. Allain TJ, Bearn JA, Coskeran P, Jones J, Checkley A, Butler J, Wessely S, Miell JP. Changes in growth hormone, insulin, insulin-like growth factors (IGFs), and IGF-binding protein-1 in chronic fatigue syndrome. *Biological Psychiatry* 1997; 41(5): 567–573.
34. Unger ER, Lin JS, Brimmer DJ, et al. CDC grand rounds: chronic fatigue syndrome- advancing research and clinical education. *MMWR Morb Mortal Wkly Rep* 2016; 65: 1434–1438.
35. Yunus MB. The role of gender in fibromyalgia syndrome. *Curr Rheumatol Rep* 2001; 3(2): 128–134.
36. Neuprez A, Crielaard JM. Fibromyalgia: state of the issue in 2017. *Rev Med Liege* 2017; 72(6): 288–294.
37. Natelson BH, Cheu J, Pareja J, Ellis SP, Policastro T, Findley TW. Randomized, double blind, controlled placebo-phase in trial of low dose phenelzine in the chronic fatigue syndrome. *Psychopharmacology* 1996; 124(3): 226–230.
38. Vercoulen JH. Swanink CM. Zitman FG. Vreden SG. Hoofs MP. Fennis JF. Galama JM. van der Meer JW. Bleijenberg G. Randomised, double-blind, placebo-controlled study of fluoxetine in chronic fatigue syndrome. *Lancet* 1996; 347(9005): 858–861.
39. Miller JB. Intradermal provocative-neutralizing food testing and subcutaneous food extract injection therapy. In: Brostoff J, Challacombe SJ (eds) *Food Allergy and Intolerance* London: Bailliere Tindall; 1987.
40. Fell P, Brostoff J. A single dose desensitization for summer hay fever. Results of a double-blind study. *Eur J Clin Pharmacol* 1990; 38(1): 77–79.
41. Pall ML. Elevated, sustained peroxynitrite levels as the cause of chronic fatigue syndrome. *Med Hypotheses* 2000; 54(1): 115–125.
42. Reichlin S. Neuroendocrine-immune interactions. *New England Journal of Medicine* 1993; 329(17): 1246–1253.
43. Harman D. Aging: a theory based on free radical and radiation chemistry. *Gerontol* 1956; 11(3): 298–300.
44. Kodama M, Kodama T, Murakami M. The value of the dehydroepiandrosterone-annexed vitamin C infusion treatment in the clinical control of chronic fatigue syndrome (CFS). II. Characterization of CFS

patients with special reference to their response to a new vitamin C infusion treatment. *In Vivo* 1996; 10(6): 585–596.

45. Thomas LD, Elinder CG,Tiselius HG, Wolk A, Akesson A. Ascorbic acid supplements and kidney stone incidence among men: a prospective study. *JAMA Intern Med* 2013; 173(5): 386–388.

46. Jiang K, Tang K, Liu H, Xu H, Ye Z, Chen Z. Ascorbic acid supplements and kidney stones incidence among men and women: a systematic review and meta-analysis. *Urol J* 2019; 216(2): 115–120.

47. Bohr C. Theoretische Behandlung der quantitativen Verhättnisse der Kohlensäurebindiung des Hämoglobins. *Centralblatt für Physiol* 1904; 24.

Chapter 5: Treatments for ME/CFS and FMS other than the Perrin Technique

1. Blythman J. *Swallow This: Serving Up the Food Industry's Darkest Secrets*. London: Fourth Estate; 2015.

2. Morris DH, Stare FJ. Unproven diet therapies in the treatment of CFS. *Archives of Family Medicine* 1993; 2(2): 181–186.

3. Myhill S, Robinson C. *The PK Cookbook: go paleoketogenic and get the best of both worlds*. Hammersmith Books, 2018.

4. Crook WG. Candida colonization and allergic phenomena. *Hosp Pract* 1994; 19(9): 20.

5. Renfro L, Feder HM, Lane TJ, Manu P, Matthews DA. Yeast connection among 100 patients with chronic fatigue syndrome. *American Journal of Medicine* 1989; 86: 165–168.

6. Girois SB, Chapuis F, Decullier E, Revol BG. Adverse effects of antifungal therapies in invasive fungal infections: review and meta-analysis. *Eur J Clin Microbiol Infect Dis* 2006; 25(2): 138–149.

7. Mulder SJ. Bacteria of food and human intestine are the most possible sources of the gad-trigger of type 1 diabetes. *Medical Hypotheses* 2005; 65(2): 308–311.

8. Krop JJ. Treatment and prophylaxis for patients suffering from environmental hypersensitivity disorder. *Folia Med Cracov* 1993; 34(1–4): 159–172.

9. Simpson JW. Diet and large intestinal disease in dogs and cats. *Journal of Nutrition* 1998; 128(12): 2717S–2722S.

10. Hasegawa M, Ohtomo M, Mita H, Akiyama K. Clinical aspects of patients with MCS – (from the standpoint of allergy). *Arerugi* 2005; 54(5): 478–484.

11. Bouziat R et al. Reovirus infection triggers inflammatory responses to dietary antigens and development of celiac disease. *Science* 2017; 356(6333): 44–50.

12. Heap LC, Peters TJ, Wessely S. Vitamin B status in patients with chronic fatigue syndrome. *Journal of the Royal Society of Medicine* 1999; 92(4): 183–185.

13. Myhill S. *Diagnosis and Treatment of Chronic Fatigue Syndrome and Myalgic Encephalitis: It's Mitochondria, Not Hypochondria.* 2nd edn. London: Hammersmith Press; 2017.

14. Castro-Marrero J et al. Does oral coenzyme Q10 plus NADH supplementation improve fatigue and biochemical parameters in chronic fatigue syndrome? *Antioxidants & Redox Signaling* 2014; 22: 8.

14a. Light KC, White AT, Tadler S, Iacob E, Light AR. Genetics and gene expression involving stress and distress pathways in fibromyalgia with and without comorbid chronic fatigue syndrome. *Pain Res Treat* 2012; 2012: 427869. doi: 10.1155/2012/427869

15. Werbach M. Nutritional strategies for treating chronic fatigue syndrome. *Alternative Medicine Review* 1998; 5: 93–108.

16. Cox IM, Campbell MJ, Dowson D. Red blood cell magnesium and chronic fatigue syndrome. *Lancet* 1991; 337(8744): 757–760.

17. Morris G, Maes M. Mitochondrial dysfunctions in myalgic encephalomyelitis/chronic fatigue syndrome explained by activated immuno-inflammatory, oxidative and nitrosative stress pathways. *Metab Brain Dis* 2014; 29(1): 19–36.

18. Porter NS et al. Alternative medical interventions used in the treatment and management of myalgic encephalomyelitis/chronic fatigue syndrome and fibromyalgia. *J Altern Complement Med* 2010; 16(3): 235–249.

19. Alraek T et al. Complementary and alternative medicine for patients with chronic fatigue syndrome: a systematic review. *BMC Complement Altern Med* 2011; 11: 87.

20. Myhill S, Booth NE, McLaren H. Chronic fatigue syndrome and mitochondrial dysfunction. *Int J Clin Exp Med* 2009; 2(1): 1–16.

21. Russell IJ et al. Treatment of fibromyalgia syndrome with Super Malic: a

randomized, double blind, placebo controlled, crossover pilot study. *J Rheumatol* 1995; 22(5): 953–958.

22. Fulgenzi A, Vietti D, Ferrero ME. Aluminium involvement in neurotoxicity. *BioMed Research International (Online)* 2014; Article ID 758323. doi.org/10.1155/2014/758323

23. Tan Z, et al. Removal of elemental mercury by bamboo charcoal impregnated with H2O2. *Fuel* 2011; 90(4): 1471–1475.

24. Regland B, Forsmark S, Halaouate L. Response to vitamin B12 and folic acid in myalgic encephalomyelitis and fibromyalgia. *PloS One* 2015; 10(4): e0124648.

25. Vanderpump MP, Lazarus, Franklyn JA et al. Iodine status of UK schoolgirls: a cross-sectional survey. *Lancet* 2011; 377(9782): 2007–2012.

26. Rowe P et al. Is neurally-mediated hypotension an unrecognised cause of chronic fatigue? *Lancet* 1995; 345: 623–624.

27. Castro-Marrero J et al. Low omega-3 index and polyunsaturated fatty acid status in patients with chronic fatigue syndrome/myalgic encephalomyelitis. *Prostaglandins, Leukotrienes and Essential Fatty Acids* 2018; 139: 20–24.

28. Puri BK, Counsell SJ, Zaman R, Main J, Collins AG, Hajnal JV, Davey NJ. Relative increase in choline in the occipital cortex in chronic fatigue syndrome. *Acta Psychiatr Scand* 2002; 106: 224–226.

29. Ren H et al. Omega-3 polyunsaturated fatty acids promote amyloid-β clearance from the brain through mediating the function of the glymphatic system. *FASEB* 2017; 31(1): 282–293.

30. Keshavarz M, Showraki A, Emamghoreishi M. Anticonvulscent effect of guifenesin against pentylenetetrazol-induced seizure in mice. *Iran J Med Sci* 2013; 38(2): 116–121.

31. Chia JKS. The role of enterovirus in chronic fatigue syndrome. *J Clin Path* 2005; 58(11): 1126–1132.

32. Roehr B. Researchers find no link between XMRV and chronic fatigue syndrome. *Br Med J* 2012; 345: e6337. doi:10.1136/bmj.e6337

33. Nagy-Szakal D. Fecal metagenomic profiles in subgroups of patients with myalgic encephalomyelitis/chronic fatigue syndrome. *Microbiome* 2017; 5: doi.org/10.1186/s40168-017-0261-y

34. Kenney MJ, Ganta CK. Autonomic nervous system and immune system interactions. *Compr Physiol* 2014; 4(3): 1177–1200.

35. Loebel M et al. Antibodies to ß adrenergic and muscarinic cholinergic receptors in patients with chronic fatigue syndrome. *Brain, Behavior and Immunity* 2016; 52: 32–39.

36. Fluge Ø et al. B-lymphocyte depletion in patients with myalgic encephalomyelitis/chronic fatigue syndrome: a randomized, double-blind, placebo-controlled trial. *Ann Intern Med* 2019. doi: 10.7326/M18-1451

37. Nguyen TC, Kiss JE, Goldman JR, Carcillo JA. The Role of Plasmapheresis in Critical Illness. *Crit Care Clin* 2012; 28(3): 453–468.

38. Tölle M, et al. Myalgic Encephalomyelitis/Chronic Fatigue Syndrome: Efficacy of Repeat Immunoadsorption. *J Clin Med* 2020; 9(8): 2443.

39. Scheibenbogen C, et al. Immunoadsorption to remove ß2 adrenergic receptor antibodies in Chronic Fatigue Syndrome ME/CFS. *PLoS One* 2018; 13(3): e0193672. doi: 10.1371/journal.pone.0193672

40. Younger J, Mackey S. Fibromyalgia symptoms are reduced by low-dose naltrexone: a pilot study. *Pain Med* 2009; 10(4): 663–672.

41. Metyas S, Chen CL, Yeter K, Solyman J, Arkfeld DG. Low dose naltrexone in the treatment of fibromyalgia. *Curr Rheumatol Rev* 2018; 14(2): 177–180.

42. Eisenstein TK. 2019 The Role of Opioid Receptors in Immune System Function Front. *Immunol* 20 December. doi.org/10.3389/fimmu.2019.02904

43. Mckay RJ, et al. Low dose naltrexone in ME/CFS and FM – the Vancouver experience. IACFS/ME Online conference August 21 2020.

44. Younger J, Parkitny L & Mclain D. The use of low-dose naltrexone (LDN) as a novel anti-inflammatory treatment for chronic pain. *Clin Rheumatol.* 2014; 33(4): 451–459.

45. Pizzorno J Jr, Murray M, Joiner-Bey M. *The Clinicians Handbook of Natural Medicine* 3rd edn. Edinburgh: Churchill Livingstone; 2016: 213–224.

46. Ven Murthy MR, Ranjekar PK, Ramassamy C, Deshpande M. Scientific basis for the use of Indian ayurvedic medicinal plants in the treatment of neurodegenerative disorders: ashwagandha. *Cent Nerv Syst Agents Med Chem* 2010; 10: 238–246.

47. Semalty A et al. Herbal drugs in chronic fatigue syndrome: an overview. *Swiss Journal of Integrative Medicine* 2012; 24: 155–168.

48. Carruthers BM, van de Sande MI, De Meirleir KL et al. Myalgic encephalomyelitis: international consensus criteria. *J Intern Med* 2011; 270: 327–338.

49. Jason L et al. The problems in defining post exertional malaise. *J Prev Interv Community* 2015; 43(1): 20–31. doi: 10.1080/10852352.2014.973239

50. Chu L. *Proceedings of the IAME/CFS conference, Fort Lauderdale;* 2016.

51. Friedberg F, Jason LA. Chronic fatigue syndrome and fibromyalgia: clinical assessment and treatment. *Journal of Clinical Psychology* 2001; 57(4): 433.

52. Fulcher KY, White PD. Randomised controlled trial of graded exercise in patients with the chronic fatigue syndrome. *British Medical Journal* 1997; 314: 1647–1652.

53. Paul L, Wood L, Behan WM, Maclaren WM. Demonstration of delayed recovery from fatiguing exercise in chronic fatigue syndrome. *European Journal of Neurology* 1999; 6(1): 63–69.

54. Crinnion W. Sauna as a valuable clinical tool for cardiovascular, autoimmune, toxicant-induced and other chronic health problems. *Alternative Medicine Review* 2011; 16(3): 215–225.

55. Soejima Y et al. Effects of Waon therapy on chronic fatigue syndrome: a pilot study. *Intern Med* 2015; 54(3): 333–338.

56. Lynch S, Seth R, Montgomery S. Antidepressant therapy in the chronic fatigue syndrome. *British Journal of General Practice* 1991; 41(349): 339–342.

57. Wilson A, Hickie I, Lloyd A, Wakefield D. The treatment of chronic fatigue syndrome: science and speculation. *American Journal of Medicine* 1994; 96(6): 544–550.

58. Klonoff DC. Chronic fatigue syndrome. *Clin Infect Dis* 1992; 15(5): 812–823.

59. Gaudiano BA. Cognitive-behavioral therapies: achievements and challenges. *Evid Based Ment Health* 2008; 11(1): 5–7.

60. Reid S, Chalder T, Cleare A, Hotopf M, Wessely S. Chronic fatigue syndrome. *British Medical Journal* 2000; 320(7230): 292–296.

61. Blenkiron P, Edwards R, Lynch S. Associations between perfectionism, mood, and fatigue in chronic fatigue syndrome: a pilot study. *J Nerv Ment Dis* 1997; 187(9): 566–570.

62. Sharpe M. Chronic fatigue syndrome. *Psychiatric Clinics of North America* 1996; 19(3): 549–573.

63. Sharpe M, Hawton K, Simkin S, Surawy C, Hackmann A, Klimes I, Peto T, Warrell D, Seagroatt V. Cognitive behaviour therapy for the chronic fatigue syndrome: a randomized controlled trial. *British Medical Journal* 1996; 312(7022): 22–26.

64. Deale A, Chalder T, Marks I, Wessely S. Cognitive behavioural therapy for chronic fatigue syndrome: a randomised controlled trial. *British Medical Journal* 1996; 312: 22–26.

65. Lloyd AR, Hickie I, Brockman A, Hickie C, Wilson A, Dwyer J, Wakefield D. Immunologic and psychologic therapy for patients with chronic fatigue syndrome: a double-blind, placebo-controlled trial. *American Journal of Medicine* 1993; 94(2): 197–203.

66. White PD et al. Comparison of adaptive pacing therapy, cognitive behaviour therapy, graded exercise therapy, and specialist medical care for chronic fatigue syndrome (PACE): a randomised trial. *Lancet* 2011; 377(9768): 823–836. doi: 10.1016/S0140–6736(11)60096–2

67. Jason LA. The PACE trial missteps on pacing and patient selection. *J Health Psychol* 2017; 22(9): 1141–1145. doi: 10.1177/1359105317695801

68. Wilshire C, et al. Rethinking the treatment of chronic fatigue syndrome – a reanalysis and evaluation of findings from a recent major trial on graded exercise and CBT. *BMC Psychology* 2018; 6: 6.

69. Jason L, Zinn ML, Zinn MA. Myalgic encephalomyelitis: symptoms and biomarkers. *Curr Neuropharmacol* 2015 Sep; 13(5): 701–734.

70. Bandler R, Grinder J. *The Structure of Magic. Vol 1: A Book about Language and Therapy* Palo Alto CA: Science and Behavior Books; 1975.

71. Iliff J, Wang M, Liao Y, Plogg B, Peng W, Gunderson GA, Benveniste H, Vates E, Deane R, Goldman SA, Nagelhus EA, Nedergaard M. A paravascular pathway facilitates CSF flow through the brain parenchyma and the clearance of interstitial solutes, including amyloid beta. *Sci Transl Med* 2012; 4(147): 147ra111.

72. Schechter D, Smith AP, Beck J, Roach J, Karim R, Azen S. Outcomes of a mind-body treatment program for chronic back pain with no distinct structural pathology – a case series of patients diagnosed and treated as tension myositis syndrome. *Alternative Therapies in Health and Medicine* 2007; 13(5): 26–35.

73. Xiang N, et al. The innate immune receptors TLR2/4 mediate repeated social defeat stress-induced social avoidance through prefrontal microglial activation. *Neuron* 2018. doi: 10.1016/j.neuron.2018.06.035

74. Gregg VH. Hypnosis in chronic fatigue syndrome. *Journal of the Royal Society of Medicine* 1997; 12: 682–683.

75. Fava GA, Ruini C. Development and characteristics of a well-being enhancing psychotherapeutic strategy: well-being therapy. *Journal of Behavior Therapy and Experimental Psychiatry* 2003; 34(1): 45–63.

76. Callahan RJ. *Five-minute phobia cure: Dr. Callahan's treatment for fears, phobias and self- sabotage.* Wilmington, DE: Enterprise Publishing; 1985.

77. Church, D. Clinical EFT as an evidence-based practice for the treatment of psychological and physiological conditions. *Psychology* 2013; 4: 645–654. doi:10.4236/psych.2013.48092

78. Shapiro F. Eye movement desensitization and reprocessing (EMDR): Evaluation of controlled PTSD research. *Journal of Behavior Therapy and Experimental Psychiatry* 1996; 27(3): 209–218.

79. Friedberg F. *Do-It-Yourself Eye Movement Techniques for Emotional Healing.* Oakland CA: New Harbinger Publications; 2001.

80. Friedberg F. Eye movement desensitization in fibromyalgia: a pilot study. *Complement Ther Nurs Midwifery* 2004; 10(4): 245–249.

81. Surawy C, Roberts J, and Silver A. The effect of mindfulness training on mood and measures of fatigue, activity, and quality of life in patients with chronic fatigue syndrome on a hospital waiting list: a series of exploratory studies. *Behavioural and Cognitive Psychotherapy* 2005; 33(1): 103–109.

82. Singleton O, Hölzel BK, Vangel M, Brach N, Carmody J, Lazar SW. Change in brainstem gray matter concentration following a mindfulness-based intervention is correlated with improvement in psychological well-being. *Front Hum Neurosci.* 2014; 8: 33.

83. Hughes LS et al. Acceptance and commitment therapy (ACT) for chronic pain: a systematic review and meta-analyses. *Clin. Journal of Pain* 2017; 33(6): 552–568.

84. Elvis AM, Ekta JS. Ozone therapy: a clinical review. *J Nat Sci Biol Med* 2011; 2(1): 66–70.

85. Mantle F, Tiran D. *Neural Therapy. A–Z of Complementary and Alternative Medicine: A guide for health professionals.* Edinburgh: Churchill Livingstone; 2009

86. Chevalier G et al. Earthing: health implications of reconnecting the human body to the Earth's surface electrons. *J Environ Public Health* 2012: 291541.

87. Hsu HH, Leung WH, Hu GC. Treatment of irritable bowel syndrome with a novel colonic irrigation system: a pilot study. *Tech Coloproctol* 2016; 20(8): 551-557.

88. Korr IM. The spinal cord as organizer of disease processes: the peripheral autonomic nervous system. Journal of American Osteopathic Association 1979; 79: 82–90.

89. Korr IM (ed.). *Sustained Sympatheticonia as a Factor in Disease: The Neurobiological Mechanism in Manipulative Therapy.* New York: Plenum; 1978; 229–268.

90. Korr IM. The sympathetic nervous system as mediator between the somatic and supportive process. *The Physiological Basis of Osteopathic Medicine* 1970; 21–38.

91. Korr IM, Denslow JS, Krems AD. Quantitative studies of chronic facilitation in human motor neuron pools. *American Journal of Physiology* 1947; 150: 229–238.

92. Korr IM, Wright HM, Chase JA. Cutaneous patterns of sympathetic activity in clinical abnormalities of the musculoskeletal system. *Journal of Neural Transmission* 1984; 25: 589–606.

93. Korr IM, Wright HM, Thomas PE. Effects of experimental and myofascial insults on cutaneous patterns of sympathetic activity in man. *Journal of Neural Transmission* 1962; 23(22): 330–355.

94. Korr IM, Wright HM, Thomas PE. Local and regional variations in cutaneous vasomotor tone of the human trunk. *Journal of Neural Transmission* 1960; 22(3): 34–52.

Chapter 6: Defining fatigue

1. 'Fatigue'. *Oxford English Dictionary.* 2nd edn, Volume V: 763.

2. Merton PA, Marsden CD, Morton HB. Is the human stretch reflex cortical rather than spinal? *Lancet* 1973; 1(7806): 759–761.

3. Perrin RN, Richards JD, Pentreath V, Percy DF. Muscle fatigue in ME/CFS and its response to a manual therapeutic approach: a pilot study. *International Journal of Osteopathic Medicine* 2011; 14: 96–105.

4. He J, Hollingsworth K, Newton J, Blamiria A. Cerebral vascular control is associate with skeletal muscle pH in chronic fatigue syndrome patients both at rest and during dynamic stimulation. *Neuroimage Clin* 2013; 2: 168–173.

5. Natelson BH, Vu D, Coplan J D, Mao X, Blate M, Kang G, Soto E, Kapusuz T, Shungu DC. Elevations of ventricular lactate levels occur in both chronic

fatigue syndrome and fibromyalgia. *Fatigue: Biomedicine, Health & Behavior* 2017; 5(1): 15–20.

6. Murrough JW, Mao X, Collins KA, Kelly C, Andrade G, Nestadt P, Levine SM, Mathew SJ, Shungu DC. Increased ventricular lactate in chronic fatigue syndrome measured by 1H MRS imaging at 3.0 T. II: comparison with major depressive disorder. *NMR in Biomedicine* 2010; 23(6): 643–650.

7. Glassford JAG. The neuroinflammatory etiopathology of myalgic encephalomyelitis/chronic fatigue syndrome (ME/CFS). *Front Physiol* 2017; 8: 88.

8. Chen W-W, Zhang X, Huang W-J. Role of neuroinflammation in neurodegenerative diseases (Review). *Molecular Medicine Reports* 2016; 13(4): 3391–3396.

9. Albrecht DS, Granziera C, Hooker JM, Loggia ML. In vivo imaging of human neuroinflammation. *ACS Chemical Neuroscience* 2016; 7(4): 470–483.

10. Morris G, Maes M. A neuroimmune model of myalgic encephalomyelitis/chronic fatigue syndrome. *Metabolic Brain Disease* 2013; 28(4): 523–540.

11. Pall M. Elevated nitric oxide/peroxynitrite theory of multiple chemical sensitivity: central role of N-methyl-D-aspartate receptors in the sensitivity mechanisms. *Environmental Health Perspectives* 2003; 111(12): 1461–1464. doi.org/10.1289/ehp.5935

12. Morris G, Berk M, Walder K, Maes M. Central pathways causing fatigue in neuro-inflammatory and autoimmune illnesses. *BMC Medicine* 2015; 13(1).

13. Gárate I, Garcia-Bueno B, Madrigal J, Caso JR, Alou L, Gomez-Lus ML, Micó JA, Leza JC. Stress-induced neuroinflammation: role of the Toll-like receptor-4 pathway. *Biological Psychiatry* 2013; 73(1): 32–43.

14. Liu JJ, Buisman-Pijlman F, Hutchinson MR. Toll-like receptor 4: innate immune regulator of neuroimmune and neuroendocrine interactions in stress and major depressive disorder. *Frontiers in Neuroscience* 2014; 8: 309.

15. Diaz JH. Hypothesis: angiotensin-converting enzyme inhibitors and angiotensin receptor blockers may increase the risk of severe COVID-19. *Journal of Travel Medicine* 2020. doi: 10.1093/jtm/taaa041

16. Simpson JB. The circumventricular organs and the central actions of angiotensin. *Neuroendocrinology* 1981; 32(4): 248–256.

17. Osterziel KJ, Hänlein D, Willenbrock R, Dietz R. Interaction between the

renin system and parasympathetic nervous system in heart failure. *Z Kardiol* 1993; 82(7): 406–410.

18. Yamawaki I, Tamaoki J, Yamauchi F, Konno K. Angiotensin II potentiates neurally mediated contraction of rabbit airway smooth muscle. *Respir Physiol* 1992; 89(2): 239–247.

19. Lazartigues E. Inflammation and neurogenic hypertension: A new role for the circumventricular organs? *Circ Res* 2010; 107(2): 166–167.

20. Üceyler N, Hauser W, Sommer C. Systemic review with meta-analysis: cytokines in fibromyalgia syndrome. *BMC Musculoskeltal Disorders* 2011; 12: 245–210. doi:1186/1471–2474-12-245

21. Albrecht PJ et al. Excessive peptidergic sensory innervation of cutaneous arteriole-venule shunts (AVS) in the palmar glabrous skin of fibromyalgia patients: implications for widespread deep tissue pain and fatigue. *Pain Med* 2013; 14(6): 895–915.

22. Naviaux RK et al. Metabolic features of chronic fatigue syndrome. *Proceedings of The National Academy of Sciences of The United State of America* 2016; 113(37): E5472–E5480.

23. Nagy-Szakal D et al. Insights into myalgic encephalomyelitis/chronic fatigue syndrome phenotypes through comprehensive metabolomics. *Sci Rep* 2018; 8(1): 10056.

24. Fukuda K, Straus SE, Hickie I, Sharpe MC, Dobbins JG, Komaroff A. The chronic fatigue syndrome: a comprehensive approach to its definition and study. International Chronic Fatigue Syndrome Study Group. *Annals of Internal Medicine* 1994; 121(12): 953–959.

25. Agarwal AK et al. Postural orthostatic tachycardia syndrome. *Postgrad Med J* 2007; 83: 478–480.

26. Jacob G, Biaggioni I. Idiopathic orthostatic intolerance and postural tachycardia syndromes. *Am J Med Sci* 1999; 317: 88–101.

27. Hoad A et al. Postural orthostatic tachycardia. *Quarterly Journal of Medicine* 2008; 101(12): 961–965.

28. Freeman R et al. Consensus statement on the definition of orthostatic hypotension, neurally mediated syncope and the postural tachycardia syndrome. *Auton Neurosci* 2011; 161: 46–48.

29. Low PA (ed.). Orthostatic intolerance. *National Dysautonomia Research Foundation Patient Conference; Minneapolis, Minnesota, USA;* 2000.

30. Medows MS, et al. The benefits of oral rehydration on orthostatic intolerance in children with postural tachycardia syndrome. *J Pediatr* 2019; 214: 96-102.

31. Beighton PH, Solomon L, Soskolne CL. Articular mobility in an African population. *Ann Rheum Dis* 1973; 32: 413–417.

32. Rowe PC et al. Orthostatic intolerance and chronic fatigue syndrome associated with Ehlers-Danlos syndrome. *J Pediatr* 1999; 135(4): 494–499.

33. Heffez DS. Is Chiari-I malformation associated with fibromyalgia? revisited. *Neurosurgery* 2011; 69(2): E507.

34. Hoh D. Spine, skull surgery may help many with CFIDS, FMS: Chiari-malformation or cervical stenosis may be common in CFIDS & Fibromyalgia. *The CFIDS Chronicle* 1999; 10–12.

35. Zhang L et al. The association of HLA-B27 and Klebsiella pneumoniae in ankylosing spondylitis: a systematic review. *Microbial Pathogenesis* 2018; 117: 49–54.

36. Higgins JNP, Pickard JD, Lever AML. Chronic fatigue syndrome and idiopathic intracranial hypertension: different manifestations of the same disorder of intracranial pressure? *Medical Hypothesis* 2017; 105: 6–9.

37. Higgins N, Pickard J, Lever A. Lumbar puncture, chronic fatigue syndrome and idiopathic intracranial hypertension: a cross-sectional study. *JRSM Short Rep.* 2013; 4(12): 2042533313507920.

38. Hulens M. et al. The link between idiopathic intracranial hypertension, fibromyalgia, and chronic fatigue syndrome: exploration of a shared pathophysiology *J. Pain Res.* 2018; 11: 3129–3140.

39. Molins CR, Ashton LV, Wormser GP, Hess AM, Delorey MJ, Mahapatra S, Schriefer ME, Belisle JT. Development of a metabolic biosignature for detection of early Lyme disease. *Clin Infect Dis* 2015; 60(12): 1767–1775.

40. Costello JM, Alexander ME, Greco KM, Perez-Atayde AR, Laussen PC. Lyme carditis in children: presentation, predictive factors and clinical course. *Pediatrics* 2009; 123: 835–841.

41. Ankri S, Mirelman D. Antimicrobial properties of allicin from garlic. *Microbes Infect* 1999; 1(2): 125–129.

42. Bedi HS et al. Bleeding risk of dietary supplements: a hidden nightmare for cardiac surgeons. *Indian Heart J* 2016; 68(Suppl 2): S249–S250.

43. Feng J, Shi W, Miklossy J, Tauxe G, McMeniman C, Zhang Y. Identification of essential oils with strong activity against stationary phase Borrelia burgdorferi. *Antibiotics* 2018; 7(4): 89.

44. de Almeida F et al. Coriandrum sativum L. essential oil: antifungal activity and mode of action on Candida spp. and molecular targets affected in human whole-genome expression. *PLoS One* 2014; 9(6): e99086.

45. Khalil M et al. Brain mast cell relationship to neurovasculature during development. *Brain Research* 2007; 1190(1): 227-227.

46. Polyzoidis S et al. Mast cells in meningiomas and brain inflammation. *J Neuroinflammation* 2015; 12: 170.

47. Iliff J, Wang M, Liao Y et al. A paravascular pathway facilitates CSF flow through the brain parenchyma and the clearance of interstitial solutes, including amyloid beta. *Sci Transl Med* 2012; 4(147): 147ra111.

48. Swedo SE, Leckman JF Rose NR. From research subgroup to clinical syndrome: Modifying the PANDAS criteria to describe PANS (pediatric acute-onset neuropsychiatric syndrome). *Pediatr Therapeut* 2012; 2: 2.

49. Swedo SE, Leonard HL, Garvey M, Mittleman D, Allen AJ, Perlmutter S, Lougee L, Dow S, Zamkoff J, Dubbert BK. Pediatric autoimmune neuropsychiatric disorders associated with streptococcal infections: clinical description of the first 50 cases. *Am J Psychiatry* 1998; 155(2): 265–271.

50. Allen AJ, Leonard HL, Swedo SE. Case study: a new infection-triggered, autoimmune subtype of pediatric OCD and Tourette's syndrome. *J Am Acad Child Adolesc Psychiatry* 1995; 34: 307–311.

51. Murphy ML, Pichichero ME. Prospective identification and treatment of children with pediatric autoimmune neuropsychiatric disorder associated with group A streptococcal infection (PANDAS). *Arch Pediatr Adolesc Med* 2002; 156(4): 356–361.

52. Murphy TK, Storch EA, Lewin AB, Edge PJ, Goodman WK. Clinical factors associated with pediatric autoimmune neuropsychiatric disorders associated with streptococcal infections. *J Pediatr* 2012; 160(2): 314–319.

53. De Luca C, et al. Metabolic and genetic screening of electromagnetic hypersensitive subjects as a feasible tool for diagnostics and intervention. *Mediators Inflamm* 2014; 924184.

53a. Mastinu A, Kumar A, Maccarinelli G, Bonini SA, et al. Zeolite Clinoptilolite: Therapeutic virtues of an ancient mineral. *Molecules* 2019; 24 (8): 1517. doi: 10.3390/molecules24081517

54. Saisch SG, Deale A, Gardner WN, Wessely S. Hyperventilation and chronic fatigue syndrome. *Q J Med* 1994; 87(1): 63–67.

55. Chen C-S, Cheng H-M, Chen H-J, Tsai S-Y, Kao C-H, Lin H-J, Wan L, Yang T-Y. Dry eye syndrome and the subsequent risk of chronic fatigue syndrome – a prospective population-based study in Taiwan. *Oncotarget* 2018; 9(55): 30694–30703. doi:10.18632/oncotarget.25544

56. Boneva RS et al. Endometriosis as a comorbid condition in chronic fatigue syndrome (CFS): secondary analysis of data from a CFS case-control study. *Frontiers in Pediatrics* 2019; 7: 195.

57. Harlow BL, Signorello LB, Hall JE, Dailey C, Komaroff AL. Reproductive correlates of chronic fatigue syndrome. *Am J Med* 1998; 105(3A): 94S–99S.

58. Puri BK, Counsell SJ, Zaman R, Main J, Collins AG, Hajnal JV, Davey NJ. Relative increase in choline in the occipital cortex in chronic fatigue syndrome. *Acta Psychiatr Scand* 2002; 106: 224–226.

59. de Morais SM, Uetrecht JP, Wells PG. Decreased glucuronidation and increased bioactivation of acetaminophen in Gilbert's syndrome. *Gastroenterology* 1992; 102: 577–586.

60. Rundo JV, Downey R 3rd. Polysomnography. *Handbook of Clinical Neurology* 2019; 160: 381–392.

61. Absinta M, Ha S-K, Nair G, Sati P, Luciano NJ, Palisoc M, Louveau A, Zaghloul KA, Pittaluga S. Human and nonhuman primate meninges harbor lymphatic vessels that can be visualized noninvasively by MRI. *eLife* 2017; 6: e29738.

62. Chang CM, et al. Chronic fatigue syndrome and subsequent risk of cancer among elderly US adults. *Cancer* 2012; 118(23): 5929-5936.

63. Allegra A, Innao V, Basile G, Pugliese M, Allegra AG, Pulvirenti N, Musolino C. Post-chemotherapy cognitive impairment in hematological patients: current understanding of chemobrain in hematology. *Expert Rev Hematol* 2020; 13(4): 393-404.

64. Colaris MJL, et al. Two hundred cases of ASIA syndrome following silicone implants: a comparative study of 30 years and a review of current literature. *Immunol Res* 2017; 65(1): 120-128.

65. Khoo T, Proudman S, Limaye V. 2019. Silicone breast implants and depression, fibromyalgia and chronic fatigue syndrome in a rheumatology clinic population. *Clin Rheumatol* 2019; 38(5): 1271-1276.

66. Dush DM. Breast implants and illness: a model of psychological factors. *Annals of Rheumatic Diseases* 2001; 60: 7.

67. Hallett M, Stone J, Carson A (eds). *Functional Neurologic Disorders: Handbook of Clinical Neurology*. Volume 139. Amsterdam: Elsevier; 2016.

68. Hives L, Bradley A, Richards J, et al. Can physical assessment techniques aid diagnosis in people with chronic fatigue syndrome/myalgic encephalomyelitis? A diagnostic accuracy study. *BMJ Open* 2017; 0: e017521. doi:10.1136/ bmjopen-2017-017521

69. Nielsen G et al. Randomised feasibility study of physiotherapy for patients with functional motor symptoms. *J Neurol Neurosurg Psychiatry* 2017; 88: 484–490.

70. Harrison R. Multiple chemical sensitivity. *Current Occupational & Environmental Medicine.* Fifth edn. New York: McGraw-Hill Education/Medical; 2014: 819–826.

71. Joshi SM. The sick building syndrome. *Indian J Occup Environ Med* 2008; 12(2): 61–64.

72. Nasterlack M. MCS, CFS, FMS, SBS and other 'modern' illnesses. *Versicherungsmedizin* 1998; 50(3): 99–103.

73. Eddington I (ed.). Aerotoxic syndrome: adverse health effects following exposure to jet oil mist during commercial flights. *Proceedings of the International Congress on Occupational Health Conference, Brisbane, Australia, 4–6 September 2000.* ISBN 0 646 401546 196.

74. Blomberg J, et al. Infection elicited autoimmunity and myalgic encephalomyelitis/Chronic Fatigue Syndrome: An explanatory model. *Front Immunol* 2018; 9: 229.

75. Oaklander AL, et al. Objective evidence that small-fiber polyneuropathy underlies some illnesses currently labeled as fibromyalgia. *Pain* 2013; 154(11): 2310-2316. doi: 10.1016/j.pain.2013.06.001.

76. Whelan RC, Gunnar Gottschalk CG, Peterson DL. ME/CFS and autoimmune-associated small fiber neuropathy. IACFS/ME online conference August 21 2020.

77. Ryabkova VA, Churilov LP, Shoenfeld Y. Neuroimmunology: What Role for Autoimmunity, Neuroinflammation, and Small Fiber Neuropathy in Fibromyalgia, Chronic Fatigue Syndrome, and Adverse Events after Human Papillomavirus Vaccination? *Int J Mol Sci* 2019; 20(20): 5164.

Chapter 7: The significance of toxins in ME/CFS

1. 'Toxin' *The New Oxford Dictionary of English*. Oxford University Press; 2001.
2. Johnson WG, Hodge SE, Duvoisin R. Twin studies and the genetics of Parkinson's disease: a reappraisal. *Movement Disorders* 1990; 5: 187–194.
3. Calne DB, Hochburg FH, Snow BJ, Nygaard T. Theories of Neurodegenerative Diseases: an overview. *Annals of the NY Academy of Sciences* 1992; 648: 1–5.
4. Veronesi B. The use of cell cultures for evaluating neurotoxicity. In: Tilson HA, Mitchell CL (eds). *Neurotoxicology.* New York: Raven Press; 1992; 21–49.
5. Tilson HA, Mitchell CL. *Neurotoxicology* Raven Press, New York, 1992.
6. Sabljic A. Chemical topology and ecotoxicology. *Sci Total Environ* 1991; 109–110: 197–220.
7. Cribb J. *Surviving the 21st Century: Humanity's Ten Great Challenges and How We Can Overcome Them.* Springer International; 2017.
8. Perrin RN. *The Involvement of Cerebrospinal Fluid and Lymphatic Drainage in Chronic Fatigue Syndrome/ME* (PhD Thesis). University of Salford, UK. 2005.
9. Zhang JJ, Lioy PJ. Human exposure assessment in air pollution systems. *Scientific World Journal* 2002; 2: 497–513.
10. Morrell S, Kerr C, Driscoll T, Taylor R, Salkeld G, Corbett S. Best estimate of the magnitude of mortality due to occupational exposure to hazardous substances. *Occup Environ Med* 1998; 55(9): 634–641.
11. Banerjee BD, Koner BC, Ray A. Immunotoxicity of pesticides: perspectives and trends. *Indian Journal of Experimental Biology* 1996; 34(8): 723–733.
12. Wallace LA, Pellizzari E, Hartwell T, Rosenzweig M, Erickson M, Sparacino C, Zelon H. Personal exposure to volatile organic compounds. I. Direct measurements in breathing-zone air, drinking water, food, and exhaled breath. *Environmental Research* 1984; 35(1): 293–319.
13. Agency for Toxic Substances and Disease Registry. *ATSDR-ToxFAQs – Benzene.* Available at: https://www.atsdr.cdc.gov/toxfaqs/tf.asp?id=38&tid=14 (Accessed: 6 August 2020).
14. Agency for Toxic Substances and Disease Registry. *ATSDR-ToxFAQs –*

Chloroform Available at: www.atsdr.cdc.gov/toxfaqs/tf.asp?id=52&tid=16 (Accessed: 6 August 2020).

15. Hoet P et al. Epidemic of liver disease caused by hydrochlorofluorocarbons used as ozone-sparing substitutes of chlorofluorocarbons. *Lancet* 1997; 350(9077): 556–559.

16. Carpenter DO. Polychlorinated biphenyls (PCBs): routes of exposure and effects on human health. *Rev Environ Health* 2006; 21(1): 1–23.

17. Gotohda T, Tokunaga I, Kubo S, Morita K, Kitamura O, Eguchi A. Effect of toluene inhalation on astrocytes and neurotrophic factor in rat brain. *Forensic Sci Int* 2000; 113(1–3): 233–238.

18. Jovanovic JM, Jovanovic MM, Spasic MJ, Lukic SR. Peripheral nerve conduction study in workers exposed to a mixture of organic solvents in paint and lacquer industry. *Croat Med J* 2004; 45(6): 769–774.

19. Sebastian A, Pehrson C, Larsson L. Elevated concentrations of endotoxin in indoor air due to cigarette smoking. *J Environ Monit* 2006; 8(5): 519–522.

20. Knobeloch L, Jackson R. Recognition of chronic carbon monoxide poisoning. *Wisconsin Medical Journal* 1999; 98(6): 26–29.

21. Clarke S, Keshishian C, Murray V et al. Screening for carbon monoxide exposure in selected patient groups attending rural and urban emergency departments in England: A prospective observational study. *BMJ Open* 2012; 2: 1–8. doi:10.1136/bmjopen-2012000877

22. Lau K, McLean WG, Williams DP, Howard CV. Synergistic interactions between commonly used food additives in a developmental neurotoxicity test. *Toxicological Science* 2006; 90(1): 178–187.

23. Latinwo LM, Badisa VL, Ikediobi CO, Odewumi CO, Lambert AT, Badisa RB. Effect of cadmium induced oxidative stress on antioxidative enzymes in mitochondria and cytoplasm of CRL-1439 rat liver cells. *Int J Mol Med* 2006; 18(3): 477–481.

24. Baars AJ. Dioxins, dioxin-like PCBs and non-dioxin-like PCBs in foodstuffs: occurrence and dietary intake in The Netherlands. *Toxicology Letters* 2004; 151(1): 51–61.

25. Yoot ML et al. Oestrogen receptor independent neurotoxic mechanism of bisphenol A, an environmental estrogen. *J Vet Sci* 2007; 8(1): 27–38. English.

26. Pahwa M et al. Glyphosate use and associations with non-Hodgkin lymphoma major histological sub-types: findings from the North American Pooled Project. *Scandinavian Journal of Work, Environment & Health* 2019; 45(6).

27. Gershon S, Shaw FH. Psychiatric sequelae of chronic exposure to organophosphorus insecticides. *Lancet* 1961; 1: 1371–1374.

28. Dunstan RH, Donohoe M, Taylor W, Roberts TK, Murdoch RN, Watkins JA, McGregor NR. A preliminary investigation of chlorinated hydrocarbons and chronic fatigue syndrome. *Medical Journal of Australia* 1995; 163(6): 294–297.

29. Reed A, Dzon L, Loganathan BG, Whalen MM. Immunomodulation of human natural killer cell cytotoxic function by organochlorine pesticides. *Hum Exp Toxicol* 2004; 23(10): 463–471.

30. Mutter J, Naumann J, Sadaghiani C, Walach H, Drasch G. Amalgam studies: disregarding basic principles of mercury toxicity. *Int J Hyg Environ Health* 2004; 207(4): 391–397.

31. Lloyd AR., Broughton C, Dwyer J, Wakefield D. What is myalgic encephalomyelitis? *Lancet* 1988; 1(8597): 1286–1287.

32. Garrel C, Lafond JL, Guiraud P, Faure P, Favier A. Induction of production of nitric oxide in microglial cells by insoluble form of aluminium. *Annals of the New York Academy of Science* 1994; 738: 455–461.

33. Haddad LM, Dimond KA, Schweistris JE. Phenol poisoning. *JACEP* 1979; 8(7): 267-269.

34. Akgündüz MÇ, Çavuşoğlu K, Yalçın E. The Potential Risk Assessment of Phenoxyethanol with a Versatile Model System. *Sci Rep* 2020; 10: 1209. doi.org/10.1038/s41598-020-58170-9

35. Weiss B. Neurobehavioural toxicity as a basis for risk assessment. *Trends in Pharmaceutical Science* 1988; 9: 59–62.

36. Needleman HL, Schell A, Bellinger D, Leviton A, Allred EN. The long-term exposure to low doses of lead in children. An 11 year follow up report. *New England Journal of Medicine* 1990; 322: 83–88.

37. Drasch G, Schupp I, Hofl H, Reinke R, Roider G. Mercury burden of human fetal and infant tissues. *Eur J Pediatr* 1994; 153(8): 607–610.

38. Drasch G, Roider G. Dental amalgam and pregnancy. *Geburtshilfe Frauenheilkd* 1995; 55(6): M63–M65.

39. Drasch G, Aigner S, Roider G, Staiger F, Lipowsky G. Mercury in human colostrum and early breast milk. Its dependence on dental amalgam and other factors. *J Trace Elem Med Biol* 1998; 12(1): 232–237.

40. Al-Saleh I et al. Heavy metal concentrations in the breast milk of Saudi women. *Biological Trace Element Research* 2003; 96(1–3): 21–37.

41. UK Parliament Environmental Audit Committee. Toxic Chemicals in

Everyday Life. 16 July 2019. www.parliament.uk.
https://publications.parliament.uk/pa/cm201719/cmselect/
cmenvaud/1805/180502.htm (accessed 1 October 2020).

42. Cheng X et al. Corrosion resistant Zeolite coatings by in situ crystalisation. *Electrochemical and Solid-State Letters* 2001; 4(5): B23–B26.

43. Croquet V et al. 1,1, 1–trichloroethane-induced chronic active hepatitis. *Gastroenterol Clin Biol* 2003; 27(1): 120–122.

44. Wallace L, Pellizzari E, Hartwell T, Zelon H, Sparacino C, Perritt R, Whitmore R. Concentrations of 20 volatile organic compounds in the air and drinking water of 350 residents of New Jersey compared with concentrations in their exhaled breath. *Journal of Occupational Medicine* 1986; 28(8): 603–608.

45. Friedberg F et al. *CFS/ME: A Primer for Clinical Practitioners.* International Association of Chronic Fatigue Syndrome/Myalgic Encephalomyelitis (IACFS/ME); 2014.

46. Hardell L, Hallquist A, Mild KH, Carlberg M, Pahlson A, Lilja A. Cellular and cordless telephones and the risk for brain tumours. *European Journal of Cancer Prevention* 2002; 11(4): 377–386.

47. Leszczynski D. Mobile phones, precautionary principle and future research. Letter; *Lancet* 2001; 358(9294): 1733.

48. Hotopf A, David A, Hull L, Ismail K, Unwin C, Wessley S. Role of vaccinations as risk factors for ill health in veterans of the Gulf War: cross sectional study. *British Medical Journal* 2000; 320: 1363–1367.

49. Shaheen S. Shots in the desert and Gulf War Syndrome. *British Medical Journal* 2000; 320: 1351–1352.

50. Hooper M. The most toxic war in Western military history. Evidence submitted to the House of Commons Select Defence Committee. *7th Report of Defence Select Committee: Gulf Veteran's Illnesses;* 1999.

51. Nicolson GL. Chronic infections as a common etiology for many patients with chronic fatigue syndrome, fibromyalgia syndrome, and Gulf War illnesses. *International Journal of Medicine* 1998; 1: 42–46.

52. Haley RW, Kurt TL. Self-reported exposure to neurotoxic chemical combinations in the Gulf War: a cross-sectional epidemiologic study. *JAMA* 1997; 277: 231–237.

53. Fukuda K, Straus SE, Hickie I, Sharpe MC, Dobbins JG, Komaroff A. The

chronic fatigue syndrome: a comprehensive approach to its definition and study. International Chronic Fatigue Syndrome Study Group. *Annals of Internal Medicine* 1994; 121 (12): 953–959.

54. Ismail K, Everitt B, Blatchley N, Hull L, Unwin C, David A, Wessley S. Is there a Gulf War syndrome? *Lancet* 1999; 353(9148): 179–182.

55. Hyams KC, Wignall FS, Roswell R. War syndromes and their evaluation from the US civil war to the Persian Gulf War. *Annals of Internal Medicine* 1996; 125: 398–405.

56. Spence A. Khan F, Belch JJF. Enhanced sensitivity of the peripheral cholinergic vascular response in patients with chronic fatigue syndrome. *American Journal of Medicine* 2000; 108: 736–739.

57. Puri BK, Counsell SJ, Zaman R, Main J, Collins AG, Hajnal JV, Davey NJ. Relative increase in choline in the occipital cortex in chronic fatigue syndrome. *Acta Psychiatr Scand* 2002; 106: 224–226.

58. Rogers S. *Tired or Toxic.* Syracuse, New York; Prestige Publishing 1990.

59. Hanin I. The Gulf War, stress and a leaky blood-brain barrier. *Nature Medicine* 1996; 12: 1307–1308.

60. Witte ST, Will LA, Olsen CR, Kinker JA, Miller-Graber P. Chronic selenosis in horses fed locally produced alfalfa hay. *Journal of the American Veterinary Medical Association* 1993; 1202(3): 406–409.

61. Schwarz B, Salak N, Hofstotter H, Pajik W, Knotzer H, Mayr A, Hasibeder W. Intestinal ischemic reperfusion syndrome: pathophysiology, clinical significance, therapy. *Wien Klin Wochenschr* 1990; 111(14): 539–548.

62. White JF. Intestinal pathophysiology in autism. *Exp Biol Med* 2003; 228(6): 639–649.

63. Burke V, Gracey M. Effects of salicylate on intestinal absorption: in vitro and in vivo studies with enterotoxigenic micro-organisms. *Gut* 1980; 21(8): 683–688.

64. Schumann K. Safety aspects of iron in food. *Ann Nutr Metab* 2001; 45(3): 91–101.

65. Jett DA, Kuhlmann AC, Farmer SJ, Guilarte TR. Age-dependent effects of developmental lead exposure on performance in the Morris water maze. *Pharmacol Biochem Behav* 1997; 57(1–2): 271–279.

66. Offit K, Groeger E, Turner S, Wadsworth EA, Weiser MA. The 'duty to warn' a patient's family members about hereditary disease risks. *JAMA* 2004; 292(12): 1469–1473.

67. Tilson HA, Mitchell CL. *Neurotoxicology.* Raven Press, New York; 1992.
68. Kammuller ME, Bloksma N, Seinen W (eds). *Autoimmunity and Toxicology: Immune Disregulation Induced by Drugs and Chemicals.* Amsterdam: Elsevier; 1989.
69. Czaja AJ, Donaldson PT. Genetic susceptibilities for immune expression and liver cell injury in autoimmune hepatitis. *Immunol Rev* 2000; 174: 250–259.
70. AG Motulsky. Ecogenetics: genetic predisposition to the toxic effects of chemicals. *Am J Hum Genet* 1992; 50(4): 881–882.

Chapter 8: The stages leading to ME/CFS and FMS

1. Iliff J, Wang M, Liao Y, Plogg B, Peng W, Gunderson GA, Benveniste H, Vates E, Deane R, Goldman SA, Nagelhus EA, Nedergaard M. A paravascular pathway facilitates CSF flow through the brain parenchyma and the clearance of interstitial solutes, including amyloid beta. *Sci Transl Med* 2012; 4(147): 147ra111.
2. Xie L et al. Sleep drives metabolite clearance from the adult brain. *Science* 2013; 342: 373–377.
3. Louveau A et al. Structural and functional features of central nervous system lymphatic vessels. *Nature* 2015; 523(7560): 337-341. doi: 10.1038/nature14432
4. Aspenlund A et al. A dural lymphatic vascular system that drains brain interstitial fluid and macromolecules. *Journal of Experimental Medicine* 2015. doi:10.1084/jem.20142290
5. Absinta M, Ha S-K, Nair G, Sati P, Luciano NJ, Palisoc M, Louveau A, Zaghloul KA, Pittaluga S. Human and nonhuman primate meninges harbor lymphatic vessels that can be visualized noninvasively by MRI. *eLife* 2017; 6: e29738. https://elifesciences.org/articles/19738 doi.org/10.7554/elife.29738.001
6. Lee H, Xie L, Yu M, Kang H, Feng T, Deane R, Logan J, Nedergaard M, Benveniste H. The effect of body posture on brain glymphatic transport. *J Neurosci* 2015; 35(31): 11034–11044.
7. Perrin RN. Chronic fatigue syndrome: a review from the biomechanical perspective. *British Osteopathic Journal* 1993; 11: 15–23.
8. Perrin RN, Edwards J, Hartley P. An evaluation of the effectiveness

of osteopathic treatment on symptoms associated with myalgic encephalomyelitis. A preliminary report. *Journal of Medical Engineering and Technology* 1998; 22(1): 1–13.

9. Keenan P. Brain MRI abnormalities exist in chronic fatigue syndrome (Editorial). *Journal of Neurological Sciences* 1999; 171: 1–2.

10. Lange G, Deluca J, Maldjian JA, Lee H, Tiersky LA, Natelson BH. Brain MRI abnormalities exist in a subset of patients with chronic fatigue syndrome. *Journal of Neurological Sciences* 1999; 171(1): 3–7.

11. Costa DC, Brostoff J, Tannock C. Brainstem spect studies in normals, ME/CFS and depression. *Nucl Med Commun* 1995; 15: 252–253.

12. Farrell M, Richards JG. Analysis of the reliability and validity of the kinetic communicator exercise device. *Med Sci Sports Exer* 1986; 18(1): 44–49.

13. Hutchinson A, Pinching L, Chambers T, Waterman J, Wayne N (eds). *A Report of the CFS/ME Working Group to the Chief Medical Officer.* HMG; 2002.

14. Fukuda K, Straus SE, Hickie I, Sharpe MC, Dobbins JG, Komaroff A. The chronic fatigue syndrome: a comprehensive approach to its definition and study. International Chronic Fatigue Syndrome Study Group. *Annals of Internal Medicine* 1994; 121(12): 953–959.

15. Sharpe M, Archard L, Banatvala J. A report: chronic fatigue syndrome: guidelines for research. *Journal of the Royal Society of Medicine* 1991; 84: 118–121.

16. Carruthers B. Definitions and aetiology of myalgic encephalomyelitis (ME): how the Canadian Consensus Clinical Definition of ME works. *Journal of Clinical Pathology* 2007; 60(2): 117–119.

17. Gasser HS. Properties of dorsal root unmedullated fibres on the two sides of the ganglion. *Journal of General Physiology* 1955; 38: 709–728.

18. Kinmonth JB. *The Lymphatics.* 2nd edn. London: Edward Arnold; 1982; 80.

19. Kinmonth JB. Some aspects of cardiovascular surgery. *Journal of the Royal College of Surgeons of Edinburgh* 1960; 5: 287–297.

20. Kinmonth JB, Sharpey-Schafer. Manometry of human thoracic duct. *Journal of Physiology* 1959; 177: 41.

21. Vodder E. *Le drainage lymphatique, une nouvelle méthode thérapeutique.* Paris, France: Santé Pour Tous; 1936.

22. Browse NL. Response of lymphatics to sympathetic nerve stimulation. *Journal of Physiology* 1968; 19: 25.

23. Still AT. *Philosophy of Osteopathy.* Published by the Author, Kirksville, Mo; 1899.

24. Still AT. *The Philosophy and Mechanical Principles of Osteopathy.* Kansas City USA: Hudson-Kimberly; 1902; 47.

25. Sutherland WG. *The Cranial Bowl.* Mankato, Minnesota: Free Press Company; 1939.

26. Wales AL (ed.), Sutherland WG. *Teachings in the Science of Osteopathy.* Sutherland Cranial Teaching Foundation, Fort Worth, Texas; 1990.

26a. Du Bouley GH. Further investigations on pulsatile movements in the cerebrospinal fluid pathways. *Acta Radiol Diagn* 1972; 13: 497-523.

26b. Feinberg DA, Mark AS. Human brain motion and cerebrospinal fluid circulation demonstrated with MR velocity imaging. *Radiology* 1987; 163(3): 793–799.

27. Perrin RN. Lymphatic drainage of the neuraxis in chronic fatigue syndrome: a hypothetical model for the cranial rhythmic impulse. *Journal of the American Osteopathic Association* 2007; 107(06): 218–224.

28. Dreha-Kulaczewski S et al. Inspiration is the major regulator of human CSF flow. *Journal of Neuroscience* 2015; 35(6): 2485–2491.

29. Puri BK, Gunatilake KD, Fernando KA, Gurusinghe AI, Agour M, Treasaden I. Increased tenderness in the left third intercostal space in adult patients with myalgic encephalomyelitis: a controlled study. *J Int Med Res* 2011; 39(1): 212–214.

Chapter 9: Osteopathy

1. Puri BK. *Chronic Fatigue Syndrome: A Natural Way to Treat ME.* London: Hammersmith Press; 2004.

2. Myhill S. *Diagnosis and Treatment of Chronic Fatigue Syndrome and Myalgic Encephalitis: It's Mitochondria, Not Hypochondria.* 2nd edn. London: Hammersmith Books; 2017.

3. Ali A, McCarthy PL. Complementary and integrative methods in fibromyalgia. *Pediatr Rev* 2014; 35(12): 510–518.

4. Puri BK, Holmes J, Hamilton G. Eicosapentaenoic acid-rich essential fatty acid supplementation in chronic fatigue syndrome associated with symptom remission and structural brain changes. *Int J Clin Pract* 2004; 58(3): 297–299.

4a. National Institute of Health and Care Excellence (NICE). Myalgic encephalomyelitis (or encephalopathy)/chronic fatigue syndrome: diagnosis and management. NICE Guidance – In development [GID-NG10091] DRAFT 20 November 2020. London UK. www.nice.org.uk/guidance/indevelopment/gid-ng10091/consultation/html-content-2

5. Wales AL (ed.) *Teachings in the Science of Osteopathy.* Fort Worth TX: Sutherland Cranial Teaching Foundation; 1990.

6. Still AT. *Philosophy of Osteopathy.* Kirksville MO: Published by the Author; 1899.

7. Still AT. *The Philosophy and Mechanical Principles of Osteopathy,* Kansas City MO: Hudson-Kimberly; 1902; 47.

8. Sutherland WG. *The Cranial Bowl,* Mankato Minn: Free Press Company; 1939.

9. Woods JM, Woods RH. A physical finding relating to psychiatric disorders. *J Am Osteopathic Assoc* 1961; 60: 988–993.

10. King HH, Lay EM. Osteopathy in the cranial field. In: Ward RC (ed.) *Foundations for Osteopathic Medicine.* 2nd edn. Baltimore MD: Lippincott Williams & Wilkins; 2003; 985 –1001.

11. Magoun HI. *Osteopathy in the Cranial Field.* 2nd ed. Kirksville MO: The Journal Printing Company; 1966.

12. Upledger JE, Vredevoogd JD. *Craniosacral Therapy* Chicago, Ill: Eastland Press; 1983.

13. Nelson KE, Sergueef N, Glonek T. Recording the rate of the cranial rhythmic impulse. *J Am Osteopathic Assoc* J2006; 106(6): 337–341.

14. Norton JM, Sibley G, Broder-Oldach R. Characterization of the cranial rhythmic impulse in healthy human adults. *Amer Acad Osteopath J* 1992; 2: 9–12,.

15. McAdoo J, Kuchera ML. Reliability of cranial rhythmic impulse palpation. *J Am Osteopath Assoc* 1995; 95: 491.

16. Hanten WP, Dawson DD, Iwata M, Seiden M, Whitten FG, Zink T. Craniosacral rhythm: reliability and relationships with cardiac and respiratory rates. *J Orthop Sports Phys Ther* 1998; 27: 213 –218.

17. Perrin RN. Lymphatic drainage of the neuraxis in chronic fatigue syndrome: a hypothetical model for the cranial rhythmic impulse. *Journal of the American Osteopathic Association* 2007; 107(06): 218–224.

18. Perrin RN. Chronic fatigue syndrome: a review from the biomechanical perspective. *British Osteopathic Journal* 1993; 11: 15–23.

19. Perrin RN, Edwards J, Hartley P. An evaluation of the effectiveness of osteopathic treatment on symptoms associated with myalgic encephalomyelitis. A preliminary report. *Journal of Medical Engineering and Technology* 1998; 22(1): 1–13.

20. Perrin RN, Richards JD, Pentreath V, Percy DF. Muscle fatigue in Chronic Fatigue Syndrome/Myalgic Encephalomyelitis (CFS/ME) and its response to a novel manual therapeutic approach. *Int J Osteopath Med* 2011; 14(3): 96–105.

21. Perrin RN. *The Involvement of Cerebrospinal Fluid and Lymphatic Drainage in Chronic Fatigue Syndrome/ME* (PhD Thesis). University of Salford, UK; 2005.

Chapter 10: Treating the patient

1. Hartman L. *Handbook of Osteopathic Technique.* 3rd edn. London: Chapman and Hall; 1997.

2. Stoddard A. *Manual of Osteopathic Technique.* 3rd edn. London: Hutchinson; 1982.

3. Chaitow L. *Fibromyalgia Syndrome: A Practitioner's Guide to Treatment.* London: Elsevier Health Sciences; 1999.

4. Pellegrino MJ. *Understanding Post-traumatic Fibromyalgia.* Columbus OH: Anadem Inc; 1996.

5. Yunus MB. Central sensitivity syndromes: a unified concept for fibromyalgia and other maladies. *JIRA* 2000; 8: 27–33.

6. Zhang HW et al. Long-term ambient hydrocarbons exposure and incidence of ischemic stroke. *PLoS One* 2019; 14(12): e0225363. doi: 10.1371

7. Still AT. *The Philosophy and Mechanical Principles of Osteopathy.* Kansas City, Mo: Hudson Kimberly; 1902: 47.

8. Dreha-Kulaczewski S et al. Inspiration is the major regulator of human CSF Flow. *Journal of Neuroscience* 2015; 35(6):2485–2491.

9. Ali M. *The Neck Connection.* Sugar & Spice Resources Ltd. USA; 2011.

10. Sutherland WG. *The Cranial Bowl,* Mankato Minn: Free Press Company; 1939.

11. Wales AL (ed.). *Teachings in the Science of Osteopathy.* Fort Worth TX: Sutherland Cranial Teaching Foundation; 1990.
12. Lee H, Xie L, Yu M, Kang H, Feng T, Deane R, Logan J, Nedergaard M, Benveniste H. The effect of body posture on brain glymphatic transport. *J Neurosci* 2015; 35(31): 11034–11044.
13. Russell A et al. Persistent fatigue induced by interferon-alpha: a novel, inflammation-based, proxy model of chronic fatigue syndrome. *Psychoneuroendocrinology* 2019; 100: 276-285. doi.org/10.1016/j.psyneuen.2018.11.032
14. Iliff J, Wang M, Liao Y, Plogg B, Peng W, Gunderson GA, Benveniste H, Vates E, Deane R, Goldman SA, Nagelhus EA, Nedergaard M. A paravascular pathway facilitates CSF flow through the brain parenchyma and the clearance of interstitial solutes, including amyloid beta. *Sci Transl Med* 2012; 4(147): 147ra111.
15. Ankri S and Mirelman D. Antimicrobial properties of allicin from garlic. *i.Microbes Infect* 1999; 1(2): 125–129.
16. Bouic PJ, Lamprecht JH. Plant sterols and sterolins: A review of their immune-modulating properties. *Altern Med Rev* 1999; 4(3): 170–177.
17. Ionescu G et al. Oral citrus seed extract in atopic eczema: in vitro and in vivo studies on intestinal microflora. *Journal of Orthomolecular Medicine* 1990; 5: 3.
18. Perrin RN, Edwards J, Hartley P. An evaluation of the effectiveness of osteopathic treatment on symptoms associated with myalgic encephalomyelitis: a preliminary report. *Journal of Medical Engineering and Technology* 1998; 22(1): 1–13.
19. Albright F, Light K, Light A, Bateman L, Cannon-Albright LA. Evidence for a heritable predisposition to chronic fatigue syndrome. *BMC Neurol* 2011; 11: 62.

Chapter 11: ME/CFS and FMS: your questions answered

1. Cserr HF, Knopf PM. Cervical lymphatics, the blood-brain barrier and immunoreactivity of the brain: a new view. *Immunology Today* 1992; 13: 507–512.
2. Perrin RN. *The Involvement of Cerebrospinal Fluid and Lymphatic Drainage*

in Chronic Fatigue Syndrome/ME (PhD Thesis). University of Salford, UK; 2005.

3. Devanur LD, Kerr JR. Chronic fatigue syndrome. *J Clin Virol* 2006; 37(3): 139–150.
4. Browse NL. Response of lymphatics to sympathetic nerve stimulation. *J Physiol* 1968; 19: 25.
5. Perrin RN, Edwards J, Hartley P. An evaluation of the effectiveness of osteopathic treatment on symptoms associated with myalgic encephalomyelitis. A preliminary report. *Journal of Medical Engineering and Technology* 1998; 22(1): 1–13.
6. Shevchuk NA. Possible use of repeated cold stress for reducing fatigue in chronic fatigue syndrome: a hypothesis. *Behav Brain Func* 2007; 3: 55.
7. Mizuno K, et al. Effects of mild-stream bathing on recovery from mental fatigue. *Med Sci Monit* 2010;16(1): CR8-CR14.
8. Schacterle RS, Komaroff AL. 2004. A Comparison of Pregnancies That Occur Before and After the Onset of Chronic Fatigue Syndrome. *Arch Intern Med* 2004; 164(4): 401–404.
9. Schacterle S, et al. A comparison of pregnancies that occur before and after the onset of chronic fatigue syndrome. *Arch Intern Med* 2004; 164: 401–404.
10. Underhill R et al. Prevalence of chronic fatigue syndrome and chronic fatigue within families of CFS patients. *J CFS* 2006; 13(1): 3–13.
11. Stejskal VD et al. Metal-specific lymphocytes: biomarkers of sensitivity in man. *Neuro Endocrinol Lett* 1999; 20(5): 289–298.
12. Genuis SJ, Genuis SK. Human exposure assessment and relief from neuropsychiatric symptoms: case study of a hairdresser. *J Am Board Fam Pract* 2004; 17(2): 136–141.
13. Racciatti D, Vecchiet J, Ceccomancini A, Ricci F, Pizzigallo E. Chronic fatigue syndrome following a toxic exposure. *Sci Total Environ* 2001; 270(1–3): 27–31.
14. Perrin R, Riste L, Hann M, Walther A, Mukherjee A, Heald A. Into the looking glass: post-viral syndrome post COVID-19. *Medical Hypothesis* Published online 27 Jun 2020. doi: 10.1016/j.mehy.2020.110055
15. Friedberg F et al. *CFS/ME: A Primer for Clinical Practitioners.* Chicago: IACFS/ME; 2014.

Appendices

1. Ocon AJ. Caught in the thickness of brain fog: exploring the cognitive symptoms of chronic fatigue syndrome. *Frontiers in Physiology* 2013; 4: 63.
2. Ravindran M et al. Dyspnea in chronic fatigue syndrome (CFS): comparison of two prospective cross-sectional studies. *Glob J Health Sci* 2012; 5(2): 94–110.
3. Alp ÇA, Sivri A. Respiratory function and dyspnea in fibromyalgia syndrome. *Journal of Musculoskeletal Pain* 2000; 9(1): 7–15.
4. Rowe PC, Underhill RA, Friedman KJ, Gurwitt A, Medow MS, Schwartz MS, Speight N, Stewart JM, Vallings R, Rowe KS. Encephalomyelitis/chronic fatigue syndrome diagnosis and management in young people: a primer. *Front Pediatr* 2017; 5: 121.
5. Albrecht PJ et al. Excessive peptidergic sensory innervation of cutaneous arteriole-venule shunts (AVS) in the palmar glabrous skin of fibromyalgia patients: implications for widespread deep tissue pain and fatigue. *Pain Med J* 2013; 14(6): 895–915.
6. De Luca C et al. Metabolic and genetic screening of electromagnetic hypersensitive subjects as a feasible tool for diagnostics and intervention. *Mediators Inflamm* 2014; 924184.
7. Chao CH, Chen HJ, Wang HY, Li TC, Kao CH. Increased risk of organic erectile dysfunction in patients with chronic fatigue syndrome: a nationwide population-based cohort study. *Andrology* 2015; 3(4): 666–671.
8. Rutherford G, Manning P, Newton JL. Understanding muscle dysfunction in chronic fatigue syndrome. *J Aging Res* 2016. doi: 10.1155/2016/2497348
9. Chandola HC, Chakraborty A. Fibromyalgia and myofascial pain syndrome – a dilemma *Indian J Anaesth* 2009; 53(5): 575–581.
10. Saury JM. The role of the hippocampus in the pathogenesis of myalgic encephalomyelitis/chronic fatigue syndrome (ME/CFS). *Medical Hypotheses* 2016; 86: 30–38.
11. Higgins JNP, Pickard JD, Lever AML. Chronic fatigue syndrome and idiopathic intracranial hypertension: Different manifestations of the same disorder of intracranial pressure? *Medical Hypotheses* 2017; 105: 6–9.
12. Hives L, Bradley A, Richards J et al. Can physical assessment techniques aid diagnosis in people with chronic fatigue syndrome/myalgic

encephalomyelitis? A diagnostic accuracy study. *BMJ Open* 2017; 0: e017521. doi:10.1136/ bmjopen-2017-017521

13. Murugan K et al. Migraine headaches in chronic fatigue syndrome (CFS): comparison of two prospective cross-sectional studies. *BMC Neurol* 2011; 11: 30.

14. Buddenkotte J, Steinhoff M. Recent advances in understanding and managing rosacea. *F1000Res* 2018; 7.

15. Chandola HC, Chakraborty A, Rutherford G, Manning P, Newton JL. Understanding muscle dysfunction in chronic fatigue syndrome. *J Aging Res* 2016. doi: 10.1155/2016/2497348

16. Chandola HC, Chakraborty A. Fibromyalgia and myofascial pain syndrome – A dilemma *Indian J Anaesth* 2009; 53(5): 575–581.

17. Gurbuzler L et al. Voice disorder in patients with f ibromyalgia. *Journal of Auris Nasus Larynx* 2013; 40.

18. Cardoso R. Lumini-Oliveira J. Meneses RF. Associations between autonomic nervous system function, voice, and dysphonia: a systematic review. *Journal of Voice* 2019; in press.

19. Tomic S, et al. Lipid and protein oxidation in female patients with chronic fatigue syndrome. *Arch Med Sci* 2012; 8(5): 886–891.

Index

Also from Hammersmith Health Books

What You Need to Know About Pernicious Anaemia and Vitamin B$_{12}$ Deficiency

By Martyn Hooper

'Every doctor should read this book.'
Dr Chris Steele MBE, resident doctor – ITV's This Morning

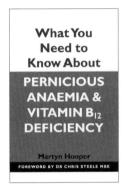

Martyn Hooper, the founder and chair of the Pernicious Anaemia Society, brings together the essential knowledge that sufferers and their families and friends need to understand, and withstand, vitamin B$_{12}$ deficiency and pernicious anaemia. Martyn discusses the many uncertainties and difficulties associated with the condition, what these may mean for sufferers, the huge variations in individual experience, and how to live as fully as possible despite having the condition.

Also from Hammersmith Health Books

Why Am I So Exhausted?
understanding chronic fatigue syndrome

By Martin Budd

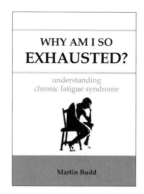

Naturopath Martin Budd explains that chronic fatigue is very rarely caused by a single disease, but by several, generally interrelated health problems. He shows how the multiple causes can be identified and treated; describes how the physical effects of long-term stress can lead to health problems and how this can result in sufferers' problems being interpreted as 'all in the mind'; and he includes detailed patient case histories that show how complex chronic fatigue syndrome can be.

Also from Hammersmith Health Books

Fighting Fatigue
a practical guide to managing the symptoms of CFS/ME

By Sue Pemberton, Catherine Berry and Janie Spencer

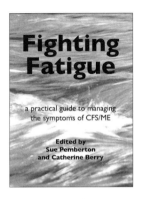

This practical manual comes from a nationally recognised centre for chronic fatigue and is jointly written by health professionals and their patients. They give straightforward and specific expert advice, accompanied by real life stories, on managing different aspects of everyday life that can affect energy and they show how to put this advice into practice. They understand the way fatigue affects concentration and therefore break their guidance into easy-to-follow steps that can be worked through at the reader's own pace. Unlike other available books, this does not cover causes, symptoms or the controversy around whether the condition is real. It is purely about how to get better.

Also from Hammersmith Health Books

Crypto-infections
Denial, censorship and suppression – the truth about what lies behind chronic disease

By Dr Christian Perronne

With a Foreword by Dr Jack Lambert

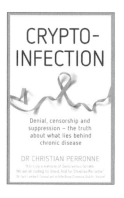

The accepted message is that humankind has largely conquered infectious disease with a mixture of antibiotics and vaccines yet it is becoming clear that chronic hidden or latent infections (crypto-infections) lie behind many of today's big killers, including heart disease, dementia and cancer. As an exemplar of how the organisms responsible can hide in plain sight, causing devastation while the medical world is in denial, Borrelia burgdorferi – the bacterium responsible for Lyme disease – has led Dr Perronne to clash with his fellow specialists in infectious disease (ID) and challenge the status quo. From his experience as one of France's – and the world's – leading ID specialists, he examines the threats that both Lyme in particular and crypto-infections in general pose and how we can rise to the challenge.